D1388181

Paediatric Oncology

Acute Nursing Care

In memory of my dad, who saw the beginning but sadly not the end, greatly missed.

FG

To the children of Piam Brown Ward in Southampton who taught me so much. To my daughters who are always there for me.

ME

Paediatric Oncology:
Acute Nursing Care

Edited by

Faith Gibson RGN, RSCN, Onc Cert, Cert Ed, MSc
(Cancer Nursing)

Senior Lecturer/Nurse Researcher,
South Bank University and Great Ormond Street Hospital for
Children NHS Trust, London

and

Margaret Evans RGN, RSCN, DipN (Lond),
BSc (Hons)

Macmillan Lecturer in Paediatric Oncology Nursing,
University of Southampton, Southampton

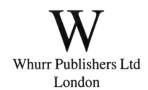

Whurr Publishers Ltd
London

© 1999 Whurr Publishers
First published 1999 by
Whurr Publishers Ltd
19b Compton Terrace, London N1 2UN, England

British Library Cataloguing in Publication Data
A catalogue record for this book is available from the British
Library.

ISBN 1 86156 047 8

Printed and bound in the UK by Athenaeum Press Ltd,
Gateshead, Tyne & Wear

Contents

Contributors

Nikki Bennett-Rees RGN, RSCN, Dip ANC (Paed Onc), Sister, Bone Marrow Transplant, Great Ormond Street Hospital for Children NHS Trust, London.

Hilary Brocklehurst RGN, RSCN, Bone Marrow Transplant Coordinator, Southampton University Hospitals NHS Trust, Southampton.

Philippa Chesterfield RGN, RSCN, RCNT, Onc Cert, BSc (Hons), Paediatric Macmillan Nurse, Southampton University Hospitals NHS Trust, Southampton.

Sharon Denton RGN, RSCN, Staff Nurse, Paediatric Surgery, St James's University Hospital, Leeds.

Gillian Dixon RGN, RSCN, Dip HE (Health Studies), Staff Nurse, Paediatric Surgery, St James's University Hospital, Leeds.

Chris Henry RGN, ONC, FETC, Cert Family Therapy, Sister, Adolescent Ward, Royal National Orthopaedic Hospital, Stanmore, Middlesex.

Rachel Hollis RGN, RSCN, BA (Hons), Clinical Nurse Specialist, Paediatric Oncology, St James's University Hospital, Leeds.

Louise Hooker RGN, RSCN, Cert Health Ed, MSc, Lecturer Practitioner in Paediatric Oncology, Southampton University Hospital NHS Trust, Southampton.

Monica Hopkins RGN, RSCN, HV Cert, NDN, BN, MSc (Nursing), Advanced Nurse Practitioner, Paediatric Oncology, Alder Hey Children's Hospital, Liverpool.

Lindy May RGN, RSCN, MSc, Sister, Neurosurgery, Great Ormond Street Hospital for Children NHS Trust, London.

Sarah Palmer RGN, RSCN, Dip ANC (Paed Onc), BN (Hons), Sister, Paediatric Oncology Day Ward, Southampton University Hospitals NHS Trust, Southampton.

Jane Pownall RGN, RSCN, Sister, Young Oncology Unit, Christie Hospital, Manchester.

Linda Scott RGN, RSCN, Ward Manager, Young Oncology Unit, Christie Hospital, Manchester.

Karen Selwood RGN, RSCN, RM, BSc (Hons), Advanced Nurse Practitioner, Paediatric Oncology, Alder Hey Children's Hospital, Liverpool.

Louise Soanes RGN, RSCN, BSc (Hons), Senior Lecturer, Paediatric Oncology, South Bank University, London.

Jane Watson RGN, RSCN, Neuro-oncology Liaison Nurse, Great Ormond Street Hospital for Children NHS Trust, London.

Gaynor Young RGN, RSCN, DMS, Manager/ Clinical Nurse Specialist, Paediatric Oncology, Southampton University Hospitals NHS Trust, Southampton.

Acknowledgements

Because we wanted to ensure that this book was accurate, detailed and reflected current practice, we invited a range of health care professionals to comment on the content at the draft and proofreading stages. We included specialist nurses, doctors, pharmacists, psychologists and play specialists. We would like to thank the following professionals for their diligence and for generously giving up their time to the book: Tracey Bannister, Angela Bowman, Karen Bravery, Bernadette Brennan, Steve Cannon, Hilary Dawson, Dave Doughty, Tracey Forrester, Rao Gattamaneri, Marjorie Gordon-Box, Sharon Hayden, George Kissen, Janice Kohler, Ian Lewis, Rebekah Lwin, Erica Mackie, Anthony Michalski, Susan Morgan, Wendy Nelson, Karen Pearson-Banerjee, Barry Pizer, Jo Sweeney, Pauline Sutherland, Roly Squire and Paul Veys. In addition, we thank students undertaking the ENB219 and 237 courses for commenting on the section related to bone tumours. In this section, we would also like to thank the illustrator, Mr Ron Hosking.

Many thanks also to our various friends, colleagues and family members who have believed in us and maintained our enthusiasm by offering constant encouragement.

Finally, we would like to express a special thanks to Ivan Thomas for his untiring devotion to this book. He helped us maintain a sense of humour, provided expert back-up computer skills, tempted us with culinary delights and provided warm encouragement through what sometimes seemed an arduous process.

Preface

It seems that the publication of this book is timely. There are no purely practical paediatric oncology nursing texts in the UK and there are few in the USA at the moment. As nurses in the UK we have often been frustrated by the lack of UK-specific texts and this was therefore an opportunity for us to make a contribution to the literature by documenting the current state of the art in paediatric oncology nursing in the UK. We hope that this book will fill this gap in the market, especially as it is dealing with areas that have received little attention, such as bone marrow transplantation or the nursing care of a child with a bone tumour. One of our aims is that this book will complement other more theoretical texts which have followed a more medical model.

This book is written for clinical nurses who may (or may not) be experienced in, but who are interested in pursuing the speciality of, paediatric oncology. It will most certainly be included as recommended reading for oncology courses. It could also appeal to a wider audience, for example, professions allied to medicine.

The style of the authors varies slightly, and there may be occasional inconsistencies in the terms that have been used. However, variations do exist between centres, and we hope that these do not detract from the content of the book.

We would like to stress that the aim of this book is to inform nursing practice so that overall quality of care to children and families is improved by increasing the knowledge of practitioners and thus positively influencing a child's cancer experience. Although the notion of 'family-centred care' (with the emphasis on empowerment and negotiation) may not have been stated specifically, we hope that it is clear that this forms the backbone of our philosophy. Likewise, implicit within the book is the recognition that each family is unique, that culture is central to every individual, and that truly person-centred and holistic care can only be provided if we acknowledge these issues.

Foreword

Progress in the management of children's cancer has presented many challenges for nurses over the years. Treatment advances and the growing numbers of long-term survivors have dramatically changed the knowledge base required to enable nurses to adapt and expand both their affective and technical skills to meet the needs of the children and their families. Nurses have broadened the scope of their practice to incorporate many aspects of the child's clinical, physical and psychological management in whichever setting the child is nursed. They work with, and value being part of, large multi-disciplinary teams.

Paediatric oncology nurses have been at the forefront of developing what the UKCC refers to as 'higher-level practice'. By sharing expertise they have taken forward the art and science of paediatric oncology nursing: the Royal College of Nursing's Paediatric Oncology Nursing Forum, established in 1984, has facilitated the 'networking' and sharing which has played a pivotal role in practice developments.

Clinical advances in future years will mean that the needs of children and families will continue to change. From the firm foundation they have established, paediatric oncology nurses will go on meeting challenges, with quality of life for the child and family always remaining the primary goal.

This book reflects that goal and stands as a marker of the state of the art of paediatric oncology nursing at this time.

Sue Burr OBE, FRCN
Royal College of Nursing's Adviser in Paediatric Nursing
November 1998

Introduction

There is no doubt that paediatric oncology has seen much progress over the past 20 years or so and childhood cancer is no longer seen as a terminal illness. Much of this progress has been due to a collaborative approach to studies and clinical trials, coordinated by the United Kingdom Children's Cancer Study Group (UKCCSG) and the Medical Research Council (MRC); and to meticulous record keeping at a national level. A multiprofessional approach to care has also made a contribution, as have major advances in supportive care, in which nurses have had a central role.

As a result of a steady improvement in survival rates (currently standing at about 65% for five-year event-free survival) the focus of care has turned to creating the best possible chance of cure. However, many difficult ethical dilemmas are created as a result of this approach. Technical skills are becoming increasingly sophisticated and could become, in the worst cases, a way of dehumanising practice when the price paid (in terms of quality of life for the sick child) is too high. Serious consideration must always be given to this issue.

A diagnosis of cancer puts a strain on the most stable family and, in the present climate of rapid social change, such families are less common. The cancer diagnosis creates much greater stresses for family members who may not always feel strong enough to make decisions by themselves. Nurses are therefore challenged as never before to look beyond the disease and the treatment, and to act as advocates for children and their families during times of decision-making throughout the trajectory of illness and beyond.

There are several ways in which nurses have taken the initiative in this speciality. The Royal College of Nursing Paediatric Oncology Nurses Forum (PONF) has been a powerful force in ensuring that nurses have a stronger voice. Negotiation with UKCCSG means that nurses are now included in decision-making groups, such as the New

Agents Group (NAG) and tumour-specific groups, and in working parties designed to improve practice in specific areas, for example, palliative care or the needs of teenagers. Education programmes (ENB240, R62 and now diploma/degree courses) are providing nurses with the knowledge, skills and attributes that are essential to enable them to take a pivotal role within the multiprofessional team.

Nurses have been influential in setting up and managing late-effects clinics which are crucial in dealing with the effects of treatment. The role of the Advanced Nurse Practitioner is being given serious consideration and two such positions have been established in Liverpool. These must pave the way for further developments.

The book is divided into four self-contained sections and the ordering of the chapters within each is similar so that the reader will be able to focus on a particular area of interest without scanning the whole text. References are provided at the end of the four sections. There are common threads which run through each chapter, for example, psychosocial issues or health education. Where appropriate, knowledge derived from other disciplines is used, evidence that nursing care is now planned and delivered from a sound knowledge base that also encompasses medicine, pharmacology, psychology, etc. Although this is an 'acute care' text it is important to keep in mind links with the community and so these have been emphasised where appropriate.

The contributors are expert practitioners in their fields. Their knowledge and expertise has been harnessed to produce this book. Wherever possible a practical approach, focusing on the detailed management of care, is underpinned by theory so that research is always prominent. At the same time, it is recognised that there is merit to purely anecdotal knowledge which is a product of experience. This is often reflected in the 'Nursing Notes' which appear throughout the text.

We are most grateful to all those who have contributed to this book and who have worked long and hard throughout a lengthy and sometimes frustrating process. It would clearly not have been possible without a sustained effort and much 'blood, sweat and tears'. We are proud of their achievement and hope that this is not the end of their writing careers. We look forward to reading their ongoing contributions which will continue to chart the domain of nursing practice in paediatric oncology.

There is a bookshop in California called The Tattered Cover. We sincerely hope that the cover of this book will become tattered very soon!

Margaret Evans and Faith Gibson

SECTION ONE
CHEMOTHERAPY

Chapter 1
Principles of chemotherapy

Gaynor Young

Cell Cycle

To understand the principles of chemotherapy and how it works it is important to have a basic understanding of the normal cell cycle. Figure 1.1 represents the proliferative phase of the cell cycle. This is the period when a cell is actively involved in reproduction. The G^1, or first gap, post-mitotic phase is that in which RNA and protein synthesis takes place; in the S phase DNA synthesis occurs; during the G^2, or second gap, pre-mitotic phase the mitotic spindles are constructed and RNA synthesis continues; finally, in the mitotic (M) phase, cell division and creation of two identical daughter cells takes place. On completion of this cycle, cells either re-enter the cycle at G^1 or move out of the cycle into the G^0, or resting, phase (Barton Burke et al., 1991; Renick-Ettinger, 1993). The term 'resting phase' for this period is something of a misnomer, for although the cells in this phase are not actively dividing, they are employed in specific functional activities. Normal cells spend most of their time in the G^0 phase and are only recruited back into the cell cycle in response to stimuli, such as growth factors or hormones, present on their surface membrane. These stimuli trigger a cell back into cycle by binding with surface receptors of the target cell in response to an identified demand for that particular cell type. The G^0 phase is also, therefore, a type of cell reservoir which is able to pull normal cells back into the proliferative cycle in response to the needs of an organism (Bingham, 1978; Barton Burke et al., 1991; Renick-Ettinger, 1993; Pinkerton et al., 1994).

Under normal circumstances this process is a well-balanced activity in which cell reproduction, activity and death are finely tuned in response to the feedback mechanisms of an organism (McCalla & Davis, 1978). However, although cancer cells and normal cells have similar cycles, cancer cells are not reproduced in response to any balanced feedback mechanism, rather, they continue to divide uncontrollably — affecting the ability of an organism to maintain normal function.

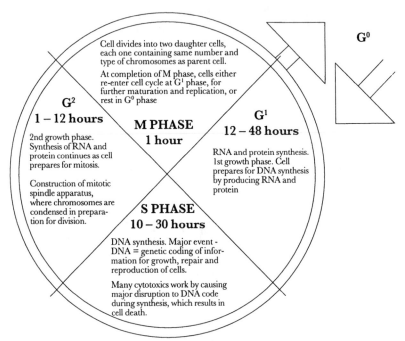

Cell Cycle Phase-specific Agents affect cells in specific phases of the cell cycle.

Cell Cycle Non-phase-specific Agents affect cells in specific phases of the cell cycle, including the G⁰ phase.
These agents are some of the most effective against slow-growing tumours.
However, because DNA is the target site for these drugs, maximum cell kill is not possible when cells are in the S phase at the time of administration.

Sources: Bingham, 1978; Barton Burke et al., 1991; Renick-Ettinger, 1993; Pinkerton et al., 1994.

Figure 1.1: The proliferative phase of the cell cycle

Chemotherapeutic agents appear to be most effective against cells during the proliferative cycle (Hardy & Pinkerton, 1992). This knowledge has enabled the development of drugs which either act specifically during one phase of the cell cycle (cell cycle phase-specific) or which have some effect during all phases of the cell cycle (cell cycle non-phase-specific) (Figure 1.2).

Cell cycle non-phase-specific chemotherapeutic agents (specifically the alkylating agents and platinum derivatives) are also effective against cells in the G^0 phase which are not actively dividing and have

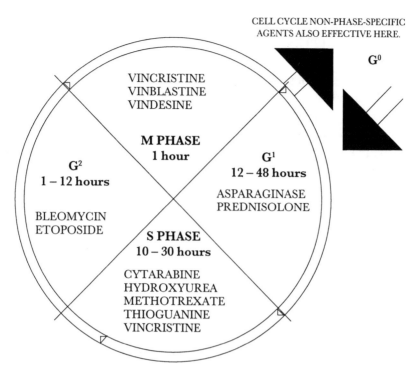

CELL CYCLE NON-PHASE-SPECIFIC AGENTS ALSO EFFECTIVE HERE.

G^0

VINCRISTINE
VINBLASTINE
VINDESINE

M PHASE
1 hour

G^2
1 – 12 hours

G^1
12 – 48 hours

ASPARAGINASE
PREDNISOLONE

BLEOMYCIN
ETOPOSIDE

S PHASE
10 – 30 hours

CYTARABINE
HYDROXYUREA
METHOTREXATE
THIOGUANINE
VINCRISTINE

CELL CYCLE NON-PHASE-SPECIFIC AGENTS INCLUDE:

ALKYLATING AGENTS	NITROSUREAS	ANTIBIOTICS	MISCELLANEOUS
BUSULPHAN	CARMUSTINE	DACTINOMYCIN	DACARBAZINE
CISPLATIN	LOMUSTINE	DAUNORUBICIN	PROCARBAZINE
CHLORAMBUCIL	SEMUSTINE	DOXORUBICIN	
CYCLOPHOSPHAMIDE	STREPTOZICIN	MITOMYCIN	
MELPHALAN		MITOZANTRONE	
		BLEOMYCIN	

Sources: Bingham, 1978; Knopf et al., 1984; Barton Burke et al., 1991; Renick-Ettinger, 1993; Pinkerton et al., 1994.

Figure 1.2: Action of chemotherapeutic agents during the cell cycle

been found to be particularly effective against slow-growing tumours (Knopf et al., 1984).

Cell Cycle Time

The overall objective in any cancer treatment plan is patient survival and the irradication of tumour cells, with minimal disruption to normal cell activity. It is known that tumours have a steady, progressive growth pattern which is affected by cell cycle time, growth fraction and cell loss. Chemotherapy has a greater effect on rapidly dividing cells. Cancer cells appear to have an initial rapid, proliferative phase during which time cells will be cycling quite quickly from mitosis to mitosis.

The time it takes for each cycle to complete ('generation time') varies between 24 and 120 hours, depending upon cell type, with most ranging between 48 and 72 hours (Barton Burke et al., 1991).

In adults most cell populations are non-proliferative and many are fully differentiated. In the developing foetus, infant, child and teenager, however, cell populations are expanding, with proliferation of cells governed by feedback mechanisms which trigger growth or cessation of growth as the individual attains various developmental stages and optimal organ size (McCalla & Davis, 1978). Because of this, it is possible to understand why certain toxicities present in the paediatric patient receiving chemotherapy and why paediatric malignancies appear to be more responsive to treatment (Barton Burke et al., 1991; Renick-Ettinger, 1993).

Growth Fraction

The growth fraction represents the number ('fraction') of cells that are cycling at any one time. During early tumour development (when tumour bulk is small) there is a high fraction of cycling cells and tumours are able to double their size quite rapidly (i.e. rapid cell division combined with a high fraction of cells going through the proliferative cycle equals rapid tumour growth).

As tumours grow in size, the blood, oxygen and nutrient supply become compromised and space for growth is restricted. During this time the cell growth fraction is low and the cycle time is slowed, therefore cell growth ('doubling time') is decreased.

Because chemotherapy is more effective against rapidly dividing cells, it may be less effective when tumours have reached this stage. However, it may be possible to increase both cell growth fraction and cell cycle time again by achieving an initial tumour reduction, either through the use of chemotherapy, radiotherapy or surgery. This would stimulate trigger mechanisms on the cell surfaces to recruit cells back into cycle in an attempt to replace the lost bulk. Once this has been achieved, chemotherapy once again becomes effective against reduced tumour bulk, with a high growth fraction of rapidly dividing cells (Barton Burke et al., 1991; Renick-Ettinger, 1993).

Cell Kill Hypothesis

The cell kill hypothesis is based on the theory that a given concentration of antineoplastic agent will kill a constant percentage of tumour cells. In theory, this constant *percentage* cell kill, rather than a constant cell *number* kill remains unchanged as subsequent treatments are given. As each treatment is given the number of tumour cells remaining is reduced, but the percentage of cells killed remains the same. Ultimately, the aim is to irradicate all the tumour cells or reduce the number of tumour cells surviving to such a small total population that the body's own immune system is able to deal effectively with them. Factors which have greatest influence on this theory include: the number and doses of repeated therapy; the time between repeated doses; and the doubling time of the tumour. Factors which limit this process are: drug toxicity; patient tolerance and recovery from toxicity; and cell mutations which render some tumour cells resistant to the chemotherapeutic agent (Renick-Ettinger, 1993; Kaufman & Chabner, 1996). In practice, there are some exceptions to this hypothesis:

- Following debulking of a large, slow-growing tumour, which may initially have shown poor or limited response to chemotherapy, the cell division rate may increase and more cells may be recruited from the G^0 phase. Fractional cell kill would be increased rather than remain constant in this situation.
- Tumours in the later stages of growth (which have undergone a mutation from their cloned originator cells) may comprise a mixture of cell types and may include cells which show very different characteristics, including different drug-response characteristics. Fractional cell kill would be decreased under these circumstances, as all the drug-sensitive cells are destroyed early, leaving only drug-resistant cells behind; these are then able to continue to proliferate (Kaufman & Chabner, 1996).

Cytostatic and Cytotoxic Therapy Principles

Cytostatic agents are used to arrest cell development by holding cells in a specific phase of their growth cycle. *Cytotoxic* agents kill cells. Some cytotoxic agents may act as cytostatic agents when given in lower doses, and some cytostatic agents may become cytotoxic when given in higher doses (Gussack, Brantley & Farmer, 1984). By combining the principles of recruitment, cytostasis and cytotoxicity, theoretically, a higher percentage of tumour cells can be killed.

Cytostatic agents are used to hold cells in a specific cell cycle phase, increasing the percentage of cells made vulnerable to cell cycle phase-specific cytotoxic agents (for example, cytarabine has a cytostatic effect, causing cells to arrest at the G^1/S phase boundary; this then renders them vulnerable to S phase-specific agents, such as methotrexate, vincristine or thioguanine (Hill, 1978)). As the overall tumour cell population is depleted more cells are recruited back into the growth cycle from the G^0 phase, once again increasing the population of tumour cells exposed to cell cycle phase-specific cytotoxic agents (Barton Burke et al., 1991).

Pharmacokinetics and Pharmacodynamics

Pharmacokinetics is the study of the movement of drugs in the body, including the processes of absorption, distribution, localisation in tissue, biotransformation and excretion (Renick-Ettinger, 1993). For these reasons pharmacokinetics plays an important role in the successful application of cancer chemotherapy. Although some tumours may be known to be sensitive to a given cytotoxic agent, that agent may still fail to achieve a response. An understanding of how a patient's body is able to deal with a given agent, in terms of absorption, metabolism and elimination, and of how these factors may be adversely affected by hepatic and renal dysfunction (common toxicities of some of the more frequently used chemotherapeutic agents) is essential in determining dose, timing and route of administration.

Individual patients may demonstrate variable responses to therapies due to particular physiological or cellular status. Interference with absorption (due to nausea/vomiting, alteration in gut motility), distribution (due to weight loss/gain, decreased body fat, pleural effusions/ascites), elimination (due to hepatic or renal impairment) and protein binding (due to hypoalbuminaemia or concomitant medications) may all affect the bioavailability of the drug adversely.

Pharmacodynamics studies the relationship between drug concentrations and their effects on the body. For example, it may be possible to give a particular drug either as a bolus or as an infusion and achieve a completely different therapeutic or toxic effect (for example, the potential to reduce the development of cardiomyopathy caused by anthracycline antibiotics when these drugs are given as a slow infusion rather than as a bolus). Abnormalities in the pharmacokinetics of a drug will have a 'knock on' effect on its pharmacodynamics (Renick-Ettinger, 1993).

An understanding of these two principles underlines the importance of careful and regular monitoring of the patient before each course of treatment, and flexibility in prescribing to ensure modifications of doses are calculated based on changes in the physiological status of the patient. Combining these two principles ensures that it is possible to give the optimal treatment for each patient (Renick-Ettinger, 1993; Kaufman & Chabner, 1996).

Considerations when Planning Chemotherapy Treatments

Drug resistance

The principles of cancer chemotherapy are based upon empirical evidence of responses by particularly chemosensitive cancers to chemotherapy. Some of the earlier treatment trials for acute lymphoblastic leukaemia involved the use of single-agent drugs which were found to be effective, at least initially, inducing remission in approximately 60% of cases. Unfortunately, remission was not maintained through continued use of that same single-agent drug and consequently almost all patients had relapsed within 6–9 months. This suggests that there may be a form of drug resistance within the cancer cells, which may be present at the outset ('intrinsic resistance') or may be a learned response by those cells as treatment progresses ('acquired resistance') (Balis et al., 1993).

It has been identified that those cancer cells which do show evidence of drug resistance express high numbers of a protein (P-glycoprotein) on the cell membrane (Kartner & Ling, 1989). This protein seems to act as a pump, rapidly pushing through and eliminating the chemotherapeutic agents from within the cell, preventing their therapeutic effect. Chemosensitive tumours have very little, if any, P-glycoprotein on their surface membrane (see Chapter 6 for more detail).

It is thought that multidrug-resistant cells (MDR) have a gene amplification of MDR transcribed into their RNA, which results in the production of high levels of P-glycoprotein (Goldstein et al., 1989). Some agents are known to be more sensitive than others to this glycoprotein and they include the antitumour antibiotics, epipodophyllotoxins and the vinca alkaloids.

It is thought that the incidence of drug resistance to specific single agents may exceed 50% in some cases (Balis et al., 1993). Ultimately, the potential of the cancer cells to acquire sufficient drug resistance to render a drug ineffective has to be a primary consideration when planning and developing chemotherapeutic protocols. Unfortunately, the ability to predict accurately specific tumour and patient sensitivity to a given drug continues to elude researchers.

It is possible to conduct retrospective analysis of tumour drug resistance which provides quite accurate results (by use of mice or *in vitro* tests). However, prospective studies are not yet available routinely. Drug selection, therefore, continues to be made on the basis of results of previous clinical trials, tumour type and extent of disease, rather than on known tumour drug sensitivity (Kaufman & Chabner, 1996).

Toxicities

Another important consideration is the fact that chemotherapy agents are essentially non-selective, i.e. they have the same cytotoxic effect on both normal and malignant cells. This cell toxicity is often dose-limiting and restrictive.

Normal cells need to have the opportunity for recovery between treatments to avoid life-threatening or life-quality threatening toxicities which may be unacceptable to patients, both in the short and long term. Even in the presence of drug resistance, unacceptable toxicities may occur because of the toxic effects of chemotherapy on normal cells. The combination of intrinsic drug resistance and adverse toxicity identifies the need for careful balancing of cause and effect when planning treatments. It is quite probable that many patients, even with the advent of modern treatment protocols, receive drugs which may be ineffective in terms of tumour response but produce unacceptable toxic effects (Balis et al., 1993).

In the palliative stages of disease, where cure is no longer the aim of treatment, careful consideration of the toxic effects of drugs used for symptom control needs to be weighed against the quality of life achievable for each individual patient. Patient choice is always an important aspect of treatment planning, but in the palliative stages it is crucial that the child and family have an understanding of all options available. Toxicity deemed acceptable during active therapy, may prove unacceptable for the dying child.

Treatment Approaches

The ultimate aims of treatment for all patients are cure and quality of life. The potential to fulfil these aims depends on a number of variable factors including: type, stage and spread of disease; scientific, technological and professional resources available; treatment options and known responses; and informed patient choice.

Approaches to treatments have evolved over time as experience has shaped future trends. With collaboration at national and international level, experience is shared more widely, facilitating a unified approach to treatment, research and development and data collection.

In active therapy (where cure is achievable) established and proven chemotherapeutic agents are utilised to achieve maximum tumour cell kill with minimal toxicity to the patient. The boundary between these aims is a very fine line. As treatment strategies continue to develop and supportive measures improve there is a move towards the use of more and more intensive treatment.

When cure is no longer a realistic goal and palliative support is being considered, established chemotherapeutic agents may be used in different ways to support the patient and manage symptoms. Any adverse toxicity at this stage may well be deemed unacceptable by the patient and carers and intensive therapies can no longer be justified. New drugs may also be utilised, with informed consent, to help manage symptoms for the individual patient but also to help with the development of future therapies. The single consistent goal in either situation is the maintainance of good quality of life for the patient.

Single Agent versus Combination

The efficacy of combinations of chemotherapeutic agents was first recognised over 40 years ago in the treatment of acute lymphoblastic leukaemia (ALL). Compared with single-agent therapy, combinations of drugs were seen to increase not only the percentage of patients achieving complete remission but also the duration of the remission achieved (Kaufman & Chabner, 1996). As previously discussed, remission was achieved but not maintained in patients receiving single-agent drug therapy, whereas 95% of patients who received four- and five-drug combinations maintained long term remission (Balis et al., 1993).

This rate of relapse with single-agent drug therapy was probably the result of cell line mutations producing a cell line with resistance to the agent being used. Higher doses of these agents were then used in an attempt to irradicate tumour cells; this, in turn, resulted in severe and often lethal toxicities (Hubbard, 1981).

Long term remission and cure in the treatment of childhood leukaemia were first realised in the late 1950s with the application of treatment regimes containing combinations of the most effective single-agent drugs. The primary rationale for the introduction of combination therapy was to overcome the potential for cell line resistance to single-agent drugs in use, the incidence of which often exceeded 50% (Goldie & Coldman, 1984; Devita, 1989). It also became apparent that these single-agent drugs were less toxic and were seen to have a synergistic effect, enhancing the antitumour effect when used in combination with others (Barton Burke et al., 1991; Balis et al., 1993).

Not all tumours respond to a particular single-agent drug, due either to intrinsic or acquired resistance, and it is impossible to predict which tumour will respond to which single-agent therapy. A patient may therefore receive a drug which is the conventional therapy for that particular malignant disease, but which is ineffective for that individual (Balis et al., 1993). This could result in further treatments being compromised, either due to unacceptable toxicity from the ineffective treatment or the development of resistant or multidrug-resistant cell lines. It is hoped that the use of combinations of the most effective single-agent drugs with independent cell killing properties will reduce this risk and a greater chance of achieving a response will be ensured (Kaufman & Chabner, 1996).

Principles for Consideration

- The potential for cross resistance must be an important consideration when planning combination therapies. One specific cell line mutation may produce resistance to many different chemotherapeutic agents.
- Each single-agent drug used in combination must have a proven record of efficacy when used alone against the malignancy being treated.
- Each single-agent drug used in combination must complement the mechanisms of action of the others being used, i.e. cell cycle phase-specific and cell cycle non-phase-specific, specific phase activity and different phase active drugs, cytostatic and cytotoxic agents.
- Each single-agent drug used in combination should produce different toxic effects which occur at different times to minimise morbidity (Barton Burke et al., 1991).

Adjuvant Chemotherapy

Adjuvant therapies are used in addition to other modes of therapy, i.e. surgery, chemotherapy or radiotherapy, to enhance treatment outcomes (Renick-Ettinger, 1993). The most common application for the use of adjuvant chemotherapy is the treatment of paediatric solid tumours, specifically those which have a high risk of relapse at metastatic sites but which show no evidence of residual disease following local treatment with surgery or radiotherapy (Balis et al., 1993).

Before adjuvant chemotherapy was used routinely, relapse at metastatic sites occurred in 60–95% of children with localised solid tumours following local therapy with surgery or radiotherapy. Adjuvant chemotherapy aims to prevent metastatic recurrence by eliminating micrometastatic deposits which may be present in the lungs, bone, bone marrow, lymph nodes and other sites. It is believed that adjuvant chemotherapy works because a larger fraction of tumour cells are actively proliferating following initial tumour debulking with surgery or radiotherapy and are therefore more susceptible to the cytotoxic effects of the chemotherapy used. The smaller burden of tumour cells remaining following initial debulking also reduces the risk of drug resisitant cells being present (Goldie & Coldman, 1984; Balis et al., 1993).

The drugs most likely to be curative when used for adjuvant therapy are those which have produced the most effective response when used in advanced metastatic or recurrent disease (Wittes, 1986).

Neo-adjuvant Chemotherapy

One natural progression from the application of adjuvant chemotherapy is the use of neo-adjuvant chemotherapy. Chemotherapy is used before definitive localised therapy in an attempt to shrink the tumour bulk, facilitating less radical surgical or radiotherapeutic interventions, and providing earlier treatment of micrometastatic disease (Balis et al., 1993). Utilised in this way it is also possible to identify those chemotherapeutic interventions which are effective against a particular tumour in a particular patient. Further courses of chemotherapy are often prescribed once recovery from definitive localised treatment is attained.

Dose-intensive Regimes

Multidrug resistance and treatment toxicities are two of the most important factors for consideration when developing chemotherapeutic protocols. As previously described, the development of combination treatment therapies has moved some way towards overcoming these problems. However, it is still possible for tumour cells to develop resistance to some combination therapies.

The growth fraction hypothesis (described earlier) postulates that tumours in the early stages of development or those with reduced bulk following initial treatment have a higher fraction of cells in the proliferative growth cycle which are more susceptible to chemotherapeutic agents (Barton Burke et al., 1991). It is also evident that the optimal dose of an agent (to achieve maximum tumour cell kill) is restricted because of the severe or lethal toxicity produced. With the development of more sophisticated and effective supportive therapies there is the potential to achieve greater tumour cell kill by combining aggressive treatment regimes with these supportive measures.

Between each block of intensive treatment there is a period of rest or 'recovery' to allow the normal cells of the body to recover. Normal cells have a greater capacity for recovery than malignant cells and it is this ability for recovery which governs the frequency of intermittent dosing schedules (Hardy & Pinkerton, 1992). Timing is all-important. If too much time is left between dosing schedules, tumour cells have a better opportunity for recovery and, potentially, the development of mutated drug-resistant cells. If too little time is left between dosing schedules the toxic effect on normal cells becomes unacceptable (Hardy & Pinkerton, 1992). It has also been shown that dose reduction to overcome problems with toxicity has, in some cases, led to an increased risk of relapse (Balis et al., 1993; Kaufman & Chabner, 1996).

Goldie and Coldman (1986) suggest that early treatment with maximum doses of effective chemotherapeutic agents, repeated as frequently as possible, will produce maximum tumour cell kill whilst preventing multidrug resistance. This theory is now an important consideration in the design of more intensive treatment protocols, for example, in the treatment of childhood leukaemia it has been shown that remission and cure rates are improved when two intensive blocks of therapy are given as opposed to one.

Strategies have been developed which allow dose-intensive therapies to be given with minimal delay between each block of therapy. These include:

- Use of bone marrow or peripheral stem cell transplant to 'rescue' the patient following treatment.
- Use of colony-stimulating factors to stimulate haematopoeitic regrowth and reduce episodes of neutropenia.
- Regional treatments, such as intra-arterial or intrathecal admin-

istration, to achieve high dose concentrations at local tumour sites whilst minimising systemic drug exposure.

- Use of established drugs in new ways, such as long term continuous infusions, which allow more drug to be given over a period of time.
- Use of high dose drug combinations which have varying toxicities at varying times. This enables more drugs to be given in a shorter period of time. For example, myelosuppressive agents given on day 1 of each cycle, followed by non-myelosuppressive agents at approximately day 8 of a 21-day cycle. This allows for bone marrow recovery between cycles whilst ensuring continued suppression of tumour growth throughout the cycle (Barton Burke et al., 1991; Balis et al., 1993; Renick-Ettinger, 1993; Kaufman & Chabner, 1996).

Classification of Drugs

In general, chemotherapeutic agents are classified according to their chemical structure and cell cycle activity. There are six major classes of drugs (see Table 1.1):

- Alkylating agents
- Plant alkaloids
- Antimetabolites
- Antitumour antibiotics
- Hormones – corticosteroids
- Miscellaneous agents

Alkylating agents

These are a group of reactive chemicals which act through the covalent bonding of an alkyl group, by substituting the hydrogen atoms in the cellular molecules. This causes cross-linking and DNA strand breaks. Through this process damage is caused to the DNA template, RNA, DNA and protein synthesis is inhibited and replication is unable to take place. The most affected of the nucleic acid bases is guanine, but cytosine and adenine are also known to be affected.

Alkylating agents are classed as cell cycle non-phase-specific and are effective against cells in all phases of the cycle, including the G^0 phase. This means that they have the capacity to effect tumour

Table 1.1: Classification of cytotoxic drugs

Drug	Action	Common uses
Alkylating agents		
Busulphan	causes DNA cross links; cell cycle non-phase-specific	leukaemias
Carboplatin	causes intrastrand and interstrand cross links by reacting with nucleophilic sites on DNA	brain tumours neuroblastoma germ cell tumours
Carmustine (BCNU)	causes DNA cross links and strand breaks	brain tumours lymphomas
Chlorambucil	causes DNA cross links and strand breaks	–
Cisplatin	causes intrastrand and interstrand cross links and prevents cell replication by denaturing the double helix	testicular and germ cell tumours osteosarcoma brain tumours neuroblastoma
Cyclophosphamide	causes DNA cross links	lymphomas leukaemias sarcomas neuroblastoma
Dacarbazine (DTIC)	causes DNA cross links and strand breaks; inhibits DNA and RNA synthesis	neuroblastoma sarcomas Hodgkin's disease
Ifosfamide	causes DNA cross links with DNA and binds to proteins	sarcomas germ cell tumours
Lomustine (CCNU)	causes DNA cross links and strand breaks; inhibits DNA and RNA synthesis	brain tumours lymphomas
Melphalan	causes DNA cross links, strand breaks and miscoding RNA synthesis	neuroblastoma sarcomas rhabdomyosarcoma leukaemias Hodgkin's disease
Nitrogen mustard	interstrand and intrastrand cross links, miscoding, breakage and failure of replication	brain tumours Hodgkin's disease
Procarbazine	affects pre-formed DNA, RNA and protein	brain tumours Hodgkin's disease
Streptozicin	interstrand DNA cross links	–
Thiotepa	chromosome cross links with inhibition of nucleoprotein synthesis	brain tumours

(contd)

Table 1.1: (contd)

Drug	Action	Common uses
Plant alkaloids		
Etoposide (VP16)	inhibits DNA synthesis in S and G^2 phases causing single strand breaks in DNA	leukaemia lymphomas testicular tumours neuroblastoma sarcomas brain tumours
Teniposide (VM26)	inhibits DNA uptake of thymidine thereby impairing DNA synthesis; works in late S and early G^2 phases	leukaemia lymphomas testicular tumours neuroblastoma sarcomas brain tumours
Vinblastine	binds to microtubular proteins causing mitotic arrest during metaphase. May also inhibit DNA, RNA and protein synthesis; active in S and M phases	histiocytosis Hodgkin's disease testicular tumours
Vincristine	Binds to microtubular proteins causing mitotic arrest during metaphase; active in S and M phases	leukaemia lymphomas most solid tumours
Antimetabolites		
Cytarabine	pyrimidine analogue incorporated into DNA; slows synthesis and causes defective links and erroneous duplication of early DNA strands; S phase-specific	leukaemias lymphomas
Methotrexate	dihydrofolate reductase enzyme inhibitor; results in the inhibition of the precursors of DNA, RNA and cellular proteins; S phase-specific	leukaemias lymphomas osteosarcoma
6-Mercaptopurine	thiopurine antimetabolite which inhibits *de novo* purine synthesis by converting to monophosphate nucleotides; S phase-specific	leukaemias
6-Thioguanine	thiopurine antimetabolite which inhibits *de novo* purine synthesis by converting to monophosphate nucleotides; S phase-specific	leukaemias

(contd)

Table 1.1: (contd)

Drug	Action	Common uses
Antitumour antibiotics		
Doxorubicin (adriamycin)	binds to DNA base pairs; inhibits DNA, RNA and protein synthesis; S phase-specific	leukaemias lymphomas solid tumours
Bleomycin	induces double and single strand breaks in DNA; inhibits DNA synthesis	lymphomas testicular and other germ cell tumours
Dactinomycin (actinomycin D)	inhibits DNA and RNA synthesis by binding to the guanine portion of DNA; DNA is then unable to act as a template for DNA and RNA; G^1 and S phase-specific	Wilms' tumour sarcoma
Daunorubicin	intercalates DNA blocking DNA, RNA and protein synthesis	leukaemias
Epirubicin	causes DNA strand breaks	lymphomas leukaemias
Idarubicin	inhibits RNA synthesis; S phase-specific	leukaemias
Mitozantrone	inhibits DNA and RNA synthesis through intercalation of base pairs; cell cycle non-phase-specific	lymphomas sarcomas
Corticosteroids		
Prednisolone	unclear how it works; thought to be due to receptor-mediated lympholysis	leukaemias lymphomas
Dexamethasone	unclear how it works; thought to be due to receptor-mediated lympholysis	leukaemias lymphomas brain tumours
Miscellaneous agents		
L-asparaginase	hydrolysis of serum asparagine; G^1 phase-specific	leukaemias
Amsacrine	intercalates and binds DNA and inhibits topoisomerase II and RNA synthesis; S phase-specific	leukaemias

Sources: Burke et al., 1991; Plowman & Pinkerton, 1992; Pizzo & Poplack 1993; Chabner & Longo, 1996.

shrinkage, causing more cells to be recruited back into the active proliferative cycle where they become susceptible to the cell cycle phase-specific agents. This also means that the alkylating agents are effective against both slow-growing and rapidly proliferating tumours.

Plant alkaloids

These are a group of compounds developed from plant extracts which includes the vinca alkaloids (derived from the shrub *Vinca rosea* or periwinkle) and the epipodophyllotoxins (derived from the root of the mandrake plant).

The vinca alkaloids, vincristine and vinblastine, act as mitotic inhibitors and work by crystallising the microtubular mitotic spindle proteins during metaphase, thus arresting mitosis.

The epipodophyllotoxins, etoposide and teniposide, are analogues of the antimitotic agent, podophyllotoxin. These drugs act in a slightly different way to the vinca alkaloids in that they cause single and double strand DNA breaks, rather than inhibiting microtubule mitotic spindle proteins.

The plant alkaloids are classed as cell cycle phase-specific, the vinca alkaloids being effective during the M phase and the epipodophyllotoxins exerting greatest effect in the premitotic G^2 phase.

Antimetabolites

These are a group of agents which act by mimicking the essential metabolites necessary for DNA and RNA synthesis. They are so structurally similar to the metabolites of which they are analogues that they are able to deceive the cells into incorporating them into the metabolic pathways.

They are effective either through inhibition of cellular macromolecular synthesis and their building blocks, or through their incorporation into the metabolic pathways which results in a defective end-product.

The antimetabolites are classed as cell cycle phase-specific and are effective in the S phase. They are most cytotoxic against cells which are synthesising DNA and are therefore most effective against rapidly proliferating rather than slow-growing tumours.

Antitumour antibiotics

This is a group of naturally occurring substances, isolated from micro-organisms, which have been found to have both antimicrobial and cytotoxic properties. Although each of the antitumour antibiotics uses a different mechanism to produce a cytotoxic effect they all either bind or react with DNA or interfere with RNA synthesis. This group of drugs includes the anthracyclines doxorubicin and daunorubicin, bleomycin and dactinomycin.

The anthracyclines act as intercalators, i.e. portions of the drug are inserted between base pairs on the double helix of DNA. Through this action, the anthracyclines interact with enzymes responsible for regulating DNA shape, replication, transcription, repair and recombination. This results in breaks in the DNA strands.

Bleomycin works by binding to DNA and producing double and single strand breaks.

Dactinomycin primarily binds to DNA by intercalation, inhibiting replication and transcription. It can also effect single strand breaks in DNA through enzyme intercalation.

The antitumour antibiotics are classed as cell cycle non-phase-specific.

Hormones — corticosteroids

The corticosteroids, although not classically defined as specific anti-cancer agents, have a significant role to play in the treatment of certain paediatric malignancies. They have a diverse clinical effect, but most specifically in relation to malignancy, their lympholytic effect and recruitment potential has made them particularly useful in the treatment of ALL, lymphoma and Hodgkin's disease. There is also some evidence to suggest that they may also recruit malignant cells from the G^0 phase into active division.

Miscellaneous agents

In normal tissues the non-essential amino acid, asparagine, is produced through synthesis of aspartic acid and glutamine by the enzyme, asparagine synthase. This results in a continual production and release of asparagine into the circulation. Normal cells are therefore able to synthesise their own asparagine, which is needed to maintain normal growth and development.

Tumour cells are unable to synthesise their own asparagine to facilitate protein synthesis because they lack an enzyme necessary for this synthesis to take place. Instead they rely on this continual circulating pool of asparagine produced by normal cells. By introducing a catalyst, the enzyme L-asparaginase, into this circulating pool of amino acids, asparagine is converted into aspartic acid and ammonia. This effectively starves the tumour cells through rapid depletion of circulating asparagine and inhibits tumour cell protein synthesis.

Chapter 2
Administration of chemotherapy

Louise Hooker and Sarah Palmer

Safe Practice with Cytotoxic Drugs

A number of studies have shown that cytotoxic drugs can produce mutagenic, carcinogenic or teratogenic effects in personnel handling them (Selevan et al., 1985; Hemminki, 1985; McDonald et al., 1988). This has been correlated to contamination via unprotected working practices, demonstrated by the presence of cytotoxic agents in the urine (Hirst et al., 1984) and measures of urine mutagenicity (Falck et al., 1979; Cloak et al., 1985) in nurses and other professionals whose work involves contact with cytotoxic drugs. Poor comparability between the studies and their conflicting results (Cloak et al., 1985) complicates any attempt to reach conclusions about the degree of risk with any certainty, as there is wide variation in the measures used (Vennitt et al., 1984) and different working practices and safety precautions reported (Valanis & Shortridge, 1987). Also, everyday contact with environmental and dietary mutagens (Caudell, 1988) confounds any calculation of the increased risk posed by administering cytotoxic drugs. However, the mutagenicity of cancer chemotherapy agents is undeniable, and they pose an occupational hazard which can be minimised by following safety precautions (Siddall, 1988). Incidences of localised reactions to contamination, such as contact dermatitis, skin irritation and corneal damage, have also been reported (Williams, 1985), as have more systemic symptoms, such as nausea, hair loss, malaise and dizziness (Caudell, 1988). There is evidence to support the effectiveness of precautions in reducing mutagens in the urine, and the associated health-related problems (Vennitt et al., 1984; Skov et al., 1992). Individuals whose working life includes contact with chemotherapeutic agents are taking unnecessary risks if they do not follow guidelines for safe practice.

To provide information and guidance, policies for safe practice with cytotoxic agents have been widely produced by hospitals and national bodies (Health and Safety Executive, 1988a, 1988b; RCN, 1989). However, efforts to ensure compliance are complicated by inconsistencies between different policies and the reticence of some individuals to take safe practice seriously (Valanis & Shortridge, 1987; Gullo, 1995). Anyone involved with the preparation, administration, handling and disposal of cytotoxic drugs requires adequate information and training. This obviously involves the educational and practical preparation of nursing, medical and pharmacy staff, for example, through registered oncology nursing courses, or chemotherapy training programmes (Pike & Gibson, 1991; RCN, 1994). However, safe practice involves not only the protection of those directly involved in administration and patient care, but also consideration of other people in the chemotherapeutic environment who may not be aware of the risks and are therefore unable to take appropriate steps to protect themselves. By virtue of their professional knowledge and role, nurses have a duty of care to others. Subsequently, they have a responsibility to support the creation and maintenance of a safety culture, where protection of themselves and their colleagues, patients and their families and other visitors is accorded due respect.

Safe practice during pregnancy

As the full effects of cytotoxic drugs on the foetus are unknown, it is advisable that pregnant women or those planning a pregnancy should not have contact with these drugs. This applies to all hospital staff as well as the child's parents and carers. Skov et al. (1992) state that conclusive evidence is now emerging that alkylating antineoplastic drugs can cause cancer and most are reprotoxic, resulting in an increased risk of miscarriages and malformations in pregnant health workers handling these particular drugs.

Safe practice with cytotoxic drugs, using recommended protection and excellent technique, should theoretically prevent exposure and therefore rule out the risk to the foetus. However, for ethical reasons, it is unlikely that research will ever be conducted to provide conclusive proof that absolutely no risk to the foetus exists if precautions are taken. The theoretical risk of birth defects and miscarriage is ruled out if exposure to these drugs does not occur. This may not be totally possible when caring for paediatric oncology patients. Ideally, staff should routinely be allowed the option of working on a different ward where their work does not involve administering cyto- toxic drugs during pregnancy. To what extent this can happen in practice is unclear, however the evidence seems to indicate that by taking the recommended precautions, pregnant staff can continue to work safely in a paediatric oncology environment, although many individuals choose not to prepare or administer chemotherapy during the first trimester of pregnancy. Each staff member should decide to what extent she continues to work with cytotoxic drugs and her decision should be supported by her management team.

Pregnant women are also advised to take care to prevent skin contact with the body fluids and excreta of children receiving chemotherapy. Mothers or other women caring for such children may need to be reminded to wear the correct gloves when changing nappies, and to take the recommended precautions when preparing and administering oral chemotherapy to their child. If a child's mother usually takes responsibility for home administration of chemotherapy, alternatives should be discussed if she becomes pregnant.

Reconstitution and Preparation of Chemotherapeutic Agents

The principle behind all the recommended safety precautions is to provide physical barriers between the cytotoxic drugs and the possi- ble routes of contamination: inhalation, absorption, ingestion and inoculation. General issues of safe practice will be outlined here, with specific details being discussed with respect to each of the differ- ent routes of drug administration.

- *Inhalation* of aerosols can easily occur without the knowledge of the handler; aerosols may be inhaled in liquid or powder form, causing local inflammation of mucous membranes or systemic effects following entry into the blood via the pulmonary circulation.
- *Absorption* can occur through contact with the skin, cornea or mucous membranes, from airborne particles or droplets (Galassi, 1996). Some agents can cause rashes, blistering or local necrosis. Fat-soluble drugs may be absorbed directly into the bloodstream (Darbyshire, 1986).
- *Ingestion* can take place if traces of drug enter the mouth via the hands, or by food or drinks placed in the area of preparation becoming contaminated.

- *Inoculation* via accidental puncturing of the skin, or if an unhealed, exposed skin injury comes into contact with the drug.

Ideally, all cytotoxic drugs should be prepared centrally in a pharmacy department, using a laminar airflow cabinet, by designated staff who have received training in this area. In the event that cytotoxic drugs have to be prepared in the ward environment, recommendations for drug preparation include a well-ventilated but draught-free room, with a closed door, limited access and running water. No food or drink should be allowed in the preparation room. It is important that the preparation worksurface can be easily cleaned and is impermeable, and that reconstitution is carried out on a disposable or easily washed tray, to contain any spillages. A paper towel placed on the tray will absorb any fluid and make safe disposal easier.

When preparing cytotoxic drugs, protective clothing must be worn by all personnel involved in the procedure, namely face mask, plastic apron, safety glasses or visor and waterproof long sleeves with cuffs (armlets), over which thick latex or vinyl gloves should be worn. When giving drugs to a child, a balance should be maintained between ensuring reasonable protective measures are taken, and the potential for alarming the recipient. By considering logically the possible routes of contamination for the method of administration and related procedures, an approach that is both sensible and safe can usually be achieved. The importance of correct and thoughtful administration practices can minimise the risk of accidental contamination. Whatever protection is worn during drug administration, the child and parents require explanation of the reasons for its use, and children may enjoy playing 'dressing up' with (unused) protective clothing to help normalise the measures taken.

Storage

If cytotoxic drugs are not intended for immediate administration they should be clearly labelled with the name, dose and volume of the drug supplied, method of storage (locked refrigerator or cupboard at room temperature), expiry date and time, and a statement that the drug is cytotoxic. Drugs should then be stored in accordance with local policy.

Disposal of waste

The management and disposal of used or contaminated equipment, body fluids, spillages and unused drugs should be addressed, as these are a potential source of drug exposure. Official guidelines, such as those used for the disposal of hazardous wastes, should be followed.

Equipment

'Sharps' (needles, ampoules and vials) should be disposed of in the approved container according to local policy. Empty syringes are either disposed of in the sharps container or with other dry clinical waste to be incinerated, including administration sets, bags and disposable protective clothing. Non-disposable equipment should be washed in warm soapy water and dried after use.

Unused drugs and solutions

Whenever possible, cytotoxic drug waste of any kind should be disposed of by high temperature incineration (1000°C) (RCN, 1989). Unused doses of drugs should be returned to the dispensing pharmacy at the earliest opportunity for possible re-use or disposal. Part-used doses of drugs should be disposed of as hazardous clinical waste, but only if their container can be securely resealed for storage and transportation. Staff should wear protective clothing when disconnecting cytotoxic infusions, disposing of equipment and waste and washing non-disposable equipment. These procedures should not be delegated to others (e.g. trainee nurses) without first providing adequate education.

Spillage

Any spillage of a cytotoxic drug must be cleared up immediately, but if the handler is pregnant it is recommended that this is carried out by another member of staff. Access to the spillage area should be restricted. Protective clothing must be worn; thick latex or vinyl gloves, waterproof armlets, plastic apron and safety glasses or visor. Absorbent paper towels should be used to clean up the spillage and the area washed down thoroughly with copious amounts of soap and water. All the waste should be disposed of in an identified cytotoxic disposal bag for incineration. If airborne powder or aerosol is involved it is recommended that a face mask or particulate respirator is also worn to prevent inhalation and that damp paper towels are used for wiping surfaces.

Contamination

If contamination of the skin or eyes occurs then immediate action must be taken. Skin should be washed thoroughly with copious amounts of soap and water and then dried. Eyes should be irrigated with 0.9% sodium chloride and eye wash using free-flowing irrigation to the eye. An eye bath should NOT be used as the contained fluid may spread the cytotoxic agent around the enclosed area within the eye bath. Further medical attention should be sought immediately if any visible trauma to the skin or eyes develops and reference to any individual drug recommendations should be followed. Any incidents should be reported, and supported by written documentation according to local hospital incident policy, and also to Occupational Health. The incident must be investigated so that precautionary measures can be taken to prevent further recurrence. If contamination to clothing or bed linen occurs, these should be changed immediately and treated according to the local policy for soiled linen.

Parents giving chemotherapy in the home need information about management of accidental spillage. According to the above guidelines, contaminated clothing or bed linen can normally be washed in a domestic machine, but if this is not possible, or in the event of excessive contamination, local risk waste procedures should be employed (RCN, 1989).

Body fluids

Body fluids may contain potentially hazardous amounts of cytotoxic drugs or their active metabolites and most drugs are eliminated by renal or faecal excretion. Body fluids should therefore be handled promptly and with caution, wearing gloves and an apron at all times. Care should also be taken when handling vomit, wound drainage fluid and blood (Health and Safety Executive, 1988a, b).

As a general rule, body fluids should be assumed to be contaminated during chemotherapy and for a minimum of two days and up to seven days afterwards, although each drug has a different excretion rate (Table 2.1). The excretion pattern varies as well; for example, some drugs are excreted unchanged in the urine; for others only a trace appears in the urine (Gullo, 1988). It is important that parents are made aware of this fact so that they can be supplied with gloves for changing nappies and/or soiled bed linen and for dealing with their child's body fluids, both in and out of hospital.

Table 2.1: Cytotoxic drugs requiring extended precautionary periods for handling excreta after administration			
Drug	Route of administration	Time in urine (days)	Time in faeces (days)
Bleomycin	injection	3	?
Cisplatin	i.v.	7	?
Cyclophosphamide	any	3	5
Dactinomycin	i.v.	5	7
Daunorubicin	i.v.	2	7
Doxorubicin	i.v.	6	7
Epirubicin	i.v.	7	5
Etoposide	any	4	7
Melphalan	oral	2	7
Mercaptopurine	oral	3	?
Methotrexate	any	3	7
Mitozantrone	i.v.	6	7
Thiotepa	i.v.	3	?
Vinca alkaloids	i.v.	4	7

Source: Cass & Musgrave, 1992.

The rate of excretion of cytotoxic drugs is dependent on:

- The particular drug
- Dose, route, duration of therapy, renal and/or hepatic function
- Concomitant drug therapy, which may influence elimination rates (Cass et al., 1997).

There are some drugs which have an extended excretion pattern and therefore appropriate precautions should be taken where indicated, i.e. continuing to treat body fluids as if contaminated for an extended period.

Chemotherapy Administration

Chemotherapy can be given by nearly all accepted drug routes. However, only the most common methods of administration for paediatric patients will be discussed and other routes are mentioned only briefly. All drugs should be given in accordance with local operational policies and procedures. The basis of good practice in the administration of chemotherapy is *safety* and *patient comfort*. Nurses giving chemotherapy must therefore ensure that they are familiar with the treatment protocol *and* the needs of the child and family.

A thorough nursing assessment must be undertaken before cytotoxic drugs are given. Meeske and Ruccione (1987) suggest that when preparing to administer chemotherapy to a child the following should be considered:

- The child's diagnosis and disease presentation
- Pre-existing conditions
- Existing chemotherapy-induced toxicity
- The child's past experience with the prescribed drugs
- Anticipation of side effects (probability, timing, prevention strategies and assessment methods)
- Preparation of the child and the family.

Potential and actual problems and planned strategies to overcome them should be documented. The involvement of the child and the family in this process can help them to understand the treatment and assist in the process of negotiating the family's desired level of involvement in care. If the agreed roles of the parents, the child and professionals are clearly recorded and these records are made available to the family, the likelihood of confusion, uncertainty and error should be reduced.

Before starting chemotherapy all children must be assessed to see if they are fit enough to commence treatment. For example, it is necessary to check the child's blood count, temperature, weight and general well-being. If the child is clinically unwell on nursing assessment, he should be referred to a doctor for a full medical assessment before proceeding with chemotherapy. Monitoring the child's full blood count is a routine test to determine both the degree of bone marrow suppression resulting from the effect of the cytotoxic drugs and to initiate supportive measures as required (see Chapter 3 for more detail).

The delay between courses of chemotherapy is determined by the specific treatment regime, but usually requires the neutrophil count to have reached $>1 \times 10^9/l$ and the platelet count to be $>100 \times 10^9/l$. However, not all drug administration is dependent on the blood count and therefore each treatment protocol should be considered individually. The dosage of drugs is calculated on the body surface area of the child. This is obtained by measuring the height and weight of the patient and calculating the surface area by use of a nomogram (m^2). Careful monitoring of the child's body surface area must take place throughout the course of treatment as significant changes in height and particularly weight can occur and would alter the dose.

Investigations and tests are carried out before the administration of specific drugs to establish a results baseline. The investigations are then repeated after administration of the cytotoxic drugs. Any short term side effects as a result of the drugs can be monitored and, if necessary, modifications to the drug dosage or even the drugs being given can be made to the next block of treatment. Examples of these tests are: blood biochemistry (to detect electrolyte imbalance and abnormal liver function); audiology tests (to check for ototoxicity); glomerular filtration rate (GFR) and tubular re-absorption of phosphate (TRP) (to detect renal toxicity); and echocardiogram (to detect cardiotoxicity). It is vital that the results of recent tests are found to be satisfactory before any further chemotherapy is given (Table 2.2).

Table 2.2: Investigation results that should be checked before administration of specific drugs (non-haematological toxicities)

Drug	Side effects	Investigations
Busulphan	pulmonary fibrosis	chest X-ray
		pulmonary function test
Carboplatin	ototoxicity	audiology
	nephrotoxicity	GFR
Cisplatin	ototoxicity	audiology
	nephrotoxicity	GFR
Daunorubicin	cardiotoxicity	echocardiogram
Doxorubicin	cardiotoxicity	echocardiogram
Epirubicin	cardiotoxicity	echocardiogram
Ifosfamide	nephrotoxicity	GFR, TRP
Methotrexate	nephrotoxicity	GFR

It is important to give appropriate antiemetics before chemotherapy (see Chapter 3 for more detail) and to plan patient care accordingly. Adequate hydration of the patient is necessary to reduce the toxic side effects of some drugs (see Chapter 3 for more detail). Pre- and post-hydration fluids are often an important requirement of the treatment regime and during administration, it is therefore important that an accurate fluid balance is recorded. To ensure that safety and accuracy are maintained when administering intravenous fluids, infusion pumps and equipment are always used in paediatric oncology care (RCN PONF, 1994).

The oral route

If at all possible, oral cytotoxic drugs should not be handled, due to their possible absorption through the skin. A non- or minimal-touch technique is advised and, immediately after dealing with them, the hands should be washed with soap and water.

Unfortunately for younger paediatric patients, there are rarely any liquid oral preparations of cytotoxic drugs available due to very small national demand for them and their poor chemical stability. If suspensions of cytotoxic drugs are prepared in a local pharmacy department, it is imperative that the bottle is shaken well immediately before each administration, to ensure that the intended dose is given, as the solid drug component may settle at the bottom of the bottle.

Intact tablets are coated to protect the hands from the risk of absorption during normal (minimal) handling (Pritchard & David, 1988). Crushing or breaking tablets disrupts the coating and extra safety measures should be taken. If it is necessary to crush tablets this should ideally be carried out in a pharmacy department under controlled conditions. Drug preparation at ward level should be carried out in a draught-free room, the handler should wear a face mask and thick latex or vinyl gloves and use an enclosed tablet crusher. Crushing tablets between two spoons is strongly discouraged because of the potential risk of powder inhalation. If an enclosed tablet crusher is not available then a pestle and mortar can be used; a small amount of water should be added first to minimise dust. The powder from the crushed tablets should then be mixed carefully with a small quantity of water or juice and given to the child from an oral syringe. Alternatively, dispersible tablets can be dissolved in a syringe once the liquid is added. A separate tablet crusher should be labelled and reserved for each drug. If a single pestle and mortar is used for all drugs, it is *vital* that is it washed and dried between each use, to prevent traces of chemotherapeutic agents being administered unintentionally. For smaller doses, tablet cutters are available from pharmacy departments and care should be taken when dealing with any fragments remaining from the broken tablets.

Capsules should be opened with extreme caution as the fine powder is easily lost into the atmosphere, posing risks of both inhalation and inaccurate dosing. For small doses, the original capsules should be divided in a pharmacy department to ensure correct dosing by drug weight. Even better, doctors should prescribe a pattern of doses that avoids having to split capsules. The contents of capsules are often irritant and can cause ulceration to the mouth (Evans, 1990). For this reason the practice of opening capsules and sprinkling their contents on to a spoon is not recommended.

With the help and advice of nurses and play therapists, even quite young children can be encouraged and taught to swallow small tablets or capsules whole. These may have to be disguised, flavoured or mixed with a small amount of food or fluid (such as jam or yoghurt). Care must be taken to ensure that disguised doses are taken immediately they are prepared, under supervision, to avoid another child mistaking the medicine for a drink or a spoonful of food.

Children should be discouraged from 'crunching' tablets as particles remaining between the teeth can cause local stomatitis. It is important for the child to have a drink following an oral dose of cytotoxic drugs to remove any residual drug from the mouth and oesophagus.

To maximise the benefit of therapeutic regimes, patient compliance is essential. In adult and general paediatric populations, issues of compliance are well documented (Ley, 1988). Within paediatric oncology, professionals have assumed that the life-threatening nature of the condition creates highly motivated parents, thereby guaranteeing compliance. Measuring compliance is difficult; self-reporting is prone to bias, and the measurement of gross blood–drug levels cannot identify inaccurate timing or missed doses (Smith et al., 1979). Assays for 6-mercaptopurine metabolites are becoming widely available and their use has suggested that one in five children with acute lymphoblastic leukaemia (ALL) fails to comply fully with oral chemotherapy, and may account for 'unexplained' late relapses (Davies et al., 1993). There is increasing interest in the role of continuing (formerly known as 'maintenance') oral chemotherapy in ALL. Studies have demonstrated inter-patient variability in mercaptopurine metabolism (Lennard et al., 1990). Subsequently, efforts to ensure that each child receives the maximum dose that he is able to tolerate, rather than a standardised dose, have been suggested (Chessells, 1995). A number of factors have been correlated with poor compliance in children with cancer. These include poor understanding, forgetfulness, lack of general and specific education and large family size (Tebbi et al., 1985); lower socio-economic status (Dolgin et al., 1986); the child refusing to take medication, or seeming 'well' and not appearing to require further treatment (Smith et al., 1981); depression and anxiety of parents or child (Lansky et al., 1983), and the age of the child. The group most commonly linked with poor compliance is teenagers (Smith et al., 1979, 1981; Tebbi et al., 1985; Dolgin et al., 1986). It has been postulated that teenagers in particular may not comply with steroid therapy due to its effects on their weight and mood, and that the normal teenage risk-taking behaviours and disputes with parents about self-care responsibilities may have a negative effect upon treatment compliance (Eiser, 1996).

Nurses need to be aware of these possible risk factors and take action to support compliance with treatment. The importance of compliance with treatment regimes should be discussed openly, in a factual non-judgemental manner, in order that parents feel able to discuss any problems they may experience in giving chemotherapy to an unwilling child. Older children and teenagers may welcome the opportunity to discuss their feelings about long term oral treatment in private.

Attempts have been made to improve patients' understanding of treatment through self-medication schemes in a number of health care settings. Benefits in terms of knowledge, skills and compliance have been reported (Bird, 1990; Leadbetter, 1991). Self-medication schemes have been employed successfully in paediatric oncology units (Fradd, 1990; Woodhouse, 1990). The effect on compliance was not formally evaluated in these programmes, but parents were happy to take responsibility for giving their child oral drugs in hospital and felt that doing so would make administration at home easier (Woodhouse, 1990). Self-medication schemes, where either parents or teenagers undertake oral medication, may offer a systematic method for assessing the learning needs of the family and implementing education to meet them. By initiating self-medication schemes, however, a number of legal and professional issues are raised. These include the teaching skills, knowledge and availability of nursing staff; questions of accountability and legal liability; and developing policies that ensure safe practice, clear documentation and secure storage of drugs (Bird & Hassal, 1993).

The intravenous route

As with any intravenous drug preparation, aseptic technique is essential at all stages. Luer-lock syringes and fittings should always be used to prevent the possibility of the needle and syringe disconnecting and accidental spillage occurring. It is recommended that syringes are made of polypropylene as this material is chemically inert (Streeter & Wright, 1993). An ampoule should be opened by wrapping its neck in a piece of gauze and opening it away from the face. When a powdered drug has to be dissolved the diluent should be injected slowly down the side of the vial. Care should be taken to avoid a build up of pressure by always equalising pressure inside and outside the vial. This is achieved by use of a filter needle (i.e. cytosafe needle) or venting system to prevent contamination. The needle should be covered with an alcohol swab as it is withdrawn from the vial to minimise the amount of drug aerosol. If air bubbles occur in the filled syringe they should be carefully expelled either back into the vial or into the sheath of a clean needle. The original needle used should not be re-sheathed as there is a potential risk of a needle stick injury (RCN ONS, 1989).

Where practical, infusion bags should be attached to the lines away from the child, in the drug preparation area, in order to minimise contamination in the event of a bag being punctured. However, this is not always possible if attaching a bag to an existing infusion line. If the infusion bag is taken to the child on a tray and the procedure performed in the tray, at a low level, safety can be maintained. Under no circumstances should it be necessary to attach an infusion bag to a line whilst it is hanging from the 'drip stand'; doing so poses an unnecessary risk to the nurse and the child if the bag was accidentally punctured.

It is less traumatic, less stressful and safer for children to have a long term central venous access device (CVAD) or implantable port (porta-cath) inserted before administration of chemotherapy (see Chapter 3 for more details). These 'lines', however, can become dislodged although they are inserted surgically. Care must be taken to ensure patency and to prevent extravasation occurring. Infusion lines need to be taped up securely to stop them becoming dislodged and to prevent young children from tampering with them. Children playing with scissors should always be supervised. Infusion lines should be kept well away from teething babies or bored toddlers, as they may develop the habit of chewing them for comfort.

Small cloth bags are often made in which to place the ends of the infusion lines whilst not in use, for comfort and to keep them out of the way. During prolonged infusions, lines should not be allowed to hang directly from the exit site, as they can exert traction on the skin exit site and tunnel of an externalised line, or on the access needle of an implanted port. This can cause irritation and predisposes accidental removal. A 'safety loop' attached to the skin of the chest, back or to the child's clothing can be devised to take the strain of movement. It is important that the child and the family are reminded to keep infusion lines off the floor, to minimise the risk that someone will trip over them. The use of 'telephone cord' spiral extension leads can offer greater freedom of movement to young children, but nurses and parents should be extra-careful not to trap or trip over these longer lines. Babies and young children can be dressed in vests that fasten between the legs to keep lines out of reach, but care should be taken to avoid the connection being near the nappy, due to the risk of faecal contamination.

When central venous access is not possible or a short course of treatment is prescribed, e.g. for Hodgkin's disease, peripheral access is used. Efforts should be made to reduce the trauma of repeated peripheral venepuncture. Children and teenagers may benefit from being coached in coping techniques, such as relaxation and guided imagery, counting games, story- or joke-telling or bubble blowing, which serves both as a distraction and slow breathing exercise. Computer games can prove very absorbing and children or teenagers can learn to distract themselves whilst playing with one hand.

Nursing note:

It is important to remember that distraction techniques are not intended to 'trick' the child into being unaware of the procedure. Rather, they are strategies that enable the child to be actively involved in coping with the threat, and mastering their anxiety. For this reason, working with the child/teenager to develop methods that they can practise and become familiar with may prove more effective than trying a different approach on each occasion.

Techniques that employ the child's own preferred coping style, whether he prefers to focus upon what is happening or to be distracted from it, have been shown to be most effective (Fanurik et al., 1993). Remedial work with children who have established needle phobia proves more challenging, and may require the input of a psychologist trained in systematic desensitisation or hypnosis. However, every nurse, play specialist and parent can help to reduce the likelihood of problems developing by learning simple distraction games which children can practise in hospital or at home and use when needed. By developing and maintaining a routine when venepuncture is required, nurses can help the child to understand what to expect and rehearse the procedure between treatments, in a safe environment. Young children may benefit from playing with the equipment involved, and injecting their teddy or doll can help then express their feelings through 'make-believe' play. A small play kit, including syringes, cotton wool, disinfecting swabs, blood bottles and plasters, can be given to the child to play with at home. Under close supervision, even young children can be allowed to touch and learn about needles and cannulae, removing the mystique and hopefully some of the fear through familiarisation.

The development and widespread use of local anaesthetic cream ('magic cream') such as Eutectic Mixture of Local Anaesthetics (EMLA) or Amitop has benefited many children undergoing venepuncture. Prolonged analgesia, from 30 minutes to a few hours is achieved if the cream is applied liberally to the designated area for a minimum of 45 minutes (maximum effect being achieved after 60–90 minutes) and an occlusive dressing placed over it (Buckley & Benfield, 1993). This can easily be done by parents or children at home, before they leave for the hospital, once they have been educated about appropriate sites for venepuncture. It may prove wise to apply cream to more than one site, to offer the person under-taking the cannulation a choice of veins. However, excessive or prolonged applications should be avoided, particularly in very young children, due to risk of absorption of prilocaine metabolites to toxic levels (methaemoglobinaemia) which can cause cyanosis (Gajraj, 1994). Although the risk of toxicity is slight with normal clinical use (Scott, 1986). Steps should be taken to avoid children tampering with the dressing and ingesting the cream, or rubbing their eyes; a light bandage over the occlusive dressing (Gajraj, 1994) or gloves can help to keep the cream undisturbed.

It has been suggested (Goede & Betcher, 1994) that children and parents should be warned to avoid accidental skin damage, as sensa-tion may be lost for some hours following application of the cream. Local anaesthetic creams may be less effective on black skin, and until this is substantiated or refuted by further research, nurses should be aware of this possibility (Hymes & Spraker, 1986). In some children, skin blanching, and rebound erythema may be observed and is caused by the vasoconstrictive effects of the cream (Buckley & Benfield, 1993). Avoiding prolonged application time may reduce this effect, which also can make visualising the vein more difficult. Sensitivity reactions may be produced by either the creams or the occlusive dressings, and some children become distressed in anticipation of the injection when the cream is applied. In any situation where the cream is not proving helpful, a discussion with the parent and the child, if old enough, is indicated in order to devise a more acceptable strategy.

> **Nursing note:**
>
> **Children who are sensitive to the occlusive dressings, but not the local anaesthetic cream, can still benefit from its use if household 'clingfilm' is placed over the cream and sealed with hypoallergenic tape.**

Ethyl chloride ('cold spray') can be sprayed locally on to the injection site. This evaporates rapidly, numbing the peripheral nerve endings in the skin. For pre-injection use, the skin should be sprayed from a distance of about 30 cm for 3–5 seconds, taking care not to frost the skin. Skin puncture should take place just as the liquid film begins to dry (Syntex Pharmaceuticals, 1994). This spray has the benefit of effective local anaesthesia being achieved within 0.5–2 minutes, lasting up to 3 minutes, offering greater flexibility and avoiding undue anticipatory anxiety for some children. Certain safety precautions need close attention, however. Ethyl chloride is supplied in breakable glass vials and is highly flammable. Mixtures of the gas with 5–15% of air are explosive; it must be stored at less than 15°C and protected from light (Reynolds, 1996). Care must be taken to avoid prolonged spraying on a small skin area, as this can cause frostbite. Inhalation of the vapour can induce general anaesthesia and there are reports of ethyl chloride abuse causing confusion, hallucinations, ataxia and short term memory loss (Nordin et al., 1988).

Any painful procedure requires careful planning, and children should be encouraged to be involved in the discussions concerning alternative methods. The effectiveness of the chosen method can be evaluated using standard paediatric pain tools (Wong & Baker, 1988) shortly after the procedure is completed. Discussion with parents about the child's behaviour at home can illuminate nursing assessment of the ongoing effects of treatment upon the child. The child may have bad dreams, become withdrawn, distressed on the way to hospital or become aggressive towards parents or siblings. Although these may be considered coping mechanisms, repeated reports of any such signs of distress should be discussed with a psychologist if the child seems to be suffering ongoing emotional trauma. It is important to remember that parents may not volunteer this information as they may think such distress is unavoidable, or feel that they have failed in some way. It is therefore important to ask specific questions, to facilitate and normalise the discussion of these issues.

When peripheral administration of chemotherapy is necessary, it is important that an appropriate site is chosen, with good venous access, and one insertion made, if possible. Sites to be avoided are: areas of poor venous circulation; sites previously exposed to radiation; the wrist; antecubital fossa; or bruised, sore areas. The cannula should be well taped in place and the limb splinted to prevent it being dislodged, but not so as to obscure the injection site in order to observe for signs of extravasation. The patency of the vein should be checked before, during and after administration of a cytotoxic drug by testing for backflow of blood. If, at any time, there is no blood return or resistance is felt when trying to give a drug, administration should cease immediately. If the child is to receive several cytotoxic drugs through the same peripheral site the vesicant drugs and bolus injections must be given first. Care should be taken to dilute the drug adequately according to the manufacturer's recommendations in order to avoid high tissue concentrations and the method of administration should be carefully checked, i.e. infusion, bolus. Peripheral infusion of vesicant drugs should be undertaken with extreme caution and continuous supervision is recommended; for this reason overnight administration is not advisable if it can be avoided.

Nursing note:

If anthracycline infusions via peripheral lines cannot be avoided, it may be advisable to increase the dilution, or administer a concurrent 'piggy-back' infusion of compatible fluids. This may reduce the venoconstriction and phlebitis caused by these drugs, and reduce the risk of vein damage and consequent extravasation. Either strategy must first be discussed with medical and pharmacy staff.

The vein should always be flushed well after the administration of a drug, choosing a compatible fluid. Great care needs to be taken when using intravenous infusion devices to administer cytotoxic drugs peripherally, particularly vesicants, and especially with children who are too young to verbalise their discomfort. It is essential that agreed pressure alarms are set on infusion pumps when administering any fluids but especially solutions of cytotoxic drugs. Children receiving treatment for cancer are often immunocompromised and are therefore at greater risk of developing infections. It is important therefore that all venous access sites are observed carefully whilst a cannula is *in situ* and after removal, as the skin integrity has been broken and this is a potential site for infection to develop.

Extravasation

Extravasation is the escape of fluid from the vessel or passages which ought to contain it. In this context, chemotherapeutic agents escaping the blood vessel wall (vein) into the surrounding interstitial tissue, can lead to intense tissue inflammation and pain. Very young children are particularly at risk as they cannot communicate pain in the same way as older children. The primary aim must be to prevent extravasation. Only appropriately trained staff should administer cytotoxic drugs and they should be aware of which drugs are vesicants (Table 2.3). The guidelines suggested by the Oncology Nursing Society (1992) state that nurses should receive formal training in chemotherapy administration, extravasation prevention, its early recognition and timely management before assuming responsibility for antineoplastic drug administration.

Table 2.3: Vesicant and irritant drugs		
Vesicants	Irritants	Non-vesicants
(associated with severe local necrosis)	(may be associated with local necrosis)	(uncommonly associated with local necrosis)
Amsacrine	Carboplatin	L-asparaginase
Carmustine	Cisplatin	Bleomycin
Dactinomycin	Dacarbazine	Cyclophosphamide
Daunorubicin	Etoposide	Cytarabine
Doxorubicin	Methotrexate	Ifosfamide
Epirubicin	Mitozantrone	Melphalan
Idarubicin	Teniposide	Thiotepa
Vinblastine		
Vincristine		
Source: Stanley, 1993.		

Close observation of the site throughout administration is essential. Should extravasation occur the first signs are usually tenderness or a burning, stinging pain, with induration, swelling or leaking at the injection site, followed by erythema. Close observation for these signs and symptoms should take place. Extravasation is not always immediately visible and therefore the monitoring of an administration site several hours or even days later is important to detect any adverse reactions. Delayed extravasation injuries occurring weeks after chemotherapy administration have been observed with vindesine (Dorr, 1990).

If extravasation has occurred, skin ulceration, blistering and necrosis may follow, leading to further problems, such as significant scarring around tendons, nerves and joints with possible contractures and loss of limb function. Necrosis and tissue ulceration may occur a considerable time after extravasation has taken place and in severe cases a plastic surgeon should be contacted as soon as possible when signs of skin deterioration occur. It is estimated that one-third of vesicant extravasations actually result in ulceration (Dorr, 1990).

There are a certain number of conflicting recommendations about the management of extravasation but a definite policy needs to be drawn up locally so that action can be taken immediately. The policy must be clear, simple and easy to follow (Table 2.4). All personnel who administer cytotoxic drugs must be aware of the policy and an extravasation kit must be available at the time of administration.

Table 2.4: Management of extravasation*		
Chemotherapeutic agent		
Vinca alkaloids Aim: dilute and spread drug	Other vesicants Aim: localise drug	Irritants –
Give subcutaneous hyaluronidase 1500 units in 1 ml normal saline around affected area in 0.1–0.2 ml aliquots	Give subcutaneous steroids: dexamethasone 8 mg/2 ml WFI** or hydrocortisone 100 mg/2 ml WFI around affected area in 0.1–0.2 ml aliquots	Observe site after one hour, if erythema apparent apply 1% hydrocortisone cream topically; continue as long as erythema lasts
–	Apply 1% hydrocortisone cream topically; continue as long as erythema lasts	
Apply warm compress for at least one hour Elevate extremity; minimise swelling; encourage movement Give analgesia if required Consider referral to plastic surgeon	Apply ice pack/cold compress for first 24 hours Elevate extremity; minimise swelling; encourage movement Give analgesia if required Consider referral to plastic surgeon	Apply ice pack/cold compress for first 24 hours Elevate extremity; minimise swelling; encourage movement Give analgesia if required
*Stanley, 1993; Bertelli et al., 1994; UKCCSG, 1998. **WFI = Water for injections.		

There are some general principles that should apply to the management of extravasation and further refinement may be made at local level:

- Stop infusion/injection immediately leaving the cannula or needle in place
- Aspirate as much of the drug back as possible and draw back blood from the suspected infiltration site
- Remove the cannula or needle
- Take action to reduce localised skin damage.

Written documentation of the event must follow with all clinical details noted. The description of the affected site should be noted and should include diameter of the erythematous area and its appearance.

Liposuction and saline flush-out are two techniques used to remove extravasated material while conserving the overlying skin. Gault (1993) found that analysis of the flush-out material confirmed that the extravasated material was actually removed. Most of this study group (86%) healed without any soft tissue loss at all. The early referral and treatment of extravasation injuries is therefore recommended.

Intrathecal route

Leukaemia, lymphoma and other malignant cells have the ability to penetrate into the central nervous system (CNS) and circulate within the cerebral spinal fluid (CSF). This means that some children require cytotoxic drugs intrathecally via a lumbar puncture, either as prophylactic or therapeutic treatment, as many of the drugs given by other routes are unable to cross the blood-brain barrier in sufficient concentrations. Drugs for intrathecal use must be reconstituted with preservative-free diluent to avoid neurotoxicity. Some cytotoxic drugs, such as the vinca alkaloids, are extremely neurotoxic and if they were given intrathecally in error would cause severe and almost universally fatal myeloencephalopathy (Rowinsky & Donehower, 1996).

> **Nursing note:**
> **For safety reasons it is considered best practice that only those drugs specifically intended for intrathecal use are available in the treatment room during a lumbar puncture procedure.**

In the UK, performing a lumbar puncture is at present a doctor's role, but it has been an area of nursing responsibility for some years in paediatric oncology settings elsewhere (Meeske & Ruccione,

1987). Accessing the CNS must be conducted as a sterile procedure to minimise the risk of introducing infection. Before the cytotoxic drugs are injected a few drops of CSF are taken and later tested for the presence of malignant cells and for infection. An Ommaya reservoir or similar device (Galassi, 1996) may be employed to administer intraventricular chemotherapy in order to facilitate prolonged CNS-directed therapy for recurrent, refractory or chronic CNS disease. These reservoirs function in much the same way as implantable venous access ports, with a resealable membrane placed under the scalp. This is attached to a catheter that passes through a hole in the skull and leads to the lateral ventricle of the brain. Although a surgical procedure is required to place the reservoir and catheter, many individuals have benefited from the relief these devices offer in avoiding the distressing effects of repeated lumbar punctures, particularly if access is very difficult due to spinal abnormality, or in children who develop a CSF leak from repeated puncturing of the meninges, or who experience severe headaches following the procedure.

Children experience post-lumbar puncture headaches only rarely in comparison to adults, the incidence and severity increasing throughout adolescence. Teenagers and younger children who have previously experienced headaches are advised to lie flat for at least two hours following a lumbar puncture, although each individual will usually discover the 'optimum' duration of lying horizontally by trial and error. Adequate analgesia and a quiet environment with dimmed lights can reduce the pain experienced. When performed as a day care procedure, it is important to ensure that an in-patient bed is available for children who suffer particularly severe headaches, as they may find the only way to avoid intense pain is to lie flat for 12 hours or more after a lumbar puncture.

Most children find the experience of a lumbar puncture extremely distressing (Harris et al., 1994) and in the UK it is common practice to administer a light general anaesthetic to help them through this procedure. Expecting children to undergo repeated invasive and painful procedures without any supportive intervention apart from enforced physical immobilisation is generally considered to be unacceptable in the UK (Eden, 1994). Efforts are made to find the most effective, yet practical anaesthetic approach for each oncology unit. This concept, however, is not always supported in other countries. Some centres use ketamine to anaesthetise children under ten years of age, but it is not recommended for older children as there is a high incidence of hallucination and other transient psychotic sequelae. Entonox by inhalation can be used for older children to bring about relief of pain during a lumbar puncture. This is self-administered 'on demand' and can be very effective if the child is taught correct use and given support and supervision throughout the procedure. Children can also benefit from distraction strategies, and relaxation techniques may help them to manage this procedure under local anaesthetic.

Nursing note:

For some children, it seems that it is the pain of the needle piercing the skin that causes most distress, in these cases effective local anaesthesia can be achieved by applying EMLA to the skin site at least one hour before the lumbar puncture (Buckley & Benfield, 1993). Some individuals may require a conventional local anaesthetic injection of lignocaine, but unbuffered lignocaine has a low pH, and causes intensely painful stinging when it is injected. Buffering is not undertaken by the manufacturers as this reduces the shelf-life of the drug, but it can be undertaken immediately prior to use. The advice of a pharmacist should be sought regarding the strength and volume of sodium bicarbonate required to achieve painless lignocaine injection (Yaster et al., 1994).

Some individuals wish to avoid what they perceive as 'losing control' during general anaesthesia or sedation, and through combinations of one or more non-anaesthetising strategies, such as low doses of oral anxiolytics, Entonox, local anaesthesia and distraction (or involvement) techniques, nurses can enable them to achieve this whilst still minimising discomfort. Once again, it is important to work with the child or teenager to find the approach that is most acceptable to them. Play specialists, psychologists and trained nursing staff can all have a major influence in the safe and smooth management of lumbar punctures.

The subcutaneous route

Vesicant drugs are never given by this route. If at all possible, drugs are administered via alternative routes. Those which are given subcutaneously (e.g. L-asparaginase) are usually injected into the thigh. Ethyl chloride spray or EMLA cream can be applied locally to the area to numb it, but it has been found that topical anaesthesia is not very effective as only the peripheral nerve endings are numbed, whereas the pain from the injection is usually from the fluid entering the subcutaneous layer of tissue. In some centres it is considered necessary for the patient's platelet count to be $>20 \times 10^9/l$, to reduce the risk of bruising and bleeding subcutaneously from the injection. However, this is not universally considered necessary for subcutaneous, as opposed to intramuscular, injections due to the paucity of blood vessels in the subcutaneous fat layer. Distraction techniques, therapeutic play and reward schemes such as sticker charts may help young children to manage these often distressing treatments. Older children may benefit from being given a choice of injection site, keeping a chart to show where they have had their injections, counting off the injections on a calendar, or even assisting with some aspects of the procedure. In some cases it is considered that the simplest, most practical strategy is to hold the child firmly and proceed as quickly as possible (Robinson & Collier, 1997). However, it is still imperative that time is taken to prepare the child through play and/or verbal explanation before each injection, to support the involvement of the parents if they wish it, and to ensure that the child receives praise and comfort after the injection is completed. The value of play specialists in supporting children through this aspect of treatment is undeniable.

Other routes of administration

Table 2.5 shows a selection of other administration routes for chemotherapeutic agents. These are rarely, if ever, used in paediatric oncology.

Non-inpatient Administration of Chemotherapy

A number of chemotherapy regimes have been given on an outpatient basis for many years, for example, treatment for Wilms' tumour and Hodgkin's disease. The trend towards early discharge from hospital has resulted in more children being cared for at home during and between courses of treatment. For many families, the advantages offered by day care or home chemotherapy over inpatient care are clear. It is potentially less disruptive to family life; children spend more time at home and school, and parents may be able to return to work. Some of the financial costs of having a hospitalised child may also be relieved, as the need for frequent travel between home and hospital is reduced. By suggesting day care or home treatment, professionals are acknowledging the caring and coping skills of parents, and by giving them the opportunity to care for their sick child within the context of family life, may help to boost their confidence.

Table 2.5: Routes of administration for chemotherapy

Route	Indications	Use in paediatric oncology
Topical	Local treatment of malignant skin lesions	In children, the topical route is limited to application of mustine solution for skin involvement of Langerhans cell histiocytosis
Intramuscular	Same as subcutaneous route	Largely supplanted by subcutaneous route in paediatrics, due to reduced risk of bruising or bleeding
Intravesicular	Drugs instilled into the bladder to treat superficial lesions	Not routinely used in paediatrics
Intrapleural	Drugs instilled into pleural space following drainage of fluid, to treat malignant effusion	Not routinely used in paediatrics
Intra-abdominal	Drugs instilled into abdominal cavity following paracentesis, to treat peritoneal seedlings	Not routinely used in paediatrics
Intrahepatic	To treat existing liver disease or as adjuvant therapy post-surgery	Not routinely used in paediatrics
Intra-arterial	Regional perfusion of limbs or head and neck with cytotoxic agents	Not routinely used in paediatrics
Intralesional	Local control of accessible lesions, for example, Kaposi's sarcoma	Not routinely used in paediatrics

Based on information from Priestman, 1989; RCN PONF, 1994.

As well as supporting philosophies of home care and parental involvement, non-inpatient chemotherapy regimes confer financial and practical benefits for health care providers. Costs per patient are reduced (Close et al., 1995) and the availability of inpatient beds is increased. However, it is vital that such considerations do not compromise patient safety, or override a family's reasonable preference. The potential reduction in hospital-acquired infection through minimising episodes of inpatient care is of benefit to all parties.

The benefits of non-inpatient treatment must be balanced against the possible drawbacks. For families, frequent day care chemotherapy can involve a lot of travelling and can incur substantial costs in terms of time and money. In addition, families may have to make arrangements for the care of their other children during sometimes lengthy treatment days.

Families without private transport, and those who live a great distance from the hospital, may justifiably consider that day care chemotherapy presents too many practical problems, and must be given a choice about the location of treatment. Many parents find contact with other parents who share their situation to be supportive (Lynam, 1987). They may feel more isolated at home, and may not benefit from the parent network to the same extent as during inpatient treatment.

Patient safety and the efficacy of treatment is of prime importance; neither must be compromised by the decision to give non-inpatient chemotherapy. This is particularly vital when teaching parents to give intravenous drugs; poor compliance may occur due either to lack of parental understanding or children refusing treatment. Issues concerning compliance with oral therapies have been discussed and it seems reasonable to assume that many of the same factors may apply to intravenous therapy. Special attention must be paid to education and support if parents are to care confidently for their child without the degree of supervision that is available in hospital, and providing for their needs may prove difficult because they have less contact with nursing staff. Maintaining some normality in family life becomes extremely difficult when one child requires complex treatment at home, particularly if the child may become acutely unwell and require hospitalisation at any time. Health care professionals have to be sure that the care of healthy siblings is not compromised. Home care may prove particularly demanding for lone parents; the availability of support from the extended family, friends and neighbours should be assessed formally as part of the planning process.

Treatment planning

When proposing to give chemotherapy in the day care or home setting, many issues must be considered. In fact, most of the important factors are those routinely assessed when preparing for the discharge of a child from hospital after inpatient chemotherapy. Details of the specific treatment regime, the circumstances of each child and family, and the services available to them must be considered when planning any package of care (Table 2.6). Most children receiving chemotherapy are cared for by their parents at home following each treatment block, and parents are routinely expected to be capable of monitoring their child for the side effects of highly toxic therapy, with the necessary information and support. Through exploring the available options with the multidisciplinary team and the family, the nurse can optimise patient safety and family coping, by ensuring that appropriate input is provided in the best location for each child.

Table 2.6: Factors that influence decision-making about the setting for chemotherapy administration

Factor	Considerations	Decision-making team
Drugs	Preparation: reconstitution, stability, storage, safety. Administration: dose, route, schedule. Side effects: immediate, short and intermediate term	Nurses (hospital and community teams), doctors, pharmacists.
Child	Age. Diagnosis, prognosis. Physical health: symptoms and management. Treatment phase: i.e. at diagnosis, relapse, ongoing therapy, palliative care. Previous experience with chemotherapy: side effects and management. Psychological factors: anxiety, needle phobia. Preference.	Nurses (hospital and community teams), doctors, child, parents/carers, play specialist, psychologist.
Family	Support: from family and friends. Social: parents' work, child care arrangements, housing etc. Previous experience: parenting, caring for sick child, cancer, chemotherapy, 'nursing' care. Education: support/needs. Preference.	Parents/carers, nurses (hospital and community teams), doctors, social worker.
Services and facilities	Available support/advice. Professionals' skills, knowledge, experience, skill-mix, roles. Financial considerations. Legal considerations. Local policies and procedures.	Nurses (hospital and community teams), doctors.

With respect to assessing families to undertake home care, Benson et al. (1993) advocate consideration of family structure, roles of family members, communication patterns and decision-making styles. These authors make the important point that nurses must avoid being judgemental about what types of family unit are suitable for home care. Patient safety and the ability of the family to cope is what must take priority, rather than whether the home circumstances are ideal. When initiating a programme of home therapy, certain criteria for domestic or housing arrangements may be appropriate, for example, the availability of a reliable power supply, running water, access to telephone, distance from hospital/professionals, and whether the family has private transport. Although for many these amenities are taken for granted, the needs of families living in challenging domestic circumstances require sensitive assessment and care planning. When working with socially disadvantaged groups, such as families living in poverty, the homeless, refugee families and travellers, the role of the community nurse is to support them in making appropriate decisions based upon an understanding of their child's needs and their ability to meet them. The issue of parental choice is paramount and a detailed discussion of the risks, benefits and care needs should be conducted with each family as part of the planning process. Roles and responsibilities should be negotiated explicitly and documented to avoid confusion and enhance coordination of care between different health care providers.

Although care is planned in negotiation with the child and family, the decisions of the professionals about the location of treatment should be based on an assessment of the risks and benefits of the available options. The possibility always exists for coercion by one or other party: professionals may believe that home treatment is always best, and subtly exert pressure on parents; or they may be under pressure themselves from the demand for inpatient beds. Families who are desperate to avoid inpatient care may endeavour to persuade staff to permit home treatment before education and assessment programmes have been completed or in the absence of sufficient professional home support services. Pressure may also be exerted by professionals from other disciplines, and nurses require both knowledge and confidence in order to negotiate effectively and honestly with their colleagues and with families.

Chemotherapy in the day care setting

Day care services have assumed greater importance in recent years, as the potential for giving more complex chemotherapy in this setting has been recognised. The subsequent effect upon families and service providers has meant that the role of nurses working in this environment has developed a higher profile. Expanding practice boundaries have allowed nurses working in day care settings to seek greater responsibilities in many aspects of chemotherapy care, including treatment planning, drug administration, the management of side effects and family education and support (Ghadile Harris & Bean, 1991).

When planning to give a chemotherapy regime in the day care setting, careful thought is required concerning the types of drugs and their administration schedules. Drugs which are given as bolus injections or shorter infusions are obvious candidates, but it is important to consider the effect that treatment may have upon families in addition to whether it is possible to administer the treatment during the hours that the day care unit is open.

Some drugs may precipitate hypersensitivity reactions (such as anaphylactic shock following L-asparginase injection) requiring immediate medical intervention. Children receiving these agents should remain in the day care unit under supervision after every dose, until the immediate risk has passed. When giving combinations of drugs it is useful to time their administration according to when such reactions might occur. For example, it is best to give bleomycin at the beginning of the day's treatment so that the child is likely to still be in the hospital in the event of a febrile reaction (Priestman, 1989) where the problem can be can easily be identified and managed.

In order to facilitate treatment as a day care procedure, some adjustments to standard schedules may be possible. However, a scheduling alteration may also alter the efficacy and/or toxicity of the dose given (Collins, 1996). Any adjustments must be sanctioned by a pharmacist specialising in cytotoxic drugs, and supported by a prescription clearly detailing the alternative schedule. This must be signed by the doctor who prescribed the original, to safeguard the nurse giving the treatment, and to avoid potentially dangerous confusion.

Drugs prescribed as an infusion must never be administered as a bolus injection, as the large doses which are usually infused may trigger life-threatening reactions, such as speed shock or anaphylaxis, if administered rapidly (Millam, 1988). It is possible under some circumstances to infuse two drugs concurrently, to children who have double lumen central lines. This can reduce the amount of time children spend in the day care unit, but the risk of fluid overload, particularly in infants, should be considered and once again it is important that the regime is checked by the specialist pharmacist, regarding the stability and solubility of each drug in combination.

Nursing note:

Etoposide infusions are often of short duration in day care regimes, increasing the likelihood of hypotension. Monitoring blood pressure is therefore of particular importance.

Drugs that require long periods of pre- or post-hydration usually require admission to hospital, but this can be overcome in some protocols by giving a drug that requires dilution in lieu of pre- or post-chemotherapy hydration for another drug, even increasing the dilution to give more fluid over the required length of time. To ensure adequate drug excretion following chemotherapy administration, the child must remain well hydrated. This will require a high intake of oral fluids at home, so it is vital that nausea and/or vomiting is well-controlled.

For day care chemotherapy to be a safe option it is clear that the child must be well enough to be cared for at home following chemotherapy, and that rapid deterioration is not expected. In some situations the introduction of day care chemotherapy is best delayed until treatment is established, and the family have the necessary knowledge and skills to care for their child.

The effective management of nausea and vomiting is a nursing priority for successful day care administration; poor control can prove to be the limiting factor as to whether day care treatment is an acceptable alternative. The child will be travelling between hospital and home after treatment, and any nausea or vomiting will be distressing for the child and cause significant problems for parents, particularly on public transport. The provision of vomit bowls, tissues and plastic bags may be wise for the journey home even if good control is anticipated. Plastic sandwich boxes are ideal as they can be sealed after use.

Nursing note:

Children who suffer from motion sickness may be particularly prone to chemotherapy-associated nausea and vomiting (Morrow, 1985); the choice of antiemetic regime should take this into account. By careful planning of antiemetic administration during day care treatment, a dose can be usefully given immediately before travelling.

Delayed or prolonged nausea and vomiting may cause problems following outpatient chemotherapy (Hockenberry-Eaton & Benner, 1990). It is important to ensure that antiemetics are supplied for the few days following chemotherapy, that the parents know what dose adjustments are possible if required and the importance of contacting the hospital in the event that control is not achieved or the child shows signs of dehydration. After each successive course of chemotherapy, antiemetic treatment should be reviewed with the child and carer and appropriate improvements made to the regime where necessary after each course. A simple record card may enable parents to remember any problems experienced with previous courses of treatment. There is a strong case for giving the most effective antiemetics available, to ensure that control is achieved during chemotherapy and can be maintained afterwards (Pinkerton et al., 1990). Oral antiemetics are only of use if good initial control is achieved; parents may be taught to give intravenous antiemetics (Hooker, 1996) but, in practice, the choice of intravenous drug for routine home use is safely limited to those that do not precipitate extrapyramidal side effects. The use of dexamethasone in antiemetic regimes is not precluded by day case treatment, the benefits achieved using intravenous dexamethasone in hospital can be continued by giving doses orally at home.

Of the drugs which can cause haemorrhagic cystitis, only cyclophosphamide is given routinely as a day care treatment. It is of particular importance to ensure antiemetic control and adequate fluid intake following administration to reduce the likelihood of risk, and to stress the need for frequent bladder emptying to avoid urine stasis. Children with bladder tumours or who have received irradiation involving the bladder may require mesna with relatively low doses of cyclophosphamide (see Chapter 3 for more detail). Mesna can easily be given at home, either in tablet form or as an intravenous preparation well-mixed in water or juice, to prolong the duration of bladder protection. Parents are advised to look for signs of haematuria and pain on passing urine. Although 'dipstick' testing for microscopic haematuria is not usually required at the low doses of cyclophosphamide given in day care regimes, parents may be taught to undertake this if their child has a previous history of haemorrhagic cystitis or is otherwise deemed to be at high risk, to facilitate early detection and action. The services of community nursing teams can offer the family particularly valuable advice and support in the days immediately after day care chemotherapy.

Children attending for day care chemotherapy are generally well, and if cared for by a nursing team which has to meet the needs of both inpatients and day cases, may be seen as a low priority in comparison to acutely sick children. However, these children and their families need specialist input from skilled nursing staff who are able to provide physical care, education and support if treatment is to be given safely in hospital and care is to be managed effectively at home between treatments. Day care treatments can be given on inpatient wards, in entirely separate units or, perhaps more ideally, in units which run in parallel with the inpatient ward but are individually staffed for each patient group (Reams, 1990). This arrangement can provide appropriate dedicated nursing staff and the skill-mix for day care treatment, whilst maintaining the family's links with all members of the oncology team and other families during treatment and beyond.

Primary nursing in outpatient oncology settings offers continuity of care throughout prolonged treatments and beyond (Paradise & Kendall, 1985). Liaison between inpatient and day care staff is vital if the family is to benefit fully from the multidisciplinary approach to care, and for transfer from one nursing team to the other with confidence. The support of a dietician, psychologist, social worker, and play specialist working with the child and any siblings (McEvoy et al., 1985) is equally important for outpatients and their families as for inpatients. Day care nursing staff need to actively manage the input of team members if the short periods of time the family spends in hospital are to be used effectively.

The documentation of day care nursing activities must meet all statutory professional and legal requirements (UKCC, 1993). However, other than signing prescriptions for drug treatment administered, traditionally, scant attention has been paid to recording nursing input. This is often attributed to the workload in busy units, but is perhaps related more to the status of outpatient nursing when the role was confined to clerical or administrative duties, housekeeping and assisting doctors with medical procedures (Tighe et al., 1985; Behrend, 1994). As the role of the nurse has become more patient- and family-focused the professional nursing responsibilities of day care provision have been recognised and documentation of care has developed to reflect this (Bru, 1989). The real constraints upon nursing time have inspired the use of records specifically designed for outpatient use: concise, time-saving and inherently practical (Bru et al., 1985; Pickett, 1992; Behrend, 1994).

The administration of day care chemotherapy requires a significant amount of planning and organisation if it is to offer a safe, effective and efficient alternative to inpatient treatment. This administration is still considered a nursing role in many centres, although there is no reason why all clerical responsibilities cannot be successfully fulfilled by a clinic manager, with appropriate support, permitting nursing staff to focus upon issues of patient care.

The logistics of delivering family-friendly day care are often complex and involve close liaison with the family and other professionals. Much organisational effort is directed at reducing unnecessary travelling and minimising waiting time in day care facilities. For example, if the family lives a long way from the treatment centre a full blood count undertaken locally on the day before planned treatment may avoid unnecessary travelling (in the event that the count is too low for treatment to be given) or will enable the pharmacy department to have drugs prepared ready for administration. If parents are taught to sample central venous lines, they can deliver blood specimens to the hospital and the child need not make an extra visit.

Contact with families before and after day care treatment can be maintained by telephone, to monitor the child's side effects, offer support and identify problems that could be eased by arranging a home visit by a community nurse. This method of communication constitutes an important aspect of nursing care within the day care setting (Nail et al., 1986). The development of protocols for managing telephone queries has proven benefits in general paediatric outpatient departments (Steger Osterhaus, 1995) and may offer improved standards of nursing care via the telephone in oncology. Nurses giving information and advice over the telephone are as accountable for this, as they are for 'hands on' care; it is important that nurses undertaking this role have the knowledge and experience to enable them to do so.

Day care chemotherapy is not necessarily limited to treatment given on a single day. Chemotherapy can be given on consecutive days, but the travelling involved may limit the number of families for whom this is ideal. Where available, 'home from home' overnight facilities may be usefully employed in increasing the number of families who can bypass hospital admission. In this way, the journey home at the beginning and end of the day may be avoided. Depending upon the treatment regime and facilities available, it may be possible to offer the family a degree of flexibility regarding chemotherapy administration. By giving chemotherapy after school hours or by running weekend treatment sessions school work is less disrupted. Teenagers in particular may welcome this option as it also reduces the isolating effects of feeling different from their friends. Parents may also benefit from being able to visit the hospital outside working hours. Following appropriate education to support enhanced practice, 'out of hours' treatment clinics represent an ideal field for the initial development of nurse-led care and could increase the health care choices available to families.

Chemotherapy in the home setting

It is widely accepted that for children, home care is the best alternative; the potentially damaging effects of hospitalisation on children and their families are well-documented (While, 1991). Home care for terminally ill children is well established (Martinson et al., 1978; Kohler & Radford, 1985; ; Goldman et al., 1990) and the role of specialist community nurses in providing practical nursing care and ongoing psychological support has been described and constitutes an integral part of children's cancer services in the UK (Bignold et al., 1994; Evans & Kelly, 1995; Hunt, 1995). However, the single largest group of paediatric cancer patients has received home treatment for many years, in the form of oral continuing (maintenance) therapy for the treatment of ALL.

Home intravenous chemotherapy has taken longer to become established in paediatrics than in adult cancer care (Daniels, 1995). Home treatment for children is often either given or monitored by parents. The increasing emphasis on parental participation in care while the child is in hospital, and the growth of paediatric community nursing, has made home administration of intravenous chemotherapy a possibility (Jayabose et al., 1991). These authors report successful programmes involving administration of injected or infused chemotherapy to children at home, through cooperation between hospital, home care agencies and the family.

As previously mentioned, the distinction between day care and home chemotherapy administration is, to some extent, false as many of the important nursing issues are shared and the family often moves from one setting to the other during a single course of chemotherapy. Most home treatment initiatives have developed from day care settings (Teich & Raia, 1984; Reville & Almadrones, 1989) with the realisation that some aspects of treatment given in a day care environment may be given as safely at home. The practice boundaries between day care and outreach teams become blurred as parents are taught by hospital staff to give drugs and are then supported at home by community children's nurses (RCN, 1994; Evans & Kelly, 1995). This requires close communication and cooperation between nursing teams. By collaborating in the development of policies and teaching protocols and by ensuring that technical procedures are consistent throughout the oncology service, nursing teams can ensure smooth transitions between hospital and home. The issue of developing working practices across practice boundaries becomes more important as increasingly complex packages of care are devised (Thornes, 1993). Appropriate documentation of care planning and delivery is also required to enhance continuity of care and parental involvement in treatment. Parent-held records have been developed in paediatric oncology to provide an up-to-date, ongoing record that is available to all the child's carers, both family members and health care professionals (Hully & Hine, 1993; Hooker & Williams, 1996).

Home chemotherapy for children is often parent-administered chemotherapy, and is almost exclusively limited to oral drugs or low-dose bolus intravenous injection. Few examples exist of more complex regimes in the UK, although a wider range of treatments is reported to have been given at home successfully (Jayabose et al., 1991). Oral drugs constitute most parent-administered home treatment, and it is perhaps easy for the family to perceive such chemotherapy as less important than injected drugs or those given in hospital. Issues of compliance, accurate dosing and the reporting of side effects are just as important, however, and perhaps more likely to be overlooked. The significance of such issues is, perhaps, best reinforced by providing written information and ongoing support to the family giving oral chemotherapy over what may be many months.

Home intravenous chemotherapy usually requires a central venous access device, although peripherally inserted 'long lines' and even peripheral cannulae have been employed successfully. These require scrupulous monitoring by parents or nursing staff. The initiation of home chemotherapy, therefore, assumes that the parents are confident, competent carers with regard to the management of their child's central venous access device.

The routine administration of vesicant drugs should not be undertaken outside the hospital setting. Other drugs given at home are also limited by safety considerations; a risk assessment of possible reactions, side effects, other adverse events and available emergency support should be carefully made before specific home treatments are offered. Some parents may perceive a wide range of treatments that are suitable for potential home administration. It is clear that the importance of a thorough clinical review is explained to ensure that the child is well enough to receive treatment and to enable monitoring of response and side effects prior to a course of treatment. This 'check-up' may necessitate a hospital visit rather than the actual drug administration and usually takes place at the start of each course of chemotherapy, although the course may be completed by the parents at home.

Nursing note:

The use of the subcutaneous route may appear to be ideal for home therapy. L-asparaginase is the only drug in current cancer treatment regimes given regularly via this route and the possibility of anaphylaxis makes home administration an unwise and avoidable extra risk.

Low-dose, low-volume continuous infusions are under evaluation and may offer scope for more home treatment in the future. Such infusions are usually established by nursing staff, either in hospital or at home, and then monitored by the patient or the parents. Higher volume infusions of chemotherapy or hydration fluids at home have been described (Allison et al., 1996). The need for close monitoring and recording of intake and output and compliance with supportive measures throughout each treatment requires careful planning, education and support. Evaluation of patient safety and the effect of complex home treatment on the family is required before such programmes can be practised confidently more widely.

The choice of infusion pumps for home use is important. The device must be suitable for its purpose, reliable and easily understood by both the parents and other nurses who may have contact with the child during a course of chemotherapy. The use of ambulatory infusion pumps may enable the child to attend school during chemotherapy. Information and support for teachers must not be overlooked. Teenagers using ambulatory infusion devices should be taught to manage their own pumps to take advantage of the increased personal freedom that these can offer. Written information about the device and who to contact in the event of equipment malfunction should accompany every child during every course of treatment.

The family undertaking either drug administration or management of treatments at home requires appropriate teaching, supervision and assessment if safe and effective care is to be provided. In order to fulfil their professional responsibilities, nurses involved in teaching such families must take reasonable precautions to ensure that aspects of care are delegated appropriately, based on an assessment of the family and the specific task (Dimond, 1990). Best practice in teaching must be followed, with verbal information and demonstration being supported, but not substituted, by written material. It is important to remember that teaching, supervision and assessment is documented and that the parents (or child) undertake the delegated care voluntarily. Some units ask parents to sign a form before undertaking aspects of nursing care, but in the event of harm coming to the child, a signed form will not protect the nurse against claims of professional negligence if teaching is found to have been deficient (Dimond, 1990).

Written information about the drugs to be given, their actions, possible side effects, and what to do in the event of the child developing side effects should accompany each course of home chemotherapy. Chemotherapeutic agents for home administration are not usually reconstituted by the parents in the home; labelled, pre-filled syringes for each dose are supplied from the pharmacy to reduce the risk of accidental exposure in the home, and to ensure correct dosing. Issues such as storage of drugs in the home and safe practice with chemotherapy (including management of spillage, needle-stick injury, skin contamination and disposal of waste) should be included in written guidelines for parents and carers.

Nursing note:

Cytotoxic waste in the community should be managed according to Health Authority/Trust 'Risk Waste' management policies (RCN, 1994). This may involve all infusion bags, giving sets and other equipment being stored in the home for collection by community nursing staff or returned by parents to the hospital for incineration. The parents need information about safe storage in the recommended sealed bags or 'sharps' containers until collection or return.

Once at home, the family needs to know who to contact for advice and support, whether community children's nurses are available 24 hours a day or if the hospital is their primary contact. Obviously, it is vital that routes of communication are clearly defined and the guidance given to the family in different situations is agreed upon by the professionals to avoid confusion and possibly conflicting advice.

The range of home chemotherapy is often limited by the services currently available. There is a financial dimension to consider, concerning the efficient time management of limited numbers of community staff, and the various roles adopted by paediatric community nurses have an important effect upon the home chemotherapy that is available (Hunt, 1995). Day care treatment is undeniably more cost-effective in terms of human resources, as a number of children can be cared for by a single nurse if they are in the same location; home chemotherapy is likely to be restricted to the less complex treatments that do not require the continued presence of a health care professional. However, there is scope to extend the chemotherapy that can safely be given by parents, with the use of prepared infusion bags and pre-programmable ambulatory pumps. In addition, the effect of commercial home care companies has yet to be fully realised. As the boundaries of the nurse's role expand it becomes possible for them to develop and evaluate innovative approaches to drug administration that may offer benefits to families and service providers alike.

In order to achieve the best care for each family, a multi-disciplinary team approach needs to be taken to consider the available alternatives. The development of practice guidelines or 'care pathways', involving medical, nursing and pharmacy staff may enhance care delivery and support advances in home care. Safe drug administration is an absolute requirement, and only if this can be achieved is there room for flexibility.

Chapter 3
Side effects of chemotherapy

Karen Selwood, Faith Gibson and Margaret Evans

Introduction

The effects of antineoplastic agents on normal cells are described as the side effects of therapy. It is the cells which have a rapid mitotic rate, such as bone marrow, gastrointestinal mucosa, gonads and hair follicles, that are most vulnerable to these side effects. In addition, certain drugs may have a direct effect on organ(s) in the body and cause toxicity over time. In parallel with the widespread cellular/tissue damage that results in site-specific side effects the child undergoing chemotherapy may also experience generalised effects, such as fatigue, anorexia, taste changes, nausea and vomiting and pain. In order to ensure effective care of these children nurses need to be knowledgeable about both the treatment and side effects; they should have skills in assessment, technical expertise and be able to support the child and family emotionally throughout the course of treatment. Symptom management and psychosocial support must be well integrated. Most side effects are responsive to nursing intervention which will ultimately have an effect on the comfort, safety and quality of life of the child. In addition, effective nursing intervention can reduce recovery times, prevent serious complications and reduce prolonged hospitalisation.

Nurses have an important part to play in the prevention, detection and management of side effects of chemotherapy. Assessment is the first step, preceding planning, intervention and evaluation in the process of providing individual nursing care; with the care plan reflecting the physiological and emotional aspects of care, within a multidisciplinary framework. Assessment consists of the collection of data from a number of different sources: observation, measurement, communication and records (Casey, 1995a). Analysis of these data can then be expressed as a problem, need or a nursing diagnosis, resulting in the identification of the needs and responses of the child and the family concerning nursing care as well as their need for information, support and teaching (Casey, 1995b).

It is essential to involve the child and the family in all aspects of care. However, parents and other family members can only take on the role of active care-givers if they have been fully prepared and feel supported within this new and seemingly complex environment. Knowledge about treatment and side effects is necessary to ensure the active participation of family members in decision-making about treatment plans, for example, timing of drug administration or monitoring of the child's side effects. Information needs to be open and honest and may need to be repeated. Families undergoing the stress of coping with a child with cancer often do not assimilate the facts on first hearing. Teaching and reinforcement needs to be a continuous process using the child's treatment protocol and highlighting the anticipated side effects. Written information does not replace verbal communication as the family may have previous experiences, both positive and negative, that need to be discussed and taken into consideration. Ongoing support and education is crucial (Evans, 1993) to enable the family to make informed decisions about care of the child and their part in it (Casey, 1995b). Promoting a realistic view is the best option as this will foster trust in which a partnership between the parents and health care professionals will develop.

The play specialist has an important role in facilitating the child's understanding of chemotherapy as well as assessing their coping and adaptive mechanisms. Play specialists make use of instructional play (Vessey & Mahon, 1990) with younger children to provide information about hospitalisation and to teach new information; 'even very young children are able to understand the nature and implications of their disease and treatment' (Faulkner et al., 1995, p. 4). For older children and teenagers there are many published books and resources available that can facilitate understanding, possibly building on projects undertaken at school. Approaches to preparation should be individualised, to encompass cognitive abilities that may not always reflect age. Cultural issues, past experiences, coping abilities and physiological status also need to be taken into consideration (Vessey & Mahon, 1990). Parents are directly involved with the play specialist in preparing their child for chemotherapy since they know the child's strengths and fears as well as patterns of communication better than anyone else (Lansdown & Goldman, 1988).

Siblings also benefit from open and honest information that is clear and age-appropriate. Involvement in the care of the sick child and an understanding of treatment may help to resolve the strain of separation and fantasies about the hospitalised child (Martinson et al., 1990). Play specialists will have an important part to play, alongside 'sibling groups' (Stone, 1993), in providing information and offering an opportunity for siblings to express their feelings and ask questions of people other than family members.

The side effects of chemotherapy can be classified in relation to the time of onset; immediate, early or late. These classifications will be used to structure the following information. Site-specific side effects will be discussed in detail and where accompanied by general effects of chemotherapy, are highlighted. Paediatric nursing literature concerning the side effects of chemotherapy is variable. Some side effects, such as oral stomatitis, nausea and vomiting, are well documented, with research studies providing evidence on which to base practice. In contrast, other side effects, such as fatigue, have received minimal attention. This may reflect the complexities of involving children in research studies (Nicholson, 1986; Lee, 1992) as well as the inherent difficulties in qualifying and quantifying objective and subjective experiences in relation to side effects of treatment (Cotanch, 1984). Overall, the discussion that follows aims to provide a description of practice, where possible, supported by evidence from a combination of clinical practice, research and other published literature.

Immediate Side Effects of Chemotherapy

These side effects occur during or shortly after administration of the chemotherapeutic agent, usually within 30 minutes. Many are localised and transient, responding well to symptomatic treatment. However, some are systemic (the most serious being hypersensitivity reactions) occurring usually within 15 minutes of initiating therapy. Table 3.1 identifies some possible immediate side effects with their corresponding nursing implications.

Early Side Effects of Chemotherapy

Gastrointestinal tract

Mucositis

Mucositis is a general term that refers to an inflammation of the mucous membranes and is further specified according to location.

Table 3.1: Possible immediate side effects of chemotherapy and their nursing management	
• When administration is peripheral, pain and a cold sensation along path of the vein	• distinguish from extravasation • inject slowly with intermittent saline flushes • further dilute injection
• Flushing along the path of the vein, over the face or the whole body	• administer drug slowly
• Urticaria: localised or systemic	• local application of topical steroids (for systemic rash use calamine lotion, may need to introduce antihistamine)
• Alteration to taste or smell	• suck strongly flavoured sweets during the injection or infusion
• Hypersensitivity	• be aware of the agents most likely to cause problems • regular nursing observation • cease administration and recommence at a slower rate
• Anaphylaxis	• discontinue administration of the drug • maintain venous access • administer oxygen as required • administer prescribed drugs as required, e.g. adrenaline or chlorpheniramine; record the reaction, noting cause and management
• Extravasation	• stop infusion/injection • leave cannula or needle *in situ* • aspirate drug back, withdrawing blood • remove the cannula or needle • further action taken needs to follow steps of the local policy • document the incident

When occurring in the oral cavity it is referred to as *stomatitis*, in the oesophagus as *oesophagitis*. Generalised mucositis of the intestinal tract is characterised by proctitis, diarrhoea and abdominal pain. In practice, however, the terms *mucositis* and *stomatitis* are often used interchangeably (Beck, 1992).

Stomatitis

This occurs due to damage and destruction of epithelial cells usually 5–7 days post-administration of chemotherapy. Therapy affects the oral epithelial cells both directly and indirectly; directly by interfering with actual cell production, maturation and replacement; indirectly due to bone marrow depression, where neutropenia and

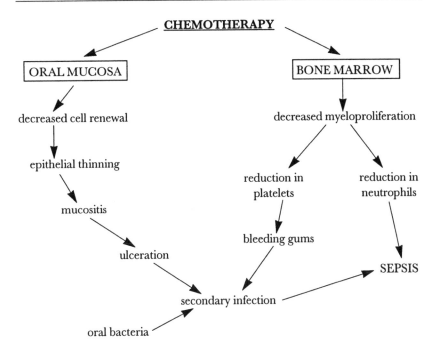

Figure 3.1: Direct and indirect effects of chemotherapy affecting the oral mucosa

thrombocytopenia increase risks from bleeding and infection. Figure 3.1 clearly illustrates the pathophysiology.

An early study by Sonis and Sonis (1979) identified that more than 90% of children experience oral problems and that this frequency was three times that of adults. Although this oft-quoted study indicated the diagnosis of the sample group it failed to identify the drugs given, the dose, length of administration and overall physiological condition of the children; all of which could have a bearing on the degree of stomatitis (Aitken, 1992). By contrast, a more recent study indicates that there are a significant number of children who experience either minimal or no problems at all (Kamp, 1988). Overall, only sporadic research has been published identifying oral complications of chemotherapy and those who are susceptible to them (Holmes, 1991a, b). The agents considered to be the most stomatoxic are the antimitotic antibiotics and the antimetabolites, as well as some of the alkylating agents, particularly in higher doses (Beck, 1992). Their effects may be increased when used in combination.

Clinical features — pain, swelling, xerostomia, inflammation, ulceration, desquamation of mucosa (gums and palate), dry and cracked lips, bleeding.

Management — the principal objective of oral hygiene is to maintain the mouth in good condition, i.e. comfortable, clean, moist and free of infection (Table 3.2).

Table 3.2: Aims of oral hygiene
• Achieve and maintain a healthy and clean oral cavity • Prevent the build-up of plaque on oral surfaces, thus helping to prevent dental caries • Keep the oral mucosa moist • Maintain mucosal integrity and promote healing • Prevent infection • Prevent broken or chapped lips • Promote patient dignity, comfort and well-being • Maintain oral function
Sources: Howarth (1977); Richardson (1987); Beck (1992); Clarke (1993)

The nurse has an important role in maintaining oral hygiene, either directly (by providing oral care) or indirectly (by providing advice and opportunities to provide self-care) (Torrance, 1990), or family care, thus contributing to the overall comfort of the child. There is certainly no dispute that regular oral care is essential in reducing the detrimental effects of a compromised oral cavity; damage caused by cancer treatments cannot be avoided but oral care may prevent infections that cause further damage to the oral tissue. Many authors, however, suggest that oral care regimes are often based on tradition, anecdote and subjective evaluation (Daeffler, 1980; Holmes, 1991a, b; Thurgood, 1994) citing limited published nursing research as the reason for this. However, it has also been suggested that even where there is research supporting practice this may be ignored resulting in a theory–practice gap (Peate, 1993). Nurses must be accountable for the care they provide and, therefore, research about oral care must be utilised to inform their practice, as indiscriminate oral care not only causes physical problems but may also have psychological ramifications. Nurses have a pivotal role in deciding which form of mouth care to provide, including which tools or solution to use and the frequency with which care is carried out (Krishnasamy, 1995). They therefore need knowledge and understanding in order to initiate appropriate oral care; care that is based on a sound scientific rationale. Decision-making may be facilitated by use of an algorithm that provides a step-by-step approach to the selection of appropriate oral care. One such framework has been introduced within a unit (Figure 3.2) and has the benefits of:

- Ensuring that all children receive appropriate oral care
- Recommending practice that is based on current research
- Decreasing conflicting information and advice given to parents as well as other members of the health care team

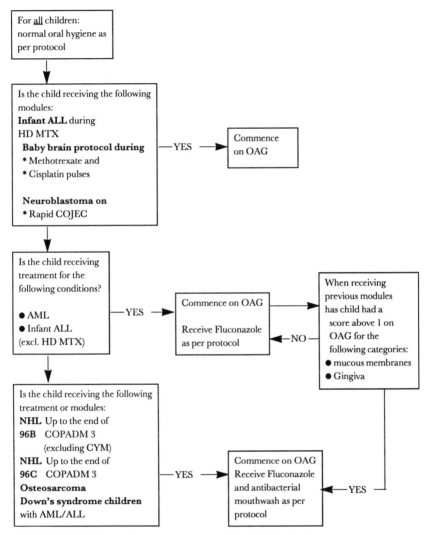

NB: Those children requiring Fluconazole and/or antibacterial mouthwash will receive them as inpatients only. i.e. all children will go home on normal oral hygiene unless specific problems to indicate otherwise.   Discuss with the doctor if: 1) There is evidence of oral fungal infection or
mucositis/ulceration prior to commencing treatment.
2) OAG (Oral Assessment Guide) > 8
  i) Discuss implementation of an antibacterial
  mouthwash if evidence of mucositis.
  ii) Commence on pain scale tool.

Great Ormond Street Hospital for Children NHS Trust (1997)

Figure 3.2: A mouthcare flowchart

- Increasing confidence and competence of nursing staff in their decision-making process (Gibson et al., 1997).

An accurate assessment is vital for effective oral care. A thorough assessment is required to:

- Provide baseline data
- Predict, prevent or minimise oral complications
- Plan effective care
- Evaluate nursing interventions (Richardson, 1987).

Following an evaluation of three oral assessment guides by Holmes and Mountain (1993), the most reliable and valid tool for clinical use has been found to be that of Eilers et al. (1988). This assessment tool divides oral status into eight areas, which are then subdivided into three categories according to the presence or absence of symptoms. Although introduced for use in an adult population this tool has been adapted (with the authors' permission) for use within a paediatric unit (Table 3.3). Assessment represents the vital 'first step' in planning effective care (Campbell et al., 1995); nursing intervention introduced to prevent, minimise or reverse changes in the oral cavity can then be individualised and the response to therapy monitored.

Nursing note:

The value of early detection would seem to be important as children may not complain until their symptoms are quite severe.

There is a great deal of conflicting information regarding which oral care regime is the most appropriate; there is much debate surrounding choice of tools, cleansing agents and frequency of oral care (Beck, 1992; Coleman, 1995). This has resulted in nurses being uncertain as to which oral care regimes they should follow. Overall, effective management will be facilitated by an appreciation of the best agents and tools available. Campbell et al. (1995) provide an excellent summary that highlights clearly the 'Do's and Don'ts' of oral care.

Holmes (1991a) concludes that the toothbrush is most effective; a small-headed, soft, multitufted, nylon bristled toothbrush is efficient at removing plaque and debris. Use of a toothbrush is recommended irrespective of platelet count, although in cases of severe stomatitis the child may not tolerate its use. In this situation, to minimise trauma, a foam stick may be introduced. Foam sticks are ineffective at removing plaque (Pearson, 1996) and therefore their use should be temporary, however, they may be the most appropriate tool to use with babies.

Table 3.3: Oral assessment scale

Category	Method of measurement	1	2	3
Teeth	observe appearance of teeth	clean and no debris	plaque or debris in localised areas (between teeth if present)	plaque or debris generalised along gum line
Voice	converse with patient, listen to crying	normal	deeper or raspy	difficulty talking, crying painful
Swallow	ask patient to swallow; to test gag reflex, gently place depressor on the back of tongue and depress	normal swallow	some pain on swallowing	unable to swallow
Lips and angle of the mouth	observe and feel tissue	smooth and pink and moist	dry or cracked	ulcerated or bleeding
Tongue	observe appearance of tissue	pink and moist and papillae present	coated or loss of papillae with a shiny appearance with or without redness	blistered or cracked
Saliva	insert depressor into mouth, touching centre of the tongue and the floor of the mouth	watery	thick or ropy	absent
Mucous membranes	observe appearance of tissue	pink and moist	reddened or coated (increased whiteness) without ulceration	ulceration with or without bleeding
Gingiva	gently press tissue	pink and firm, stippled	oedematous with or without redness, smooth	spontaneous bleeding or bleeding with pressure

Adapted from Eilers et al., 1988 with permission. Great Ormond Street Hospital for Children NHS Trust, 1997.

There is a general consensus that the use of fluoridated tooth-paste is essential as it strengthens tooth enamel and decreases the risk of dental caries (Beck, 1992). There is less agreement about the use of a prophylactic antibacterial mouthwash. The benefits of their use, such as decreased plaque and mucosal inflammation, are not disputed (Galbraith et al., 1991), however, there is no conclusion as to which mouthwash is the best one to use. Various mouthwashes are available and often appear to be used indiscriminately (Coleman, 1995). This may be borne out by the fact that most paediatric centres use 'Corsodyl' as their first choice.

Nursing note:

Lemon and glycerine swabs have been used routinely for their moisturising and refreshing properties; they were also considered to have a pleasant taste. However, there are no overall benefits in using them as they have little value in either cleaning or moisturising the oral cavity (Beck, 1992); glycerine is hypertonic, drawing moisture from the tissue and causing reflex exhaustion of the salivary process and lemon contains acid which can irritate the mucosa and decalcify the teeth (Roth & Creason, 1986).

The use of agents to control oral infections is also debated. Nystatin is active against *Candida albicans*, however, in combination with chlorhexidine, the action of both solutions is impaired (Barkvoll et al., 1989). Galbraith et al. (1991) recommend that when these two drugs are used in combination a gap of one hour should be allowed between their administration, as well as an interval between eating or drinking. This will have implications for nutrition and may interfere with compliance. Studies have demonstrated the effectiveness of a new antifungal agent, fluconazole (Chandraseka & Gatny, 1994). This agent has several advantages over nystatin. Fluconazole is taken only once a day, compared with the 4–6-hourly administration of nystatin; a capsule is available for those children who dislike nystatin or fluconozole suspension; it allows concurrent use of chlorhexidine-based mouthwashes; and it is more effective in preventing oropharyngeal candidiasis (Philpott-Howard et al., 1993). However, there is a concern that indiscriminate use of fluconazole will result in the emergence of resistant fungi (Hoppe et al., 1994) and therefore it should only be used in children who are at a high risk of developing fungal infections (Chandraseka & Gatny, 1994). Identifying those children at high risk (see Figure 3.2) will reduce indiscriminate use.

There are, as yet, no research-based guidelines indicating the optimum frequency of oral care regimes and yet the frequency of intervention is likely to be the key to success (Beck, 1992). Normal oral care should involve cleaning teeth at least twice a day, particularly after meals and at bedtime. Frequency may alter according to oral assessment and will be increased if there is evidence of oral stomatitis. In cases of severe stomatitis care should be continued during the night, otherwise any progress made during the day will be negated. Moisturisers should be applied frequently in order to maintain comfort and lubricate the lips and mucosa. Petroleum jelly seems to be the most acceptable method of preventing dry and cracked lips (Campbell, 1987).

The choice of tools or agents used should reflect current research findings but also consider the individual needs of the child; there are occasions when an optimum oral hygiene regime may need to be sacrificed when balanced against the child's general comfort. Alterations in comfort from oral complications range from mild (from cracked lips) to severe (due to prolonged stomatitis) resulting in difficulties in eating and talking. It is important to assess the amount of pain the child is experiencing to ensure that adequate pain relief is given either topical or systemically. Oral hygiene becomes very painful and will only intensify the problem. Topical mouthwashes provide local relief but their action is short-lived and they can also desensitise the mouth.

Care needs to be taken with hot foods or drinks (Lever et al., 1987). The use of anaesthetic mouthwashes in children under the age of 12 years is not recommended without supervision as there is the potential for young children to swallow the mouthwash resulting in problems with swallowing. Either oral analgesia or intravenous/subcutaneous opiates may be necessary and there should be a low threshold before commencing this pain management. This will enable the child to perform adequate mouth care and hopefully maintain a good oral intake, all of which will assist in the healing process. Involvement of a dentist or dental hygienist is essential from diagnosis and throughout treatment. These professionals are able to offer practical advice on cleaning teeth and oral hygiene; problems can then be identified early, supporting nursing staff and parents in their role. There may be an occasion for dental work to be performed in order to lessen future complications.

Most children are familiar with their parents helping them with oral care. However, parents may find having to cope with performing mouth care on their child an additional stress, particularly when the child may be experiencing pain or discomfort related to oral complications. Nursing staff can offer support and advice to parents undertaking this role; and when this role is re-negotiated the nurse will need to discuss with parents the best way to perform this role to ensure the child's cooperation. The child may be familiar with a tooth-brush but not other oral care regimes that may need to be introduced whilst in hospital. Alongside the parents, the play specialist, would be involved in preparing the child. Allowing the child to handle mouth care products, in a non-threatening environment, by either practising on a favourite toy, their parent or a nurse, may help to reduce anxiety and increase compliance: creativity and imagination taking central roles.

Preparation for teenagers is also important. They need information relating to the drugs in their protocol that may result in oral problems and when they are most likely to occur. Advice regarding the oral care regime is required with the teenager being given the responsibility to undertake this care independently, thus maintaining some control. Support and encouragement may be necessary to ensure compliance, particularly when pain and discomfort are discouraging factors.

Nursing note:

In an attempt to control their own situation some teenagers may choose not to comply with the advice and teaching that has been given regarding their oral care regime. In this situation they need to be supported in their decision, provided with opportunities to express their feelings, and encouraged to receive pain relief if assessed as being necessary.

The role of the nurse is to facilitate self-care and family-centred care, as well as educating, advising or referring children for more specialised dental assessment or treatment; maximising opportunities presented for health promotion.

Before discharge parents need to be aware of their continued role in maintaining a normal hygiene regime for the child. Written information is useful and should identify further problems that may be experienced (e.g. oral thrush) and indicate the action needed to be taken. Most children will not need to continue the use of anti-bacterials or antifungals whilst at home, however, a written record of their regime is useful should they need to be admitted to their shared-care hospital.

Taste alteration

There are 10,000 taste buds situated on the tongue and oropharynx and these have a high cell turnover which can be damaged by chemotherapy. This, with the effect on salivary glands, results in taste alteration and possibly xerostomia (dry mouth). The effect varies in individuals depending on treatment received. This effect can also be influenced by antibiotic therapy, nausea and vomiting, oral stomatitis or infection. It can also be related to the disease process (Wall & Gabriel, 1983).

Clinical features — the child may complain of experiencing different tastes, these may be bitter or metallic, especially with carmustine, dacarbazine or cyclophosphamide, or it may seem that everything tastes of cardboard, sawdust or may have no taste at all. Some children develop an increased threshold for sweet foods; in contrast, some children develop a complete aversion to some foods and this may contribute to a loss of appetite and anorexia. Such aversions may also be a learned response, associating symptoms, disease and treatment (Bernstein, 1978). Occasionally, the taste alteration may cause the child to feel nauseous and vomit, especially if it occurs when a particular drug is being administered.

Management — the family should be made aware of this potential problem in order to help adjustment to what they may perceive as the child being fussy. The family should be encouraged to experiment with different foods, cooked in a variety of ways, in an attempt to tempt the child. Serving foods warm will intensify the taste and the use of gravies will increase the moisture level thus facilitating swallowing if the child's mouth is dry. In addition, by establishing what foods the child likes/dislikes diet can be planned to maintain adequate nutritional intake. However, the fact that such likes and dislikes may alter through the course of treatment will need to be highlighted. Children often develop a liking for very odd foods, often with strong tastes (for example, pickled onions, salt and vinegar crisps and spicy foods).

A dietician should be involved to offer support and advice to the family and nursing staff during this time. It is essential to stress that this will be a transient problem and should revert back to normal when the treatment is completed. Parents have reported that taste changes appear to be cyclical, depending on the treatment the child is receiving (Wall & Gabriel, 1983). Some parents may find this extremely frustrating, especially if the child changes his or her mind frequently about what food is wanted, and tempting the child to eat can be made even more problematical. Maintaining oral care is essential to help offset the taste, keep the mouth clean from debris and maintain moisture level.

Nausea and vomiting

Chemotherapy-induced nausea and vomiting are considered to be among the most adverse of the side effects (Zeltzer et al., 1991), causing much distress to the child and the family (Hockenberry-Eaton & Benner, 1990). Despite new developments in the use of pharmaceutical agents and evidence of a wider use of behavioural techniques aimed at controlling these distressing symptoms, nausea and vomiting remain significant problems for some children (Keller, 1995). Incidence and severity is related to the emetogenic potential of the drug. Although 'league tables' exist (Table 3.4), there are other variables, such as anxiety and stress, which may contribute to the child's overall experience. The potential to induce vomiting is a complex interaction between the chemotherapeutic agent given, the dosage, how it was administered and the child's response. It is well known that individuals vary considerably in their response to cytotoxic agents (Hogan, 1990) and that susceptibility in children varies (Ward, 1988), but what appears to be consistent is the degree to which these symptoms distress children (Zeltzer et al., 1984).

Table 3.4: Emetic potential of common cytotoxic agents		
Low	**Moderate**	**High**
bleomycin	amsacrine	cisplatin
busulphan	carboplatin	cyclophosphamide*
etoposide*	cytarabine*	dactinomycin
5-fluoroucil	daunorubicin	melphalan
methotrexate	doxorubicin	
mercaptopurine	mitozantrone	
thioguanine	ifosfamide*	
vincristine		
*dose-related Source: Knopf et al. (1984)		

The physiology of nausea and vomiting has been well reviewed elsewhere (Andrews & Davis, 1993) and therefore only a summary will be provided here. Vomiting is believed to be controlled by the vomiting centre, which is localised in the lateral reticular formation of the medulla oblongata near the respiratory centre. The vomiting centre may be triggered by a number of pathways (Figure 3.3). These pathways include:

- The chemoreceptor trigger zone (CTZ). This is situated in the area postrema in the floor of the fourth ventricle. This is a highly vascular area of the brain, emetic substances circulating in the blood or cerebrospinal fluid (CSF) stimulate the receptors of the CTZ which in turn stimulate the vomiting centre. Mechanisms of CTZ communications with the vomiting centre are not fully understood.
- Via the afferent vagal and visceral nerves. These stimulate the vomiting centre in response to gastrointestinal irritation, distension or delayed gastric emptying.
- Via the cerebral cortex and limbic system. These areas are stimulated by all the senses (particularly smell and taste), anxiety, pain and increased intracranial pressure. This stimulation is thought to have a direct effect on the vomiting centre and does not involve the CTZ. This source of stimuli may be responsible for anticipatory nausea and vomiting.
- Via the vestibulocerebellar afferents. These afferents are stimulated by rapidly changing body motions, with signals from the labyrinth of the inner ear. They are thought to play a minor role.
- The sympathetic visceral pathway. Afferents from the gastrointestinal tract, heart and kidneys may be stimulated as a result of inflammation, obstruction or distension.

The most likely explanation for chemotherapy-associated nausea and vomiting is that treatment causes a release of 5-HT (serotonin) from the enterochromaffin cells of the gut mucosa (Andrews et al., 1988). The 5-HT then activates vagal afferent nerve terminals to initiate vomiting and it may also enter the systemic circulation via the portal vein where hepatic afferent neurones can be activated (Hawthorn, 1995). However, it is likely that there is more than one process involving more than one transmitter (Andrews & Davis, 1993).

Anticipatory nausea and vomiting is more complex and is thought to result from stimulation received by the vomiting centre from the cerebral cortex and the limbic system (Yasko, 1985). It is described as a classical conditioned response during which previously neutral stimuli provide the thoughts, images or reminders that become the stimulus to recall the previous experience of chemotherapy administration (Dolgin et al., 1985), a process illustrated in Figure 3.4.

Clinical features — nausea, retching and vomiting, frequently described in tandem. However, they are three separate problems that may occur in sequence, separately or in combination. The symptoms may lead to dehydration, metabolic abnormalities, poor

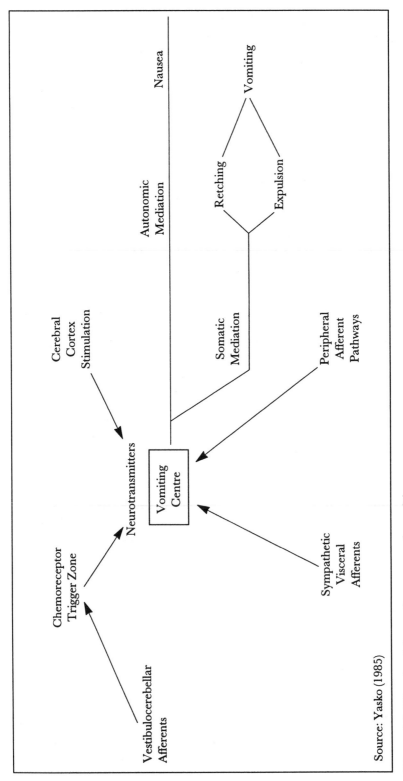

Source: Yasko (1985)

Figure 3.3: The physiology of nausea and vomiting

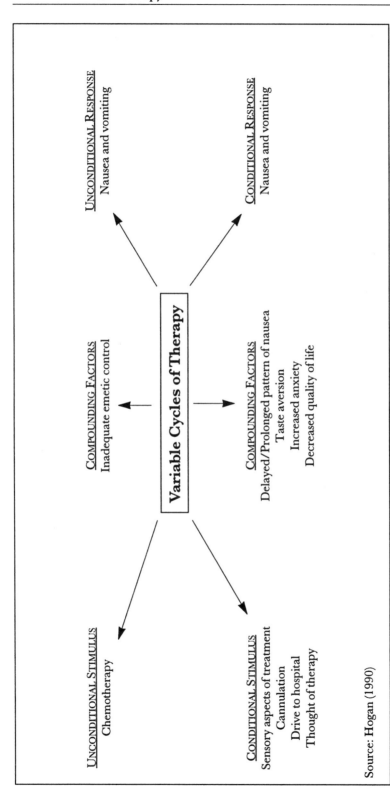

Figure 3.4: Development of anticipatory nausea and vomiting

nutritional intake with resulting weight loss and a deterioration in the general condition of the child (Hockenberry-Eaton & Benner, 1990). A disruption of normal childhood activities may result. The child may also suffer from emotional and psychological stress associated with the vomiting which can lead to non-compliance and refusal of treatment, especially in teenagers (Burish & Tope, 1992; Adams, 1993).

Management — the goal is to minimise the direct effect of treatment and to facilitate the early recovery of the child; the distress of the symptom has far-reaching consequences not only for the child but for the parents, other family members, nursing and medical staff. It is suggested that if successful antiemetic therapy is achieved during the first course of chemotherapy then nausea and vomiting may be avoided and, in practice, this appears to be the case (Billet & Sallan, 1993; Jenns, 1994). At any age children can develop learned behaviours. A negative experience with the first course of chemotherapy may result in behaviour that is difficult to reverse (Pinkerton et al., 1994). Children, especially teenagers, may develop anticipatory vomiting before or during the administration of chemotherapy if adequate control is not achieved (Dolgin et al., 1985). Non-pharmacological methods of controlling nausea may need to be explored with the family as these can assist in controlling emesis. The foundation for symptom control is an understanding of the various pharmacological and non-pharmacological interventions that are available (Keller, 1995). However, the effectiveness of interventions is rarely observed and documented methodically and this has resulted in a failure for ongoing management of these symptoms to inform 'best practice' within the variety of clinical situations. Added to this is the subjectiveness of the experience that often complicates research studies and produces difficult situations in symptom management.

Nursing note:

Children often complain that the nausea is worse than the vomiting. With some children, however, the ability to communicate this as a symptom may not always be well developed (Gibson, 1994).

Nursing management commences with assessment and this will begin by identifying the child's previous experience of nausea or vomiting, highlighting actions that have been successful in the past. Parameters then to be considered in assessing symptoms are the frequency, duration and intensity and degree of distress experienced by the child (Rhodes, 1990). Assessment could significantly influence the choice of interventions and therefore enable the nurse to decrease the direct effects of treatment (Hockenberry-Eaton & Benner, 1990). Overall, assessment should enable care to be planned and delivered more effectively as the nurse has information that relates to an individual child and his or her response to treatment. Various rating scales have been used in research studies (LeBaron et al., 1988), however, their universal use in practice has yet to be seen, although studies have shown that children as young as five years of age could use a rating scale (Zeltzer et al., 1988). In comparison, there is literature supporting the complex nature of the ability of children to self-report their symptoms, particularly in the younger age group (Abu-Saad, 1993; Gibson, 1994). Studies are needed that will result in a reliable and valid instrument to assess nausea and vomiting, qualitatively and quantitatively, as well as incorporating ease of use.

It is essential to include the child and the family when planning antiemetic intervention and with knowledge gained through teaching, the parents can be instrumental in instigating interventions and undertaking non-pharmacological approaches.

Pharmacological interventions

The administration of prophylactic antiemetics before, during and after chemotherapy should follow an antiemetic protocol or guidelines which indicate the emetic potential of the drugs with corresponding chemotherapeutic agents to be used, allowing for the individual needs of the child (Billet & Sallan, 1993; Foot & Hayes, 1994). Strict attention to a protocol will ensure effective management as knowledge of the antiemetic potential of individual drugs will be utilised more fully. As nausea and vomiting can be a result of different stimuli, a combination of agents which are synergistic may be required to achieve control.

Antiemetics are used to block the pathway to the vomiting centre. The vomiting centre contains many muscarinic, cholinergic and histamine H_1-receptors; the CTZ is rich in dopamine receptors. The CTZ responds to chemical stimuli through the activation of dopamine or serotonin receptors. The majority of currently available antiemetics are dopamine receptor antagonists, even if they have other properties (Hawthorn, 1995). Recent studies have identified other agents, those capable of antagonising 5-hydroxytryptamine (5-HT serotonin), thought to be more important in controlling emesis. Eagan et al. (1992) provide a summary of some of the earlier trials. For classification of antiemetics see Table 3.5.

Table 3.5: Classification of antiemetics		
Drugs	Site of action	Administration and side effects
Antihistamines • cyclizine • promethazine	antagonise the action of histamine at the H_1-receptor, poor as a single agent but useful in a 'cocktail' because of their sedative properties	• intravenous (i.v.) preparation • causes sedation
Substituted butyrophenone • domperidone	antagonist of dopamine receptors, also acts at peripheral sites and does not readily cross the blood-brain barrier; has direct action on gastric motility	• oral preparation or suppository • lower incidence of extrapyramidal effects
Phenothiazines • chlorpromazine • prochloperazine	dopamine receptor antagonist, block in the CTZ	• slow i.v. bolus or short infusion • sedation • dry mouth • hypotension • extrapyramidal reactions
Corticosteroids • dexamethasone	unknown, may act by blocking prostaglandin; extremely useful given in combination (synergistic action with ondansetron)	• oral and i.v. preparation • give as short infusion • immediate vomiting and anal itching when given too quickly
Cannabinoids • nabilone	action unknown, relates to central nervous system depression, may also have an anti-opioid activity	• oral preparation • drowsiness • euphoria • hypotension
Benzodiazepine • lorazepam • diazepam	may work by blocking cortical pathways to the vomiting centre, therefore particularly useful in anticipatory nausea and vomiting	• i.v. and oral preparation • drowsiness • amnesia

(contd)

Table 3.5: (contd)

Drugs	Site of action	Administration and side effects
Substituted benzamides • metoclopramide	at low doses it antagonises dopamine receptors, but at higher doses it is a 5-HT_3-receptor antagonist	• i.v. and oral preparation • given i.v. as short infusion • sedation • extrapyramidal reactions
5-HT_3-receptor antagonist • ondansetron • granisetron • tropisetron	binds to type 3 serotonin receptor 5-HT_3 in the gastrointestinal tract and central nervous system	• i.v. and oral preparation (tablet and syrup) • headache • dizziness • constipation

Nursing note:

In practice a combination of ondansetron and dexamethasone has been demonstrated to be very effective with children receiving highly emetogenic regimes. It is important to remember that when giving dexamethasone the child may already be taking steroids and so the dose may need to be altered. Dexamethasone can change the appearance of scans in children with brain tumours, however, it is still possible to give the drug, as long as its use is noted, particularly at the time of re-staging.

It is a general rule that it is easier to prevent emesis from occurring rather than to control it once it has started (Hawthorn, 1995). Where the symptom is predicted the child and the family should be informed and antiemetics given prophylactically; the timing of this will depend on the route of administration and the latency of the chemotherapeutic agent. For example, the onset and duration of emesis following cisplatin is 1–72 hours, compared to cyclophosphamide, which is 8–24 hours (Hawthorn, 1995). Antiemetics given the night before chemotherapy, particularly nabilone, may alleviate anticipatory symptoms.

Nursing note:

Some children have the added problem of travel sickness. Symptoms need to be anticipated and antiemetics administered.

It is inappropriate to prescribe antiemetics 'as required', nevertheless their successful administration will depend on the nurse caring for the child having appropriate knowledge. As yet, nurses are not able to prescribe drugs (Department of Health, 1989, 1998), however, in practice they often do when they, rightly, influence the medical team in their choice. The antiemetic(s) prescribed will depend on:

- The emetic potential of all the chemotherapy agents to be given during the course of treatment
- The child's previous response (if this is a subsequent course of treatment)
- The experience of the nurse gained previously in caring for children receiving particular chemotherapy regimes
- Knowledge of the action of the various antiemetics
- The side effect profile (in some cases an antiemetic may be chosen for its sedative effect).

Nursing note:

Teenagers may not like the sedative effect of some antiemetics as they may feel a loss of control. It is helpful if information is provided so that they are free to make a choice.

The route of administration will need to be decided. The intravenous route is often considered to be the most effective as it may be the only one available in a child who is vomiting. In some cases oral administration may be selected; oral ondansetron is as effective as the intravenous formulation (Cohen et al., 1996). Some children like the choice but, with respect to cost, the oral route should be chosen. The availability of ondansetron in syrup form since the late 1990s may increase its popularity.

Assessment of antiemetic intervention is essential to monitor effectiveness. In a child who continues to vomit, alternative antiemetics may be chosen or a 'cocktail' of agents may be effective. The pharmacist should be involved to provide advice and support; pharmacists may also be called upon in the search for information about current studies of new antiemetics or different approaches to antiemetics currently in use.

Nursing note:

In some cases ondansetron, dexamethasone and metoclopramide in combination have been found to be effective.

Extrapyramidal reactions

Antiemetics that work by blocking or antagonising dopamine receptors have the potential to cause extrapyramidal side effects. They result from excessive cholinergic activity in the extrapyramidal tract of the nervous system as a result of unintentional blockade of the post-synaptic dopamine receptors by the antiemetic drug; resulting in a disturbance of normal dopaminergic transmission causing an inability to coordinate voluntary movement, alterations in muscle tone and the occurrence of involuntary movements (Hawthorn, 1991). The child may experience varying effects: general restlessness and muscle tremor (irritable legs 'that want to keep walking'); limb dystonia (may resemble a seizure); opisthotonus (muscle spasm causing the back to be arched and the head retracted, with the muscles of the neck and back very rigid); or oculogyric crisis (rolling of the eyes together with laryngeal spasm that can result in respiratory distress). The effect is more common in children (Terrin et al., 1984), particularly in higher doses, with an increased risk related to metoclopramide (Graham-Pole et al., 1986).

This side effect can be managed by either concurrent administration of procyclidine or, following a reaction, the effect can be reversed with intravenous benztropine. However, the rate of incidence and the distressing nature of this side effect for the child and their parents has resulted in antiemetics that have extrapyramidal reactions in their side effect profile becoming unpopular in practice.

The new group of antiemetic agents, the 5-HT$_3$ antagonists (for example ondansetron) have undoubtedly significantly improved the control of symptoms (Jürgens & McQuade, 1992). However, their efficacy is limited in highly emetogenic regimes that contain cisplatin or ifosfamide (Pinkerton et al., 1990) and is ineffective in the control of delayed-onset nausea and vomiting (Bleiberg, 1992). They are favoured as their side effects are minimal and they do not cause extrapyramidal reactions (Smith, 1989).

Non-pharmacological interventions

Alternative or complementary methods of controlling nausea and vomiting can be explored, to be used independently or in conjunction with antiemetics. Behavioural approaches include:

- Hypnosis (Redd et al., 1982)
- Progressive muscle relaxation (Cotanch, 1983)

- Relaxation with guided imagery (Donovan, 1980)
- Systemic desensitisation (Morrow & Morrell, 1982).

Successful use of these techniques with children will be related to their involvement and their feelings of gaining control over a situation in which they may previously have felt helpless (Hockenberry-Eaton & Benner, 1990). Non-pharmacological interventions may be more relevant for teenagers and be successful in managing anticipatory symptoms, and as a conditioned response, they may be more responsive to psychological intervention (Zeltzer & LeBaron, 1983).

Nursing note:

Constant reassurance and understanding will be necessary when caring for a teenager who is experiencing uncontrolled vomiting. Creativity with 'cocktails' of antiemetics alongside complementary methods may be required.

In younger children simple techniques of distraction using storytelling may be useful, making the most of children's imagination and magical thinking. Providing different activities, such as play and education, can offer structure and focus the child on something other than the treatment. Also, acupressure wrist bands have shown some benefit in adults (Stannard, 1989) and children (Williss, 1991).

An understanding of complementary methods and an awareness of those members of the multidisciplinary team who can advise, assist or teach these skills (such as psychologists, play specialists and teachers) is essential.

Nursing note:

In addition to these interventions, education about diet and mealtimes is also useful. In particular, discourage the parents from eating meals by the child's bedside when he or she may be feeling very nauseated. A suitable place must be found for parents to eat their meals.

Ongoing assessment is necessary in order to evaluate the various interventions and to anticipate further problems. Parents can be relied on to report their child's symptoms accurately (Gibson, 1994) and will take on the role of 'time keeper' by prompting the nurse caring for the child in advance of the antiemetic being due. The parents can also be involved in recording fluid intake and output, whilst also encouraging the child to continue with oral fluids and diet.

In the situation of the child who continues to vomit and is unable to tolerate oral intake it may be necessary to introduce intravenous fluids to prevent dehydration and electrolyte imbalance. The dietician may also become involved to advise on maintaining adequate calorie and protein intake.

The overall distress caused by these symptoms can be minimised by adopting a sensitive approach; maintaining a constant supply of vomit bowls and providing privacy when children are vomiting. Oral care is essential, and rinsing the mouth should be encouraged after each episode of vomiting. This process will remove debris from the mouth as well as provide general comfort in terms of taste and oral freshness. The play specialist and ward teacher may need to be involved to provide gentle activities for those children not wanting to 'face the noise' of the playroom. The use of favourite tapes and the involvement of family members in reading stories may provide some distraction when the child may be feeling 'just awful'.

Before discharge after chemotherapy, some preparation is necessary, and antiemetics should be continued. If they need to be given intravenously the parents need to have been taught this skill and to feel confident to undertake this role. Written information should be provided to complement that given verbally (Ley, 1988; Davis, 1990). Community nursing teams must be made aware of the child's planned discharge in order to provide support and care as necessary.

The family should also be aware of the potential problems from delayed or continued vomiting and should be given advice about fluid hydration and the reasons for re-admission.

Nursing note:

Sometimes there is a delayed reaction following the use of cisplatinum. Families should therefore always be prescribed antiemetics to take home. If community nurses are unable to visit the family it is important to telephone them following discharge to ensure that the child's vomiting is easing.

An understanding that it may also take time to re-establish a normal eating pattern after chemotherapy may provide reassurance for a family worrying that the child is still not eating. In addition, the family needs to be aware that a constant feeling of nausea or continuous vomiting is not normal; often misguided advice from family and neighbours may suggest otherwise.

Anorexia/weight loss

Anorexia is a loss of appetite which usually occurs as a result of the child's condition or treatment. Other factors that may contribute to this symptom are:

- Nausea and vomiting
- Mucositis and/or stomatitis
- Altered taste.
- Constipation
- Diarrhoea associated with typhlitis or other infections
- Pain
- Metabolic disturbances.

In addition, an emotional response to being diagnosed and treated for a life-threatening illness may result in psychological factors that will need to be considered; depression can often be accompanied by a reluctance to eat. Young children may be unable to differentiate between disease, treatment and side effects, thus contributing to their unwillingness to eat (Hanigan & Walter, 1992).

Nutritional status has a prognostic effect upon outcome (Rickard et al., 1986). Studies have indicated that adequate nutrition is essential, as children who are well-nourished are better able to resist infection and tolerate treatment (Van Eys, 1979).

Weight loss can be a symptom of anorexia or present independently, related to infection, increased metabolism, eating problems or any one of the problems identified in relation to anorexia. Although several factors may play a part, the basic problem is often one of lack of intake of food.

Clinical features — loss of appetite, lack of desire to eat, reduced calorie and protein intake, lack of energy, muscle wasting and low albumin, and weight loss.

Management — assessment of anorexia is difficult as it involves the subjective experience of how the child is feeling and an objective measurement of food intake. A range of assessment techniques are available and include physical examination, biochemical investigations (Goodinson, 1987), dietary history and dietary assessment.

Initial assessment is required to identify any underlying cause that may be exacerbating the anorexia or weight loss, as well as providing a baseline of the child's nutritional status, eating habits (that acknowledge cultural influences) and any problems perceived by the family. Ongoing assessment includes regular monitoring of weight in addition to recording intake and output. The frequency of weighing may vary but most centres record two or three times a week and thereby avoid weighing too often, as in the case of minimal weight gain the child may become despondent and more depressed, contributing further to the anorexia. Weight loss may be one of the few indications that the child is not receiving an adequate diet and therefore other methods of ensuring an adequate nutritional intake may need to be considered.

Children need good nutrition to maintain their normal growth and development. The goals of nutritional support are to maintain this need as well as to prevent nutritional depletion and to meet the needs of an increasing demand for nutrients during treatment (Hanigan & Walter, 1992). When planning the management of symptoms consider the following:

- Identify children at risk
- Undertake clinical assessment, including dietary history
- Involve the multidisciplinary team
- Introduce a nutritional care plan
- Identify realistic goals
- Involve the child and the family in all stages through ongoing education and participation in care.

The child should be encouraged to eat by being offered small frequent meals of appetising foods. Identifying favourite foods and establishing a pattern of intake may be helpful. Well-balanced and nutritional meals should be offered but this may be difficult as children seem to crave certain foods, such as hamburgers and crisps, and at times this is all they will eat. Encouraging the children in the ward to eat their meals together at a table fosters social interaction with others and provides some routine to the day. Allowing teenagers to eat later in the evenings may encourage food intake but this will rely on flexible kitchen arrangements. Some centres have cooking facilities in the ward area where the family can prepare meals for their child allowing them to have 'home cooked food' within the ward environment. If this is not possible food can usually be brought in from home. It is important that mealtimes do not become a battle between the child and their parents. Some children may see this as a way of manipulating their parents or rebelling against their treatment and thus feel that they are maintaining control. Similarly, parents may feel that this is one area in which they can affect the outcome and also have some control (Panzarella & Duncan, 1993). Explanation is preferable to coercion. Children require time to express their feelings and may need help in making sense of their experiences.

Nursing staff will need to be prepared to assist and encourage children to eat, especially if it is becoming stressful for parents. Younger children may be encouraged to eat if they are able to feed themselves or 'pretend play' with food in the play room. Cooking can be encouraged as a school activity, if the child feels up to cooking, with the food being consumed following the activity. This gives some control back to the child, particularly in this area of their treatment.

Dieticians must be involved from the beginning of the child's hospitalisation at the time of prevention and not just intervention. They can offer support and advice, consult with the family regarding food selection, supplements and alternative means of nutritional support; oral steroids may be recommended to increase the child's appetite. Providing favourite foods and encouraging a child to eat can be an expensive process for some families who may require financial assistance.

Nursing note:

Milkshakes are a popular drink; high-calorie milkshakes can be made even more appealing with the addition of ice-cream.

Enteral or parenteral feeding is indicated when the child is unable to meet nutritional needs by mouth. Enteral feeding, via a nasogastric tube, can increase nutritional uptake if tolerated well and the gut is working to use it. When considered alongside other interventions, nasogastric feeding may be dismissed as being psychologically traumatic for the child (Rickard et al., 1986), but it has been shown to be accepted by children and tolerated well, with nutritional benefits (Smith et al., 1992). If nursing staff are negative about the use of enteral feeding this attitude may be conveyed to the child and the family and result in poor compliance. Preparation for insertion of the tube is essential and will involve the skills of the nurse, parent and play specialist. Delay tactics may be used. Preparation time needs to be sufficient without increasing levels of anxiety. Adequate time needs to be allowed for parenteral feeding, providing time for the child to express any worries and question the procedure. Equipment stored for this purpose can be used for the child to feel the tube and play with the syringes.

Enteral products can be either complete meal replacements that will require digestion, or constitute elemental diets which require minimal or no enzymatic activity prior to absorption (Irwin, 1986). The dietician is responsible for calculating calorie requirements and for balancing fluid needs. The feed is introduced gradually and tolerance assessed daily. Feeding can be given via bolus feeds or overnight via a feeding pump. If given via a bolus the child should be encouraged to eat a meal first and then receive the enteral feed as a 'top-up'. This allows mealtimes to be maintained and the child to attempt to eat normally. Overnight feeds allow the child to eat normally during the day whilst providing extra calories at night. If weight loss or anorexia continues to be a problem then enteral feeding may be continued at home, following the parents' agreement and a comprehensive teaching programme.

Nursing note:

Older children and teenagers can be taught to pass their own naso-gastric tube, thus allowing periods of freedom from the tube and maintaining some normality.

Long term use of enteral feeding in infants can lead to problems with sucking, eating and speech development. Involvement of the speech therapist can help to alleviate these potential problems.

Enteral feeding is cheaper and less invasive than parenteral nutrition. However, the choice of feeding will be determined by other factors such as:

- Nutritional requirements
- Degree of nutritional debilitation
- Disease process
- Timing in relation to treatment
- A functioning gut
- Resources available (Irwin, 1986).

Total Parenteral Nutrition (TPN) may be indicated and be given via a central venous access device or very occasionally a peripheral line. A central venous access device is preferred as administration of high glucose concentrations is required for children to obtain sufficient calories (Macleod, 1994). In addition to glucose, TPN contains water, fats, carbohydrates, electrolytes, vitamins and minerals; in some cases the fat (lipid) component is given separately (Michie, 1988). It is not without risks and these include fluid overload, metabolic, vascular and septic episodes in some patients (Michie, 1988). Initially, daily monitoring of serum glucose is necessary and once stable, following a period of TPN administration, this may become less frequent. Lipids may affect liver function and this must be checked regularly. Nursing observation will include recording intake and output, daily urine testing for glucose and regular recording of weight.

Parenteral feeding is an expensive therapy to use and ideally must be managed by a nutrition team (Fawcett, 1995). Other methods, such as enteral feeding, may need to be considered before it is implemented, especially if the gut is functioning. Several days are needed to build up to full-strength parenteral nutrition for the child to obtain maximum calories from it, and for the metabolic adaptation of infused nutrients (Macleod, 1994). Infusion pumps are used to ensure a constant rate is delivered. Once established, TPN is infused over a 12–14-hour period, allowing the child some freedom from the restraining infusion lines. During the administration of parenteral nutrition the child should continue to be offered oral fluid and food to allow oral stimulation. The involvement of a psychologist may be beneficial in offering advice on ways to encourage the child to eat.

Nursing note:

The use of a reward system such as a sticker chart may encourage some younger children to eat, but rewards need to be appropriate to the child's age and have achievable and relevant goals.

In summary, when planning interventions the following should be considered:

- Identify the child's favourite foods
- Offer small, frequent meals
- Encourage dietary supplements
- Maintain assessment and involvement of the dietician
- Manage the side effects of chemotherapy (e.g. nausea and vomiting) effectively
- Consider enteral feeding early
- Introduced TPN where appropriate.

Some children are very reluctant to eat whilst they are in hospital as they associate the ward environment with unpleasant treatments and experiences. Before discharge, the family can be reassured that eating will probably resume once the child is back at home. As part of a planned discharge paediatric community teams need to be informed in advance of the child's discharge so that follow-up care can be arranged. Visits can be planned to provide ongoing support and encouragement to the child and the parents.

Cachexia

This is a syndrome of progressive wasting associated with anorexia and metabolic alterations (Lindsey, 1986). It appears to progress with the disease and may result in profound loss in body weight and muscle tissue and a decrease in both functional status and quality of life (Grant & Rivera, 1995). It is thought to result from an imbalance between the energy needed by the body versus the energy available due to reduced intake alongside biochemical alterations. These changes may also influence the development of fatigue (Piper et al., 1987); a multifaceted phenomenon that is not yet well understood (Aistars, 1987), particularly in children.

Lindsey (1986) suggests that children who are at critical growth periods and receiving aggressive anticancer therapies are even more vulnerable to developing cachexia. Its cause is unknown, but there are several hypotheses:

- Reduced oral intake and anorexia resulting from the malignancy or treatment (Bozzetti, 1995)
- Impaired digestion and absorption (Theologides, 1979)
- Increased energy expenditure despite a decreased calorie intake, leading to progressive wasting (Lindsey, 1986)
- Alterations in carbohydrate metabolism, including decreased glucose tolerance and normal or increased fasting blood glucose. Glucose uptake by the tumour is increased and varies with the size of the tumour (Lindsey, 1986)
- Tumour–host competition for nutrients, with the aggressive tumour winning over the host (Theologides, 1979)
- Abnormal lipid metabolism with depletion of fat reserves (Sutton, 1988).

Cachexia cannot be explained as a result of starvation alone, but as part of a much more complex metabolic disorder (Theologides, 1979), with the tumour itself clearly inducing profound nutritional problems (Holmes, 1991a, b).

Children most at risk are those who are nutritionally compromised at diagnosis; those who have a large tumour burden, particularly of the abdomen; or those requiring intensive chemotherapy (Foley et al., 1993).

Clinical features — weight loss, anorexia, early satiety, weakness, muscle atrophy, fatigue, impaired immune function, anaemia, decreased motor and mental skills, decreased attention and concentration abilities, muscle wasting and loss of body fat. It eventually leads to asthenia and emaciation (Lindsey, 1986).

Management — begins with assessment. This will highlight any contributory factors that may have a role to play, for example, taste changes, anorexia, psychological or emotional responses. Assessment includes a diet and weight loss history and this information will influence the planning of individual interventions. Nutritional support is required to meet the minimal calorie and protein requirements. The child's appetite needs to be increased and weight gain established. However, reversal of the effects depends largely on eradication of the cancer and prevention of the common side effects of treatment that have a debilitating effect (Calman, 1982). In some cases, despite increased calorie intake the child may still fail to gain weight.

Nutritional support can be given orally, intravenously, or entrally; methods used alone as well as in combination. Aggressive use of total parenteral nutrition may be advocated allowing the body to cope with the chemotherapy (Wesdrop et al., 1983). The issue of altered body image also needs to be addressed as this may also have implications for the child who is unable to eat (Sutton, 1988).

Diarrhoea

Diarrhoea is defined as an abnormal increase in stool liquidity caused by rapid movement of faecal matter through the intestine. The mucosal epithelial cells (villi and microvilli) lining the intestines are characterised by rapid cell division and if they are not replaced the mucosal cells atrophy and become inflamed. The villi and microvilli shorten and become eroded and the inflamed mucosa produces large amounts of mucous which stimulates accelerated peristalsis. Malabsorption is also common. This is due not only to the diarrhoea but also to the direct effect on the absorptive surface of the intestinal lining. The villi and microvilli are responsible for both digestion and absorption of food; when damaged, absorption of nutrients, water and electrolytes does not occur (Barton Burke et al., 1991), thus compromising nutritional status.

The cause of diarrhoea may be multifactorial, related to anxiety, a change in diet, use of nutritional supplements, medication (frequent antibiotics), infection, site of tumour and chemotherapy (particularly cisplatinum and cytarabine). It can be very distressing and debilitating to the child, and cause embarrassment.

Pseudomembranous colitis is a rare complication of antibiotic treatment which is characterised by proliferation of the bacterium, *Clostridium difficile*, in the colon, leading to diarrhoea (Andrejak et al., 1996). Antibiotics (vancomycin and metronidazole) are used for the treatment of this specific problem (Andrejak et al., 1996; Wenisch et al., 1996). Cryptosporidium can also cause diarrhoea in the immunocompromised child. This can be transmitted from person to person through ingestion of contaminated water or food (Juranek, 1995). This can be treated with the administration of spiramycin. Antidiarrhoeals are not recommended as the toxins would fail to be excreted.

Clinical features — frequent loose stools, abdominal cramps, pain, flatus and rectal excoriation. The stools can be very mucousy and on occasions sections of bowel mucosa or blood may be passed. This may lead to dehydration, fatigue, electrolyte imbalance, weight loss and malnutrition, and can also result in typhlitis.

Management — assessment includes noting the child's normal bowel habits, this is vital so that the 'abnormal' can be recognised promptly. Accurate records of intake and output are maintained, noting number, amount, consistency and colour of stools. An increase in stools alone may not be a true indicator, it is more important to note an alteration to the child's normal habit. Identifying the cause can be difficult due to the range of possible contributory factors. A review of current drugs and the child's dietary history should be considered. Specimens should be sent to the laboratory for investigations virology, microscopy, culture and sensitivity and any infection treated.

Administration of an antispasmodic agent, such as hyoscine-N-butyl bromide (Buscopan), may help to relieve the pain resulting from abdominal cramps. Fluid balance charts should be maintained, weight recorded (frequency will depend on severity of clinical symptoms), observations made for signs of dehydration and electrolyte imbalance which should be treated promptly with intravenous fluids and electrolytes as needed. Early and effective interventions are necessary and short term use of parenteral feeding may be required.

Diarrhoea can also lead to the breakdown of skin and thus may increase the risk of opportunistic infections. Good general hygiene should be reinforced, teaching strict handwashing technique (Gould, 1995) when handling stools, as well as ensuring that the area is kept clean and dry and applying barrier creams as required to help prevent excoriation.

Nursing note:

A gentle oil, such as baby oil, used to clean a sore bottom is more soothing than water. Sucralfate can be applied to excoriated skin followed by an application of a barrier cream that may consist of 50% metanium/white soft paraffin.

Daily examination of the area ensures that there are no signs of local infection, tissue breakdown or anal fissures. Infection in this area can occur easily in the immunocompromised child and can be the cause of much pain and distress. Pain can be relieved with the use of anaesthetic gels alongside other analgesics that may be required.

The importance of reporting episodes of diarrhoea must be stressed to the child and the family to ensure prompt treatment. The parents can be involved in keeping accurate records of intake and output; weighing nappies and disposing of bedpans. The child and the family need to be encouraged to discuss any problems with nursing staff without feeling embarrassed. For the child, unpredictable bouts of diarrhoea may result in a feeling of loss of control and they may chose to withdraw from social activities with other children (Aitken, 1992). Diarrhoea can interfere with the activities and general lifestyle of the child and family, requiring support and understanding.

Constipation

Constipation is defined as a decrease in the frequency of the passage of hard stool caused by either a complete or incomplete action of the bowels. There is a tendency for dry stools to accumulate in the descending colon where fluid absorption continues thus dehydrating the stool even further (Holmes, 1990). Considerable discomfort may be experienced from straining and may result in anal tears which may become infected leading to abscess formation.

Aitken (1992) divides constipation into three categories: primary, resulting from external factors, such as a lack of exercise, poor diet lacking in fibre and the failure to allow sufficient time for defecation (with children in hospital a lack of privacy resulting in embarrassment can also be a cause); secondary, resulting from pathological changes, such as spinal cord compression, intestinal obstruction or electrolyte imbalance; iatrogenic, following administration of medications, such as opioids and vinca alkaloids (as a result of autonomic neuropathy).

Clinical features — passage of irregular, infrequent hard stools usually accompanied by pain and discomfort. There may be nausea, abdominal distension with decreased bowel sounds and a decreased appetite.

Management — assessment of normal bowel habits and, where possible, prevention. Accurate records are kept of the number and consistency of stools. Dietary intake is recorded. Observation would include inspection of the anal area as well as noting any complaints of abdominal pain and difficulties with bowel movements. The family needs to be encouraged to report any signs of constipation, such as irregular bowel actions, abdominal pain or a decreased appetite so that early interventions can be commenced if needed.

Educating the child and the family on the causes and prevention of constipation is vital. Dietary advice regarding a nutritional well-balanced diet with plenty of fibre and fluids should be stressed but may not always be possible with a child who is unable to eat.

Nursing note:

This may be an opportunity to promote a 'healthy diet' for all the family.

Exercise should be encouraged as this appears to stimulate the bowel and may be beneficial in helping prevent constipation.

Children and especially teenagers need to understand the importance of discussing their bowel habits and informing parents or nursing staff when they are experiencing difficulties. Some teenagers may find this difficult, although they may have developed a good relationship with one member of staff and may be encouraged to confide in them.

Ensuring that the child has privacy even from his or her parents when using the toilet or bedpan may help them to maintain normal bowel habits. It is important to acknowledge the child's embarrassment and be sensitive to individual needs.

Stool softeners/laxatives should be administered and their effectiveness monitored. These should be given prophylactically with the administration of opioids or vinca alkaloids (sometimes it is necessary to use both softeners and stimulants depending on the cause and the severity of the problem). Ongoing assessment is required in order to regulate symptoms and avoid diarrhoea. Very occasionally, suppositories or enemas are required but these should be used with great care in the neutropenic child as there is a risk of trauma to the anal area resulting in anal fissures, infection and bleeding which can be a particular problem in the child who is thrombocytopenic. Some units do not use suppositories or enemas for this reason.

Trauma caused by the child straining to pass a constipated stool can be relieved with topical anaesthetic (lignocaine) applied to the rectal area.

Nursing note:

With regard to prevention it is important to explain to families and especially teenagers that vincristine is highly likely to cause constipation and that they must report problems early. When constipation is a problem it is worth considering alternative therapies, such as reflexology.

Typhlitis

This is a necrotising colitis which is usually localised in the caecum and commonly occurs in association with prolonged neutropenia and broad-spectrum antimicrobial therapy. Bacterial invasion of the mucosa of the bowel may progress from inflammation to full thickness infarction and perforation. It occurs most frequently from *Clostridium septicum* and Gram-negative organisms, especially *Pseudomonas aeruginosa* (Lange et al., 1993) (Table 3.6).

Table 3.6: Pathological process of typhlitis

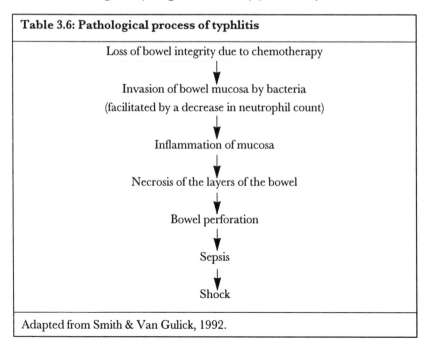

Loss of bowel integrity due to chemotherapy

Invasion of bowel mucosa by bacteria
(facilitated by a decrease in neutrophil count)

Inflammation of mucosa

Necrosis of the layers of the bowel

Bowel perforation

Sepsis

Shock

Adapted from Smith & Van Gulick, 1992.

Clinical features — pain, usually in the right lower quadrant that can be 'colicky' or constant, pyrexia, neutropenia, ascites, altered bowel habits, nausea and vomiting and shock can occur.

Management — symptoms are identified through close observation and an understanding of this complication and the associated risk factors.

Medical management may be conservative as follows:

- Nil by mouth
- Nasogastric tube
- Broad-spectrum antibiotics
- Intravenous fluids
- Pain relief.

Surgical resection of the necrotic bowel may be indicated if there is persistent gastrointestinal bleeding, perforation or deterioration in the child's overall condition (Ross & O'Neill, 1992; Lanzkowsky, 1995). There is some discrepancy concerning the role of granulocyte colony stimulating factors (G-CSF) in the treatment of typhlitis. Hanada et al. (1990) have used G-CSF successfully with antibiotics in children with leukaemia and typhlitis. In contrast, Vlasveld et al. (1990) have hypothesised that G-CSF may augment typhlitis by stimulating cytokines and thus potentially bacterial toxins, making the situation worse.

Typhlitis can be a major complication of chemotherapy and it can have considerable mortality (Smith & Van Gulick, 1992). Pizzo and Young (1989) estimate mortality from typhlitis to be greater than 50%. Nursing care needs to be supportive, to monitor changes in the child and response to treatment; and to work closely with medical colleagues in giving optimum care to the child. The family will be under considerable stress in coping with the child's malignancy as well as a serious complication and will need support and information to help them to deal with this. Awareness of the needs of the child is vital. Both the child and the family will need frequent explanations and to be involved in care as appropriate, to enable them to cope with this illness and its complications (Kinrade, 1988).

Bone marrow

Haematological problems

Chemotherapy destroys or damages the stem cells in the bone marrow. This results in neutropenia, thrombocytopenia and anaemia (see Table 3.7 for normal blood cell values in infancy and childhood). The point at which this occurs following chemotherapy depends on the lifespan of the circulating cells.

Table 3.7: Normal blood count values in childhood					
Age	Hb (g/dl)	WBC (x10/l)	Neutrophils (x10/l)	Lymphocytes (x10/l)	Monocytes (x10/l)
Birth	14.9–23.7	10–26	2.7–14.4	2.0–7.3	1–1.9
2 weeks	13.4–19.8	6–21	1.8–5.4	2.8–7.3	0.1–1.7
2 months	9.4–13.0	6–18	1.2–7.5	3–13.5	0.1–1.7
6 months	11.1–14.1	6–17.5	1.0–8.5	4–13.5	0.2–1.2
1 year	11.3–14.1	6–17.5	1.5–8.5	4–10.5	0.2–1.2
2–6 years	11.5–13.5	5–17	1.5–8.5	1.5–9.5	0.2–1.2
6–12 years	11.5–15.5	4.5–14.5	1.5–8.0	1.5–7	0.2–1.0
12–18 years	12.0–16.0	4.5–13	1.8–8.0	1.2–6.5	0.2–0.8

Adapted from Hinchliffe, 1992.

Anaemia

Anaemia is a reduction in the concentration of haemoglobin and the circulating red blood cell mass (Fischer et al., 1993). The lifespan of red blood cells is 120 days.

Clinical features — pallor, fatigue, dizziness, dyspnoea, headache, sweating, irritability, tachycardia, tachypnoea or anorexia. Some younger children are able to adapt with minimal symptoms but if they feel cold or are reluctant to eat, this may be a sign of anaemia.
Management — transfusion of red blood cells is a supportive intervention which may be used when the child's haemoglobin falls below 7–8 g/dl, or if they are symptomatic. The idea is to maintain the haemoglobin above 10 g/dl.

If blood transfusions are carried out electively, it makes it easier for the transfusion service to provide specific requirements and avoids the need for 'emergency bloods'. Cross-matching of blood is important to help to prevent reactions. Many units transfuse cytomegalovirus (CMV) negative blood products to prevent CMV infection in the immunocompromised child. Occasionally, children are found to be CMV positive in which case it is not required.

Packed cells are normally used for children. This allows the required concentration of red cells to be given in smaller volumes which may help prevent circulatory overload. The child should be monitored closely during transfusions for allergic reactions.

Febrile reactions

In the case of non-haemolytic febrile transfusion reactions (NHFTR), antibodies in the child's plasma react against transfused leukocytes in the blood (McClelland, 1996).

Clinical features — shivering (usually 30–60 minutes after the transfusion is commenced), tachycardia, fever.
Management — transfusion should be slowed or stopped and paracetamol given. The child's condition should be monitored and the child should be kept warm.

If the child has had a previous febrile reaction recurrence may be prevented by administering paracetamol before the transfusion or employing leukocyte depletion filters. Some transfusion services are investigating the use of leukocyte depletion at source, in an effort to prevent reactions but this is not common practice at the time of writing.

Allergic reactions

In this case, the child has antibodies which react with proteins in the transfused blood components (McClelland, 1996).

Clinical features — urticaria and itching within minutes of transfusion.
Management — transfusions should be slowed and chlorpheniramine given. If no further symptoms, the transfusion should be continued. If repeated reactions, chlorpheniramine should be given 30 minutes before the transfusion and the child should be watched very carefully.

Nursing note:

Children receiving treatment for cancer are often on regular steroid treatment. It is therefore best to avoid giving steroids at other times as much as possible. It seems that a simple antipyretic is now thought to be as effective as hydrocortisone and, in some cases, chlorpheniramine (McClelland, 1996).

For the management of anaphylaxis, see under 'Nursing emergencies' later in this chapter.

In cases of severe anaemia blood may need to be administered over a longer time span than usual so as not to compromise the cardiovascular system. It is important to remember, however, that blood can only stay out of the fridge for a maximum of four hours.

Some children and families find the concept of blood transfusion difficult. They may have listened to news reports about the risks associated with blood-borne diseases, such as HIV and Hepatitis B, and worry about the potential risk to their child. Reassurance about testing and about how the blood is prepared is therefore vital. In some cases families prefer the bag to be covered whilst blood is infusing as it seems to give them more confidence, especially if they do not like the sight of blood.

> **Nursing note:**
>
> There are particular difficulties with Jehovah's Witness followers. This can create serious dilemmas for medical staff and families when the giving of blood may be a life-saving measure. One option is to arrange for a 'specific issue order' which means that an application is made to the High Court to address a dispute about a child's management. In the medical context this usually means controversial medical treatment. Hendrick (1997) describes it as 'depriving someone with parental responsibility of the right to make a decision empowering the court to make it instead.'

Thrombocytopenia

After chemotherapy, the number of circulating platelets falls with the associated risk of bleeding. Platelets have a short lifespan, lasting for about a week.

Clinical features — petechiae, purpura, bruising, bleeding (especially from the nose and gums) and menorrhagia.
Management — the prevention of bleeding is important and the child and the family should be taught how to observe for signs of low platelets in which case they might need to have their blood count checked. Prevention of trauma to susceptible areas is helpful, for example, the use of a soft toothbrush or foam sticks for mouth care will help lessen trauma to the gums. It may be necessary to discourage children from activities such as roller blading until their platelet count recovers! The use of progesterone may be recommended in young women with menorrhagia to suppress menstrual bleeding.

Transfusion of platelets may be necessary to sustain the child until his own platelet production recovers, but this will depend on local policy. Some units will only transfuse platelets if the child is symptomatic or about to undergo an invasive procedure but, in general, in the absence of bleeding, platelets are given if the blood count is less than $10 \times 10^9/l$. In some cases, because transfused platelets have a short lifespan, they are given routinely before a procedure to ensure that there are an adequate number of platelets circulating.

If the child receives platelets and has a fever, infection, hepatosplenomegaly, antiplatelet antibodies or alloimmunization, their effectiveness may be decreased (Fischer et al., 1993). As with blood transfusions, there is the potential for reactions and this increases the more transfusions the child receives. The symptoms of a platelet reaction are the same as for a blood transfusion (see under 'Anaemia'). Anaphylactic shock may also occur (see 'Nursing emergencies' later in this chapter).

To minimise damage, platelets should be filtered and administered 'free-flowing', unless a peristaltic infusion pump is used. There has been some controversy about the use of infusion pumps and a study carried out by Norville et al. (1994) found that a peristaltic pump is acceptable because it does not negatively affect platelet recovery. This is a useful study as it is clearly safer and more accurate to use a pump.

Nursing note:

When giving blood and platelets, it is advisable to give platelets first. This is because blood will expand the fluid volume and could cause capillary bleeding in the thrombocytopenic child.

If teenagers want to shave, an electric razor is recommended to reduce the risk of cuts.

Tranexamic acid has been found to be useful in the community setting to arrest bleeding.

Neutropenia

Neutropenia remains a major cause of morbidity in children with cancer (Wujcik, 1993b; Rogers, 1995). The cytotoxic effect of chemotherapy increases the child's vulnerability to infection because there is a reduction in circulating white cells. This impairment to the host's defences results in an increase both in the incidence and in the severity of infection (Lehne, 1990).

Clinical features — fever may be the only sign of infection in the neutropenic child, although some children (especially infants) may present with no temperature but may have tachycardia and poor perfusion. Other signs and symptoms indicating an inflammatory response, such as erythema, swelling or pain, are absent because there are no neutrophils to contribute to pus formation (Rikonen et al., 1993).

Management — it is important that the child and the family understand how to minimise infection and know the signs to look for. Parents should be advised to check the child's temperature at regular intervals and to telephone the hospital if he is febrile. At the same time, the child should lead as normal a life as possible, so a balance must be negotiated.

Children should be treated for an infection on presentation with a fever (Albano & Pizzo, 1988; Wujcik, 1993a, b). Before this, a septic screen should be performed. This will include the following:

- Central line blood cultures (and sometimes peripheral)
- Urine sample
- Stool sample
- Swabs from any potentially infected area
- Chest X-ray.

Antibiotic therapy should be commenced with a combination of drugs to expand the spectrum of activity against as many organisms as possible during the initial treatment (Albano & Pizzo, 1988). Each unit will have a policy to follow concerning the administration of antibiotics to ensure that the 'cover' is adequate prior to the availability of blood culture results (Figure 3.5). The duration of the course of antibiotic therapy depends on the nature of the infection, the neutrophil count and the child's response (Hughes et al., 1990). Monitoring of vital signs should take a high priority in acutely unwell neutropenic children as they are at risk of septic shock. Accurate recording assists in evaluating the response to antibiotics.

Although it is important to stress from the outset that parents should be vigilant, it must be remembered that most bacterial infections that the child develops will be from his own gut. The vulnerable areas that parents need to watch are the peri-anal area, the mouth and central venous access device sites.

Nursing note:

The use of paracetamol or other antipyretics should be discouraged until antibiotic treatment is under way as this will mask symptoms. If pain relief is required an alternative, such as codeine, will need to be found. This also applies when the child is neutropenic and afebrile, for the same reason. Other cooling methods can be used, such as cooling the circulating air or removing clothing.

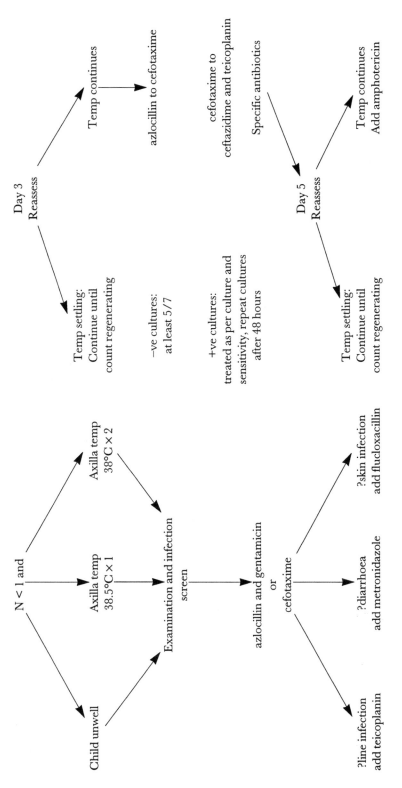

Figure 3.5: An example of the management of febrile neutropenia

Parents often worry about the child catching infections from school, but the risk of catching bacterial infections is minimal and unless they are unwell children do not necessarily need to stay away from school even when they are neutropenic. It must be stressed, however, that parents must be contactable by the school. School teachers may worry about the child, because they rarely see children with cancer. Paediatric oncology outreach nurse specialists provide a valuable service in that they are able to visit schools to make teachers aware of the potential risks to the child but will also encourage teachers to allow the child to mix with their friends without being over-protective (Larcombe et al., 1990).

Prophylaxis

There is some controversy about the use of drugs as prophylaxis for endogenous infections in the neutropenic child and some units will elect not to use any prophylaxis as the use of antimicrobials may encourage resistance (Rogers, 1995). Regimes vary according to local policy and may include oral non-absorbed agents, such as neomycin, coliston and nystatin, and systemically absorbed co-trimoxazole and fluroquinolines, such as ciprofloxacin. Rogers (1995) suggests that each of these regimes are beneficial in reducing bacterial infections due to Gram-negative rods (e.g. *Escherichia coli*, Proteus) because the intestinal flora is decreased. This may explain the emergence of resistant Gram-positive bacteria as a cause of sepsis in neutropenic patients. There are, however, no antibiotics which can provide cover for these pathogens and which can be given safely throughout neutropenia.

Prophylaxis for fungal infections is often limited to nystatin and oral amphotercin B which suppress colonising yeasts in the intestinal tract but are not absorbed and therefore offer no systemic protection against fungal infections (Rogers, 1995). Fluconazole is absorbed systemically after oral administration but there are some concerns over the limited antifungal spectrum of this drug in the neutropenic patient (Wingard et al., 1991). Itraconazole is also used, but its use is not fully established, although it is felt to provide some benefit in children with prolonged neutropenia (Cowie et al., 1994).

If the child is to receive prophylactic drugs during the neutropenic phase of his or her illness, the issue of compliance should be addressed. The child and the family should understand why they are receiving the drugs and how they should be given.

Home administration of intravenous antibiotics

It is clear that substitution of oral for intravenous drugs could be beneficial in terms of ease of administration but there is still concern about the feasibility of this approach. Lau et al. (1994) found that they were able to change a group of children from oral to intravenous antibiotics after 72 hours as long as the following criteria were met:

- Negative blood cultures
- Temperature of 38.0°C or lower for 24 hours
- Absence of clinical sepsis.

Some parents and teenagers are taught to give intravenous antibiotics at home through a central venous access device and with the support of paediatric oncology outreach nurse specialists this can be a successful way to promote early discharge with associated advantages for the family.

A study by Hooker (1996) looked at the safety and desirability of home administration of intravenous drugs and found that few clinical problems were encountered and that parents welcomed this initiative.

Wiernikowski et al. (1991) found that such a programme can be cost-effective in terms of saving bed spaces. At the same time, parents should *not* be persuaded to take their child home for this purpose.

Nursing note:

A booklet and video have been produced to guide parents and patients through the administration of intravenous antibiotics (Fay & Evans, 1997).

Other attempts to reduce the risk of infection in neutropenic children include the use of a sterile diet and protective isolation. Evidence on the effectiveness of these measures is conflicting because studies differ in the type of gut decontamination used and the level of isolation (Marcus & Goldman, 1986).

Most centres now emphasise the need to avoid foods which are likely to be contaminated with bacteria, such as re-heated foods or soft cheeses, unless in the case of bone marrow transplant patients when guidelines are much stricter (see Chapter 10 for more detail).

Isolation of neutropenic patients certainly varies from one unit to another. In some cases, children are nursed in a single room with or without filtered air whilst others are nursed on an open ward. There appears to be no conclusive evidence which will benefit the child most (Albano & Pizzo, 1988), but the psychological disadvantage of isolating children must clearly be considered. One solution to the problem is to isolate children being nursed on a general medical ward but this is not necessary on a paediatric oncology ward unless the child is likely to infect others.

The use of G-CSF for neutropenic children is now established practice in paediatric oncology when there is an overwhelming infection. It is, however, an expensive drug and its use does need to be justified in the present economic climate. G-CSF can reduce the severity and duration of neutropenia and may allow chemotherapy to be given in higher doses and at more frequent intervals. It is given either intravenously or subcutaneously but if it is given subcutaneously a higher leucocyte count is seen (Lieschke et al., 1990). In the past, leucocyte transfusions have been used for neutropenic children with documented infections that are not responding to treatment but they are not recommended for routine use (Hockenberry-Eaton et al., 1986). The use of leukocyte transfusions is now limited, due to the increasing use of G-CSF, as they can increase the risk of reactions to blood products.

Children who present with a fever but are not neutropenic need to be investigated as to the cause and treated appropriately with antibiotics and analgesia. They are usually assessed on the oncology unit if they are undergoing treatment to ensure that there is no underlying problem such as an infected central venous access device.

Several hospitals may be involved in the care of the child with cancer and liaison is vital to ensure all information is available and the same policies are followed when the child is neutropenic. Paediatric oncology outreach nurse specialists have a crucial role here in maintaining continuity and support, and in promoting shared care.

The compromised immune system

The child undergoing treatment with chemotherapy will often have lymphocytes in their blood but their function will be impaired and the immune system will not fight infections adequately. The parents are usually shown the child's blood count and the need to appreciate that monitoring of the neutrophil count, which is crucial during treatment, is highlighted.

Opportunistic infections

Pneumocystis carinii pneumonia (PCP) is identified by pyrexia, dyspnoea, a cough and a characteristic X-ray. It used to be common in children on immunosuppressive regimes but since the advent of cotrimoxazole, which is given three times a week as a prophylactic measure, the incidence has been reduced and it is now rarely seen. Cotrimoxazole should always be continued even if another antibiotic is added to treat an incidental infection.

Although the standard and most effective treatment for PCP is cotrimoxazole, bone marrow suppression and hypersensitivity sometimes limit its use and in this case pentamidine has been found to be effective (Sieve & Betcher, 1994).

Nursing note:

Although *Pneumocystis carinii* pneumonia (PCP) is rare, it is still a potentially fatal condition and it is therefore important to ensure that parents know what to look out for. The importance of taking prophylactic drugs should be emphasised.

Viral infections

Measles and chickenpox can be potentially fatal in the immunosuppressed child and the family must be aware of the danger of contact with these diseases.

Varicella (chickenpox) is an acute and highly infectious disease which is common during childhood. It is spread by direct contact or droplet infection and the incidence is at its peak from March to May. The incubation period is between two and three weeks. The characteristic vesicles usually cover most of the body, although in mild cases may be less easy to find. The infectious period is one to two days before the rash appears and until the vesicles are dry (around 21 days). This time may be prolonged in immunosuppressed children, however, and can be as long as 28 days.

Varicella can cause serious problems for the immunocompromised child as it carries the risk of dissemination of the virus to the lungs, brain, liver or skin (Rogers, 1995). The child's antibody status should always be checked at diagnosis. If they are not immune, such children should receive passive immunisation with *Varicella zoster* immune globulin (VZIG) within seven days of contact with the disease (Salisbury & Begg, 1996).

During this time if antibody levels are unavailable assays can be checked, the results of which should be available within 48 hours.

Nursing note:

There could be a false positive reading of antibodies soon after transfusion of blood products. This obviously needs to be treated with caution and re-testing for antibodies will need to be done if there is further exposure (Salisbury & Begg, 1996).

VZIG may not prevent the child developing the illness but it may reduce its severity. If a second exposure to the disease occurs after three weeks VZIG will need to be repeated (Salisbury & Begg, 1996). It is extremely important to isolate the infected child should he or she need to visit hospital, and, where possible, to keep visits to a minimum.

Some units do not use VZIG but if the child has been in contact with chickenpox a course of prophylactic acyclovir is administered instead. If the child develops chickenpox he is then treated with acyclovir and nursed in strict isolation, if hospitalised (McCalla et al., 1993). Very few children die from chickenpox since acyclovir has become available (Atra et al., 1993).

Nursing note:

If the child has been in close contact with shingles (re-activation of varicella) either VZIG or acyclovir is still needed if they have a low immunity. Shingles is as transmissible as chickenpox in immunocompromised children, but there is little evidence that it can be acquired from another child with chickenpox (Salisbury & Begg, 1996). Ensure grandparents are aware as they may not make the link between shingles and chickenpox.

Although the family must be aware of the potential dangers of chickenpox they must not become over-protective. The child should be encouraged to attend school and teachers need to be aware of the potential problems and inform the family if there is chickenpox in the class or school.

Nursing note:

There is controversy surrounding the issue of sending children who are immunocompromised to school when there is chickenpox in the class. In some centres VZIG may be given as a prophylactic measure when the child has negative titres, even though they have not been in direct contact with the disease. It should be emphasised to parents and to teachers that contact with a child whose sibling has the disease is *not* direct contact. When the child completes treatment for cancer their immunity should be checked as so many variables could have affected it.

Herpes simplex

Most *Herpes simplex* infections are due to HSV type 1 which manifests as oropharyngitis, cold sores or generalised sepsis. Clinically, the lesions appear as clear vesicle eruptions in clusters on an erythematous base but may be nondescript and atypical in appearance. HSV type 2 infection more commonly involves the genital area. Treatment is with oral or intravenous acyclovir. If it is used orally, large doses are required to maintain high levels as only 20–30% of the drug is absorbed. It also has a half-life of 3–3.5 hours which means the drug needs to be given every 4–6 hours (Sinniah & Belasco, 1992).

Measles

Measles is an acute viral disease and is transmitted by droplet infection. Clinical features include a rash, fever, conjunctivitis, coryza, Koplik spots and bronchitis. The incubation period is about 10 days. Measles is highly infectious from the prodromal period until 4 days after the appearance of the rash which usually takes 2–4 days to appear (Salisbury & Begg, 1996).

The introduction of the measles, mumps, rubella (MMR) vaccination programme in 1988 reduced the incidence of measles which was (up until that time) a major cause of mortality in children with cancer. The risk, although now minimal, is still present and measles in the immunocompromised child can lead to pneumonia and encephalitis. Passive immunisation with human immunoglobulin (HIG) should be given within six days of exposure to the disease, although its efficacy is at present controversial (Sinniah & Belasco, 1992; Rogers, 1995).

All the precautions regarding exposure to chickenpox should be taken into account with measles but the latter is a more life-threatening disease and exposure to it should be treated extremely seriously, especially if the child has a low immunity.

> **Nursing note:**
>
> **It is a good idea to provide a letter for other parents at school informing them about the need to tell the school if their children develop chickenpox. Parents should be made aware of the importance of ensuring that siblings have received the MMR vaccine.**

Immunisation

Live vaccines, such as measles, polio, rubella and BCG, are contraindicated in immunocompromised children because there is a risk of them developing the infection (Albano & Pizzo, 1988). Other immunisations, such as tetanus, diphtheria and pertussis, are not contraindicated but the response is often poor and it is best to delay them until treatment is complete. Six months to one year, depending on treatment and on local policy, should elapse before they are recommenced and, of course, this includes any that may have been missed. In some cases, children may need total revaccination. Their antibody status should be reviewed at this point.

Siblings should continue with their immunisation programme whilst their immunocompromised brother or sister is receiving treatment to minimise the risk of infecting the child with the natural disease. There is no risk of vaccine strain spread; however, the inactivated preparation of the polio vaccine (IPV) should be used to prevent cross-infection from the oral–faecal route.

Nursing note:

Parents need to be informed that the inactivated polio vaccine is given intramuscularly as opposed to orally. They may need a letter informing community staff of the need for this.

It should be made clear to parents that if the child cuts himself he must be given tetanus toxoid as short-term cover.

Cutaneous side effects

Alopecia

Chemotherapy destroys the rapidly dividing epithelial cells of the hair follicle reducing hair growth on the body and causing alopecia. The degree of hair loss depends upon the dose, the route and the nature of the treatment as well as the child's health prior to treatment (Price, 1990). Crounsel and Van Scott (1960) found that at any given time 90% of human hair follicles are in the dividing phases of the cell cycle and are therefore susceptible to the effects of chemotherapy. Hair loss can be extremely distressing both for the parents and the child and can have a severe effect on body image (see Chapter 4).

All body hair may be affected and hair loss usually begins 1–2 weeks after commencing chemotherapy with regrowth 1–2 weeks after the final course of treatment. It is more severe with drugs that have a long half-life of active metabolites, such as doxorubicin, the nitrosoureas and cyclophosphamide. Preparation and advice to the child and the family are very important.

There is very little that can be done to prevent alopecia. Scalp cooling has been tried in adults and it is thought to inhibit cellular uptake of a drug that is temperature-dependent (Dean et al., 1979) but there are inconsistencies in the method, length of time involved and how much hair is eventually retained (Tierney, 1987). Scalp cooling is only effective when certain drugs are used, for example, daunorubicin (David & Speechley, 1987). There are concerns that because hypothermia decreases the drug concentration to the scalp it may become a sanctuary for micrometastatic malignant cells (Barton Burke et al., 1991). There are contraindications to the use of scalp cooling in that it requires specific skills which are time-consuming; and, more importantly, it can be unpleasant for the child.

Skin

The child may have problems with their skin, particularly after high-dose cytarabine, which causes rashes that may be an irritant and blister. The following guidelines should be observed:

- Pay careful attention to skin hygiene to ensure that it is kept clean and free from irritation
- Apply moisturising cream as skin often becomes dry during chemotherapy
- Act promptly when rashes or abnormalities are seen
- Ensure that the child wears total sunblock when outside because the skin becomes more sensitive to sunlight during chemotherapy.

Nursing note:

This is a good opportunity to provide health education about the dangers of too much sun at any time.

Gonadal side effects

Fertility and growth are both affected by certain chemotherapeutic agents (see Chapters 2 and 5 and Chapter 8 for more detail).

Nursing Emergencies

Septic shock

This is one of the commonest causes of treatment-related mortality in childhood cancer. It is a specific clinical syndrome which is characterised by systemic sepsis with evidence of circulatory insufficiency and inadequate tissue perfusion (Wetzel & Tobin, 1992). The mechanism begins with the proliferation of micro-organisms at an infection source which then invade the blood stream and stimulate both endotoxins and exotoxins. These then have a profound influence on the physiological mechanisms of the heart, other organs and vasculature (Parrillo, 1993; Kulkarni & Webster, 1996) (Figure 3.6).

Early diagnosis and intervention are essential to pre-empt septic shock, but it can develop from any infectious disease. The most common organisms to cause septic shock are Gram-negative ones, such as Pseudomonas, Klebsiella or *Escherichia coli* (Smith & Van Gulick, 1992). Any proven Gram-negative infection should be treated with great caution.

Clinical features — raised pulse and respiration rate; hypotension or a falling blood pressure; fever, chills; decreased tissue perfusion with pallor, clammy skin and cool extremities; mental confusion, apprehension; and oliguria. In addition, there may be a current history of skin, urinary or gastrointestinal infection or the child may recently have had surgery.

Management — treatment is aimed at optimising perfusion of the critical vascular beds, particularly the kidneys, as there can be a risk of renal failure. A full septic screen is performed and broad spectrum antibiotics commenced.

Nursing note:

The onset of septic shock can be sudden with no previous signs or symptoms and the child may present in a collapsed state. There is a clear cause for concern if a child presents with cool extremities, clammy skin and increased respiratory effort.

Supportive care involves the use of oxygen therapy to maintain adequate oxygenation; correction of hypovolaemia with blood and plasma as required; and antipyretics to control the temperature (Wesley & Coran, 1986).

Nursing care comprises:

- ensuring there is reliable venous access
- observing the child's general condition carefully
- administering all medications and supportive measures promptly
- monitoring temperature, pulse, respiration
- taking blood pressure frequently
- monitoring urine output
- supporting the child and the family during this critical time
- keeping the parents informed of what is happening to their child and of the child's general condition.

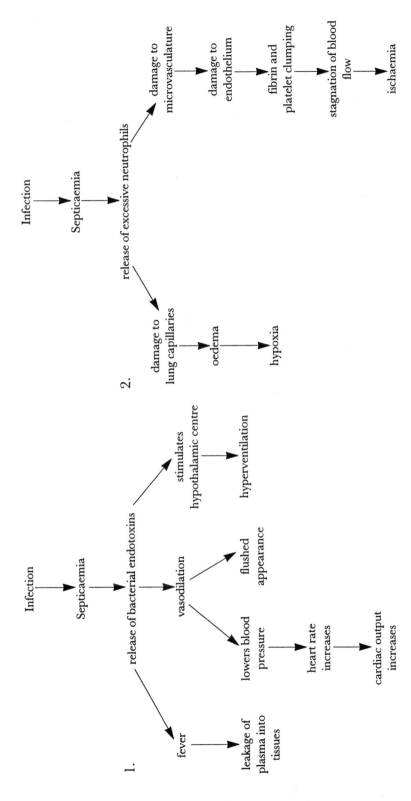

Figure 3.6: Events in septic shock: a two-stage process

The general outcome of septic shock usually relates to early recognition and speedy intervention (Darovic, 1984).

> **Nursing note:**
> **Remember that persistent tachycardia is an important sign of septic shock.**

Close observation of the child is vital as his or her condition can deteriorate quickly, requiring further support with intubation and ventilation.

Parents will need the opportunity to be involved in care and to voice their anxieties. At the same time negotiation should be emphasised as they may feel unable to continue with carrying out care in strange surroundings or when they are exhausted and anxious.

Home care

A child can deteriorate very quickly with overwhelming sepsis. It is therefore necessary to stress to families the importance of observing the neutropenic child at home for temperatures. Parents should also be made aware that they may need to seek help promptly if they are unhappy about the child's general condition, as infection can occur without fever. Paediatric oncology outreach nurse specialists and community children's nurses have an important part to play in reinforcing this information.

Advice to parents on going home after chemotherapy is to:

- Take the child's temperature regularly
- Observe respiratory rate
- Note if the child's skin colour changes
- Note if the child is lethargic or off-colour
- Ring the hospital for advice on any of the above
- Call an ambulance if the child collapses.

Disseminated intravascular coagulation (DIC)

Disseminated intravascular coagulation (DIC) can be a confusing syndrome because there are several reasons for its occurrence. It is characterised by coagulation and haemorrhage occuring simultaneously (Figure 3.7).

The management of DIC is particularly challenging when children have leukaemia because of the abnormalities in blood formation which are already present. In fact, children with leukaemia may present with features of DIC without actually having the syndrome. This syndrome occurs when the coagulation process is abnormally activated (Table 3.8).

There is overactivity in four main areas:

- The clotting mechanism, allowing extensive thrombus formation in greater amounts than can be neutralised by the body. There is conversion of fibrinogen to fibrin and aggregation and destruction of platelets.
- Fibrinolysis with destruction of clotting factors and associated haemorrhage.
- Decreased macrophage clearing function, thereby aggravating the process by limiting the removal of activated clotting factors so that obstruction and eventual necrosis of tissue occurs.
- Damage and haemolysis of red blood cells.

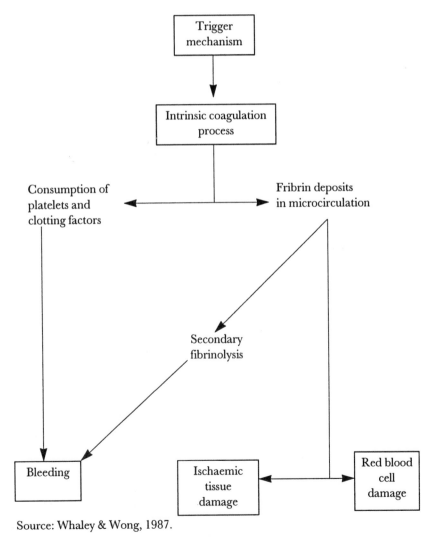

Source: Whaley & Wong, 1987.

Figure 3.7 Effects of disseminated intravascular coagulation (DIC)

Table 3.8: Laboratory findings		
	Normal	In DIC
Platelets	150–450,000	decreased
Prothrombin time (PT)	10.5–12.9 sec	prolonged
Partial thrombin time (PTT)*	24.3–36.3 sec	prolonged
Fibrinogen	200–440 mg/100 ml	<150 mg/100 ml
FDP	>10	<40
Haemaglobin (Hb)	>40	decreased

*A raised PTT, decreased platelet count and decreased fibrinogen is generally indicative of DIC.
Adapted from Kurtz, 1993.

DIC is a symptom, not a disease and is associated with an underlying condition such as Gram-negative septicaemia or newly diagnosed or relapsing acute non-lymphoblastic leukaemia, particularly promyelocytic leukaemia. It occurs less frequently in disseminated neuroblastoma and other metastatic solid tumours. It has been reported that up to 85% of patients with acute promyelocytic leukaemia (APML) have DIC (Kurtz, 1993). DIC can also be associated with transfusions or drug reactions and haemorrhage. It is therefore important to know whether the child has any allergies.

Clinical features — oozing at surface injuries; petechiae, purpura; variable degrees of haemorrhage from multiple sites; and variable degrees of circulatory failure and shock.
Management — the primary management is treatment of the underlying cause and supportive therapy (Buchanan, 1993; Bray, 1993). Venous access (usually in the form of a central line) is essential to treat these children as they may require supportive therapy quickly.

Supportive therapy includes broad-spectrum antibiotics; platelets and fresh frozen plasma (if the child has mucosal or internal bleeding); cryoprecipitate to replace specific clotting deficiencies; and red cell transfusions to correct anaemia (Bray, 1993; Buchanan, 1993).

Nursing note:

Venous access with a central line can lead to problems as it becomes another site for haemorrhage and therefore close observation of the site and surrounding tissues is essential.

The child's prognosis depends on the severity of the DIC and the prognosis of the underlying disease. Close observation of these children is essential, looking for signs of further haemorrhage. Nursing care includes:

- Monitoring for an increased thready pulse and decreased blood pressure
- Observing for petechiae (especially in less obvious places such as under the arms)
- Discouraging the child from picking their nose or blowing it too hard
- Packing nasal passages if epistaxis occurs
- Avoiding all venepunctures if possible and applying firm pressure if they become essential
- Encouraging gentle mouthcare to avoid trauma to the gums by use of a soft toothbrush or foam sticks
- Avoiding rectal drugs
- Providing psychological care and support (symptoms can be frightening, especially for younger children).

Heparin has been used for the treatment of DIC in children with APML but its usefulness has been debated. It may be suggested for use in patients with a thrombotic tendency to prevent the formation of thrombus but a delicate balance is required to prevent unnecessary haemorrhage (Kantarjian et al., 1986; Goldberg et al., 1987). The use of all-trans retinoic acid (ATRA) for patients with APML is being evaluated as it initiates cell differentiation and appears to have some effect on the potential problems of DIC (Castaigne et al.,1990).

Anaphylaxis

This is a severe life-threatening antigen–antibody response resulting from exposure to a foreign substance, an allergen. Antibodies are produced and attach themselves to the mast cells which remain in the body. Ingestion of subsequent allergens causes a reaction with the mast cells which can lead to a rapid, complex series of events from the mediators released in the body. A reaction occurs which may be exacerbated after each exposure to the allergen (Hammond, 1988; Barton Burke et al., 1991; Benjamin & Leskowitz, 1991). It can be extremely frightening for the child and the family as well as the nursing staff.

Anaphylaxis is often associated with specific drugs in paediatric oncology — L-asparaginase, etoposide (VP16), teneposide (VM26) and cisplatin. It can also occur during or after transfusion of blood products or administration of antibiotics (most commonly with second or subsequent doses of antibiotics). It can occur very quickly and the child's condition deteriorates rapidly.

Clinical features — symptoms of systemic shock (see 'Septic shock' earlier in the chapter), urticaria, paroxysmal coughing, dyspnoea, wheezing, cyanosis, vomiting and anxiety.

Management — stop the transfusion or drug, maintain venous access, give oxygen if required, give drugs as prescribed (e.g. adrenaline, chlorpheniramine), give salbutamol by nebuliser and get expert advice (McClelland, 1996).

All staff working within paediatric oncology should be aware of the potential for children to have an anaphylactic reaction to chemotherapy and be aware of local policy on how to deal with this situation. It is essential that all staff, especially if they are new to the ward, are aware of the exact location of appropriate drugs so that they are readily available. Some centres will call the arrest team if such an episode occurs, to ensure that medical assistance arrives promptly but this may not always apply. A record should be kept of reactions, including the cause and the treatment used.

Anaphylaxis is not usually dose-related but an increased frequency of allergic reactions is seen with cumulative doses, high doses, intravenous administration and single-drug administration (Hammond, 1988).

L-asparaginase should be given intramuscularly or subcutaneously in an effort to avoid reactions but the child may still suffer a delayed reaction. It is recommended that the child remains on the ward or in clinic for at least one hour post-administration so that they can be observed for any late reaction. It is for this reason that L-asparaginase is not given in the community setting but should always be adminis-tered in hospital with resuscitation facilities available.

If the child suffers a mild reaction to a drug, it should be fully docu-mented so that if the drug is given in the future all staff are made aware. The decision may be to administer hydrocortisone and chlorpheni-ramine 'cover' or avoid it completely. The family should be made aware of the drug which caused the reaction, so that they can ensure it is avoided in the future if appropriate. The family should be given instructions as to what to do in an emergency (see under 'Septic shock').

Nursing note:

Giving the family a card with the name of the drug which causes a reaction is helpful. Information can also be recorded in the parent-held record

Some centres leave a gap of six hours between the administration of intrathecal methotrexate and L-asparaginase to ensure that they are fully aware of any reactions.

Acute tumour lysis syndrome

Acute tumour lysis syndrome (ATLS) is a potentially fatal metabolic complication that occurs as a result of the rapid release of intracellular metabolites (uric acid, potassium, phosphate) from the destruction (lysis) of malignant cells in quantities that exceed the excretory capacity of the kidneys with the initiation of treatment (Cohen et al., 1980). The metabolic abnormalities that occur are hyperuricaemia (usually in the early phase), hyperkalaemia and hyperphosphataemia with resultant hypocalcaemia; all of which may occur in isolation or in combination (Allegretta et al., 1985). Complications typically manifest within 1–5 days of the start of chemotherapy (Lange et al., 1993; Lawrence, 1994). The signs and symptoms observed will be directly related to the metabolic changes that are occurring (Figure 3.8). ATLS occurs most commonly in patients who have a large tumour cell burden that is also extremely sensitive to chemotherapeutic agents, for example, B cell (Burkitt's) lymphoma, T cell leukaemias/lymphomas and children presenting with a high white cell count at diagnosis. It may also occur in children presenting with evidence of renal infiltration at diagnosis. Although rare this complication has been reported with other solid tumours.

Prevention of these problems is the main aim; adequate prehydration and regular metabolic evaluation being two of the most important features. Before commencing chemotherapy the child's renal function will be established and a baseline blood pressure recorded. The child's weight is recorded and an electrocardiogram (ECG) performed. Vigorous hyperhydration is essential and this needs to commence at least 12–24 hours prior to chemotherapy. Administration of allopurinol also commences at this time to promote the breakdown of uric acid and thus reduce urate precipitation in the renal tubules. A renal ultrasound may be performed to assess whether there are any infiltrates or problems (such as renal enlargement) that may compromise renal function once treatment has commenced.

Nursing note:

It is important to be aware that cell lysis can occur with hydration before chemotherapy commences. It may also occur with induction using a general anaesthetic for a bone marrow/lumbar puncture as the resulting hypotension leads to a general 'sluggish system' compromising the brain.

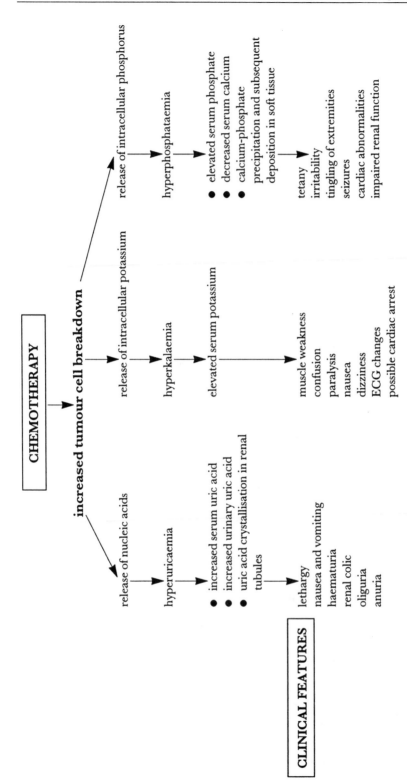

Figure 3.8: Sequence of events in acute tumour lysis syndrome (ATLS)

Liaison with other medical teams that may be involved in the child's care is important, especially the renal service who may not only provide advice regarding management but also haemodialysis; prior knowledge of the child could save time at a later stage. If the child has an extremely high white cell count leukopheresis may be considered to attempt to lower the white cell count before chemotherapy treatment commences. Although this appears to be a rare occurrence it has been shown to prevent severe ATLS in some patients (Maurer et al., 1988), but others have found that in some patients the white cell count only alters by about 30% (Cuttner et al., 1983). Leukopheresis, therefore, could benefit some patients and should be considered as a method to reduce the white cell count if the facility is available. Any child that has the potential to develop ATLS should commence treatment when adequate medical cover is available; commencing chemotherapy in the early hours of the morning ensures that any major problems expected would then occur in the afternoon.

Once treatment has started it is vital to maintain an accurate fluid balance, record weight and blood pressure frequently, undertake frequent monitoring of urea, electrolytes (in particular, potassium, magnesium and urate), calcium and phosphate, and take action upon any abnormalities (Lawrence, 1994). The frequency of monitoring the urea and electrolytes will depend on the previous results, but may be undertaken every 4–6 hours (this may vary within different units). Good urine output (*greater* than 3 ml/kg/hr) is essential, with frusemide being used to achieve this if oral intake is poor. Cardiac monitoring may be introduced to observe for peaked T waves and dysrhythmias associated with hyperkalaemia.

In relation to the overall management it may take time to organise the insertion of a central venous access device, as well as organise haemodialysis. It is for this reason that some units have introduced indicators, such as;

- Absolute indications for haemodialysis: potassium *greater* than 5 mmol/l; and/or phosphate *greater* than 2.5 mmol/l; pulmonary oedema; and anuria (ensuring that the bladder is empty, catheterising if there is a technical problem).
- Relative indications for haemodialysis: rapid rise in potassium, phosphate or urate; oliguria unresponsive to frusemide; urea *greater* than 15 mmol/l or creatinine *greater* than 150 mmol/l.

Medical management requires consideration and correction of each chemical imbalance, thus each metabolic abnormality will be addressed individually.

Hyperuricaemia

Uric acid is the end-product of the metabolism of purines, which are the building blocks of DNA and RNA; the purine bases, xanthine and hypoxanthine, are converted to uric acid by the enzyme, xanthine oxidase. The kidneys eliminate the greatest percentage of uric acid from the body with a small amount being eliminated within the faeces. The normal blood value is 0.1–0.45 mmol/l.

Urinary pH and urinary uric acid concentration are the main factors affecting uric acid solubility in the renal tubules; prolonged dehydration may be an exacerbating factor (Stucky, 1993). Uric acid is insoluble in body fluids and therefore small increases above normal blood value may result in uric acid precipitation. The child's urine needs to be alkaline to aid solubility and excretion. If the urine is acidic and there is excessive uric acid circulating due to the breakdown of tumour cells, deposits of uric acid crystals can occur in the kidneys, ureters and bladder leading to renal failure (Patterson & Klopovich, 1987). The resulting oliguric renal failure is known as uric acid nephropathy and is potentially life-threatening (Patterson & Klopovich, 1987).

Clinical features — lethargy, nausea and vomiting, haematuria, renal colic, oliguria, anuria (Allegretta et al., 1985; Patterson & Klopovich, 1987).
Management — aims to decrease uric acid production and increase the solubility of uric acid in the urine. Intravenous hydration commenced prior to chemotherapy is usually calculated at three times maintenance hydration. This will aid the kidneys to excrete the uric acid. Concurrent administration of the drug allopurinol will help decrease uric acid levels as allopurinol inhibits the enzyme xanthine oxidase which is necessary for the production of uric acid. Maintaining an alkaline urine may also help excrete the uric acid, however, there is some debate as to whether sodium bicarbonate should be included in the hydration fluid as it may enhance the deposition of calcium phosphate or xanthine precipitation in the renal tubules (Nace & Nace, 1993). Lange et al. (1993) suggest discontinuing sodium bicarbonate hydration once chemotherapy commences. Overall, alkalisation of urine is probably unnecessary if the fluid input is adequate (Pinkerton et al., 1994).

If the child develops renal failure, dialysis will be necessary, preferably haemodialysis as this achieves a more rapid reduction of plasma uric acid and prompt correction of any other electrolyte abnormalities (Nace & Nace, 1993). Within some units the insertion of a rigid dialysis catheter is selected as a precaution at the start of prehydration. These lines are more rigid and have a wider bore; thus are more suitable for haemodialysis than other types of central venous access devices.

Hyperkalaemia

Normally 98% of the body's potassium is intracellular. However, with ATLS intracellular potassium is released as the tumour cells are destroyed causing an elevation in serum potassium (Nace & Nace, 1993). Dehydration and acidosis may accentuate the problem as both result in extracellular shifts of potassium. In addition, as the kidneys play an important role in maintaining potassium balance, uric acid nephropathy or calcium deposits will affect the excretion of potassium and therefore exacerbate hyperkalaemia. Normal blood value for potassium is 3.5–5.0 mmol/l.

Clinical features — muscle weakness, confusion, paralysis, nausea, dizziness, ECG abnormalities (elevated T waves, prolonged PR, QRS and ST segments and arrhythmias) and possible cardiac arrest (Nace & Nace, 1993; Lawrence, 1994).
Management — includes decreasing potassium intake, facilitating the shift of extracellular potassium and aiding excretion. In the presence of hyperkalaemia intravenous hydration fluids, containing no added potassium, will need to be increased. Urine output may need to be maintained by use of frusemide. In theory, the child should not be given any foods containing potassium (such as bananas, fruit juices, malted drinks, Marmite, potato crisps, chocolate and milk). In practice, however, this is rarely an issue due to a general poor oral intake.

Close monitoring of electrolyte levels during induction is essential. If the level is increasing then the administration of a potassium binding resin, such as 'Kayexalate' (sodium polystyrene sulfonate) may be indicated (Patterson & Klopovich, 1987; Lange et al., 1993). This can be given orally or rectally. However, as it is unpalatable to swallow, either a nasogastric tube may need to be passed or the rectal route selected. Once it is mixed it becomes quite thick and may need further dilution to administer via the nasogastric tube or to be given *per rectum*.

Occasionally calcium gluconate or glucose and insulin may also be given intravenously to help shift the extracellular potassium back into the cells, consequently reducing serum levels, improving myocardial function and restoring a normal ECG (Lange et al., 1993). Patterson and Klopovich (1987) suggest that the child has a cardiac monitor if there are significant ECG changes, however, nursing staff need to be able to recognise abnormalities promptly for this to be of benefit. Salbutamol (either intravenously or nebulised) has also been used to lower potassium by shifting the extracellular potassium back into the cells (McClure et al, 1994). If the serum potassium continues to rise then haemodialysis would be indicated. In some units haemodialysis is introduced as a first-line measure.

Hyperphosphataemia and hypocalcaemia

Hyperphosphataemia results from the release of intracellular phosphate into the blood during ATLS. This then interacts with the extracellular calcium causing a precipitation of calcium salts and subsequent hypocalcaemia (Patterson & Klopovich, 1987). Calcium phosphate crystals precipitate in the microvascular and renal tubules which can lead to tissue damage and hypocalcaemia. Hypocalcaemia results from hyperphosphataemia and the inverse relationship between calcium and phosphate (Stucky, 1993).

Normal blood values are: *calcium* — infant 1.75–3 mmol/l, child 2–2.6 mmol/l; *phosphate* — at 1 year 1.23–2.1 mmol/l, at 2–5 years 1.13–2.20 mmol/l, above 5 years 0.97–1.45 mmol/l.

Clinical features

Usually asymptomatic from hyperphosphataemia, symptoms are related to the resulting hypocalcaemia; numbness, tingling of extremities, irritability, muscle cramping and seizures, cardiac abnormalities (prolonged QT interval) and impaired renal function (Allegretta et al., 1985; Patterson & Klopovich, 1993). On physical examination carpopedal spasm and a positive Chvostek or Trousseau's sign may be evident (Stucky, 1993).

Management — in theory, an increase in phosphate intake needs to be avoided by excluding food items such as bran, hard cheeses, nuts, dried fruit and vegetables. In practice (due to general poor oral intake) this is rarely followed. Administration of aluminium hydroxide orally will enhance excretion of phosphate in the stool but it can also precipitate constipation, and this should be avoided. Hypocalcaemia can be corrected by intravenous calcium gluconate.

Nursing implications of ATLS

Nursing staff need to be aware of the children who may develop ATLS. Preventative measures can be taken as recommended, with the child observed closely. Any abnormalities that do occur need to be reported promptly and action should be taken to prevent further complications. During this time the family is going to be under considerable stress, initially from the diagnosis and treatment and then from the possible complications. Frequent explanations should be provided on what is happening, how it is being managed and the expected outcome. Preparation should incorporate the possibility of the child being transferred to another unit, such as a renal or intensive care unit. Although such a transfer is usually temporary, none the less, it will increase the overall anxiety of the family. They will need support from all members of the multidisciplinary team to help them through this difficult period. The child will also be anxious and frightened and will need support and reassurance. During this time the child will need close observation, numerous blood tests and some unpleasant procedures. Full explanations of all of this will help the child and the family to deal with this situation.

Potential Toxicities Related to Specific Chemotherapeutic Agents

An awareness of the potential toxicities associated with chemotherapy is essential, so that children will receive treatment safely, with a minimum of problems. The child and the family will need frequent and clear explanations about why investigations are necessary.

Nephrotoxicity

Cisplatinum and methotrexate cause direct damage to the renal cells and the toxic levels of these drugs must be monitored carefully by regular baseline checks so that prompt adjustment can be made where necessary (Table 3.9).

Haemorrhagic cystitis

This occurs in 5–10% of patients receiving cyclophosphamide and in 20–40% of patients receiving ifosfamide (Balis et al., 1993). It can occur immediately, during or after administration, but can also occur months, possibly years later. The toxicity appears to be dose-related and happens when toxic metabolites, in particular acrolein, come into contact with the bladder wall (Table 3.10). Adequate pre- and post-dose hydration is essential to prevent haemorrhagic cystitis, with concurrent mesna in susceptible patients or those receiving high doses. Mesna prevents urothelial toxicity by reacting with the metabolic acrolein.

Table 3.9: Nephrotoxicity

Problem	Drug	Baseline tests	Management
Nephrotoxicity	• cisplatinum	renal function, urea and creatinine clearance, GFR	If GFR decreased, doses recalculated and reduced; change cisplatinum to carboplatinum; ensure hydration adequate, urine output adequate in relation to amount of fluid given; watch for renal failure
	• methotrexate	regular checking of blood levels and renal function	Vigorous hydration for MTX and urine kept alkaline; check MTX levels; urine pH testing for alkalinity

GFR = glomerular filtration rate; MTX = methotrexate

Table 3.10: Haemorrhagic cystitis

Problem	Drug	Symptoms	Management
Haemorrhagic cystitis	cyclophosphamide, ifosfamide	mucosal erythema, inflammation, ulceration, necrosis, diffuse small-vessel haemorrhages, reduced bladder capacity, dysuria, microscopic and macroscopic haematuria, pain	Prevention: aggressive hydration, administration of mesna, maintenance of good urine output, frequent voiding, urine tested for blood Treatment: chemotherapy stopped, mesna increased, hydration rate increased, pain relief, large gauge catheter to help pass clots if needed, bladder irrigation if needed, if no relief — endoscopy and bleeding points cauterised

Nursing note:

If there are problems with the GFR there can be a delay in clearance of the drug from the kidneys and enhancement of other toxic effects (Balis et al., 1993). Methotrexate levels must be taken frequently to ensure it is being excreted as required (Balis et al., 1993). Administration of nephrotoxic agents, such as the aminoglycoside antibiotics (e.g. gentamycin) or amphotericin B must be monitored carefully if they are given at the same time as methotrexate or cisplatin. If GFR is decreased the aminoglycosides will not be excreted effectively, leading to increased levels and possible ototoxicity (Walker, 1993). It may be advocated that gentamicin is not used at all when children are receiving cisplatin.

Nursing note:

Occasionally, the bladder goes into spasm and medication may be required to relieve it.

Mesna is oxidised in the plasma to a stable form then excreted by the kidneys where it is re-activated in the kidney tubules as needed. This then reacts with the metabolites in the urine to reduce or eliminate the toxic effects of these drugs in the bladder without interfering with the antitumour effect of the drugs (Fischer et al., 1993; Balis et al., 1993). A false positive urine test to ketones is seen when mesna is given. Mesna is stable for 24 hours. Haemorrhagic cystitis may be associated with a low platelet count and this should be checked. This can be a traumatic event and the family will need much support.

Cardiac problems

These problems are associated with the anthracyclines. Within 24 hours of administration the child can develop acute arrhythmias, conduction abnormalities and decreased left ventricular function, but these are usually transient problems (Balis et al., 1993). Some children, however, will develop problems with the minimal amount of treatment. Most cardiac problems seem to be long term and are seen after treatment has ceased. However, the anthracyclines appear to be less cardiotoxic when given as an infusion rather than a bolus (Table 3.11).

Lung problems

These are related to carmustine (BCNU) and lomustine (CCNU) or bleomycin. Initially, there is a decrease in type I pneumocytes

Table 3.11: Cardiotoxicity			
Problem	Drug	Baseline tests	Management
Cardiotoxicity	doxorubicin, daunorubicin	echocardiogram before treatment	Regular cardiac echo — if abnormality, dose altered or omitted; record of cumulative doses of drug — no more than 550 mg/m²; NEVER give as a bolus; advise re activity if problem found; all children followed up carefully

Nursing note:

The echocardiogram can also give an indication of how the cardiac function is changing over time.

The development of chelating agents (ICRF-187) which may block the cardiotoxic effects of the anthracyclines but do not alter the anti-tumour activity, may be useful in the future, especially for patients that have relapsed and ideally need more anthracycline treatment (Speyer et al., 1988; Wexler et al., 1996).

and an increase and redistribution of type II pneumocytes into the alveolar spaces, leading to pneumonitis. The alveolar septas become thickened and decreased in number, with an increase in the amount of collagen secreted by the interstitial fibroblasts (Table 3.12)

Table 3.12: Lung fibrosis			
Problem	Drugs	Baseline tests	Management
Lung fibrosis	carmustine (BCNU), lomustine (CCNU), bleomycin, busulphan	lung function test	Regular checks on lung function; watch giving radiotherapy and oxygen together, as this can exacerbate problem; inform anaesthetist so oxygen can be controlled; watch for dry hacking cough and dyspnoea

> **Nursing note:**
>
> **If pulmonary fibrosis develops the child will develop a dry, hacking cough and dyspnoea, this can lead to eventual death (Balis et al., 1993).**

Neurological problems

These are commonly seen with the vinca alkaloid drugs which have the potential to bind to microtubules. These provide a conduit for neurotransmission along the nerve axons and thus there is the potential for problems along these axons (Table 3.13).

Table 3.13: Neurological problems			
Problem	Drug	Baseline tests	Management
Peripheral neuropathy with loss of deep tendon reflexes, drop foot, motor weakness, numbness, tingling fingers, jaw pain and constipation	vincristine, vinblastine	–	Vigilance with regard to potential problems; physiotherapy; analgesia for jaw pain; advice about constipation to pre-empt problems; dose may need to be reduced.

> **Nursing note:**
>
> **In vinca alkaloid associated therapy, children present with pain in the legs and may be unable to put their foot on the ground. They may have a limp and walk on their toes; they may also have weak ankles. The child and the family should be reassured that the symptoms usually disappear when the drug is stopped. The physiotherapist should be brought in at the earliest opportunity to help with the drop foot. The child may have to wear splints at night.**

Conclusion

The care of the child undergoing chemotherapy is both challenging and rewarding for the paediatric oncology nurse. Knowledge of the actual and the potential side effects of treatment ensures that the nurse is able to assess, manage and evaluate care. The oncology nurse also needs to develop a mature and professional approach to care, in order to be able to offer appropriate advice and support to families.

Chapter 4
Altered body image

Sarah Palmer and Margaret Evans

Introduction

Altered body image is a subject which has recieved much more attention in the adult literature than it has in the paediatric literature, notably through the work of Price (1990) and Salter (1988).

The reason for this is probably due to the fact that paediatric oncology is a relatively 'young' specialism. It has been the recent emphasis on the effect of intensive treatment regimes which has brought this problem into focus.

Altered body image is associated with a feeling of loss in adults and this, in turn, affects the individual's self-concept (Lendrum & Syme, 1992). The same is true for children, but it is complicated by the fact that a positive body image is a learned concept which develops with maturity and influences the development of a positive self-concept. Thus, as Price (1993) commented, physical and psychological care are often difficult to separate (Table 4.1).

Nurses therefore need to have a knowledge of childhood development in order to understand the effect of altered body image on the individual (Table 4.2). In addition, Glen (1988) has identified several key components which influence body image in children:

- Aspects of classical and operant conditioning within the framework of cognitive development
- The child's environment
- Significant others in that environment
- Maturation of the central nervous system.

Table 4.1: Variables in the maintenance of normal body image

Body reality
   ageing (including growth spurts)
   level of fitness
   physical function/dexterity/coordination
   control of body functions (e.g. continence)
   sight/touch/hearing (the means by which we maintain a sense of body
   boundaries and contours)

Body ideal
   norms of body boundary (personal space)
   norms of body control (e.g. grace, coordination)
   fashion/advertising/social mores (e.g. weight)
   culture (different cultures value different aspects of body and appearance)
   socialisation and peer pressure (body as a symbol of social membership)

Body presentation
   wealth (capacity to adjust body through fashion, surgery, grooming,
   manicure, etc.)
   aesthetics (e.g. sense of colour coordination)
   necessary appendages (e.g. hearing aid, walking frame)
   environment (e.g. temperature extremes)

Coping strategies
   direct, possibly prevaricating
   subconscious (including grief reactions)
   approaches such as rationalisation or displacement of fears and feelings
   social skills and acceptability (the 'good patient' syndrome)

Social support network
   extensive or limited
   responsive or unresponsive
   clear or confused roles and communication
   geographically central or dispersed
   insight into body image concerns or ignorant and fearful

Adapted from Price (1993) (with permission)

Table 4.2: Eight stages of development

Ego qualities to be developed	Approximate age (years)
basic trust versus basic mistrust	0–1
autonomy versus shame, doubt	2–3
initiative versus guilt	4–5
industry versus inferiority	6–12
identity versus role confusion	13–18
intimacy versus isolation	19–25
generativity versus stagnation	26–40
ego integrity versus despair	41+

From Erikson (1965)

It is helpful if these factors are taken into consideration when assessing each child's level of understanding of their unique body image. It has also been suggested by McEwing (1996) that a knowledge of their own body and its internal parts is necessary, as well as identifying words or language used to describe the body. Children of different ages or levels of understanding may use different words to describe the same area, for example, 'tummy', 'belly', 'stomach', 'gut', 'abdomen'. Neff (1990) stated that the age of the child, as well as experience of living with a chronic illness, seems to have an important influence on the way the child feels about their body. It was found that children with cancer had more concerns about body parts as indicated in their drawings and had a greater knowledge about the functioning of their body organs than other children. Side effects of chemotherapy may be difficult to explain to a young child, as understanding may be limited to how the body works and to the effects of the drugs. For example, a child being treated for a bone tumour in the leg may be confused about the fact that they experience nausea, vomiting, develop mouth ulcers and have to have regular blood tests, in an attempt to 'get rid of the lump in your leg' (Table 4.2).

Athough changes in body image caused by cancer and its treatment are often thought of as a threat, if parents are positive about the changes this may help the child to adapt positively as well.

For all age-groups, there may be difficulties associated with returning to school and with dealing with the reactions of other people. Children can be cruel and make fun of anyone who looks odd or does not conform to the image of a group. On the other hand, it does not help the child to be singled out and treated as special. Parents and siblings may find it difficult as they very naturally want to defend the child, but they do need to build up their own confidence. Many children going through the experience of cancer confirm that it is best to return to school as soon as possible.

Teenagers and Altered Body Image

Teenagers are a particularly vulnerable group when considering altered body image in cancer care; because a positive body image is such a significant part of their identity they may require help to develop coping mechanisms (Evans, 1996).

Nurses need to have an appreciation of what coping is and how it can be facilitated (McHaffie, 1992). They may then be able to recognise if a particular teenager has found coping mechanisms which are appropriate for them as an individual, so that they can help to develop these mechanisms in a constructive way. Price (1992) has identified variables in the maintenance of normal body image showing how an appreciation of individual coping strategies as well as social support networks, help to form a background as to a person's 'stable state' before they developed cancer (Table 4.3). In the case of teenagers that stable state may be compromised because not only do they have to cope with a threat to body image imposed by adolescence but also with the threat imposed by cancer and its treatment (Evans, 1996). Gross (1991) recognised that teenagers have two main body images: their own body image in the way they think they look, and their ideal body image in the way they would like to look. Their level of self-esteem will relate to the distance between the two and cancer treatment threatens to change their body image and widen that distance.

In recent years many people have written about the concept of empowerment so that the client feels more in control of his health care (Gibson, 1991; O'Berle & Davies, 1992). This is particularly relevant for teenagers who are facing limitations and adaptations to their lifestyle and need to find a way of regaining lost control so that their self-concept is kept as intact as possible and they are then better able to deal with threats to their body image. At the same time, the young person may feel 'divided' between turning to parental comfort and nurturing and being independent.

All members of the multidisciplinary team should be aware of the needs of this particular age-group and be able to give teenagers time to express fears and emotions. They should be able to help the young people to cope with their bruised self-esteem by encouraging them to set realistic goals for themselves. Focusing on positive goals and 'getting on with life' is important, because issues such as social life, peer groups, education and privacy are all disrupted by an alteration in body image. The provision of accurate information is also important and MacGinley (1993) suggests that trust, empathy and touch should be incorporated into interpersonal skills. It is certainly true that trust leads to cooperation, especially with teenagers.

Effects of Chemotherapy Resulting in Altered Body Image

The effects of altered body image can be seen as direct and indirect. They have the potential to affect long term survival, both physically and psychologically.

Table 4.3: Psychodynamics of body image development
Pre-school years Child mapping and exploring (body reality), forming a clear picture of dimensions, size and relationship of body parts; variable progress towards a sophisticated, total body image, but moving space with a sense of body boundaries *School years* Increasing reference to peers as social mirror, with regard to the acceptability of body presentation — a period of body ideal formation against the norms of other children *Adolescence* Explorations, advanced much further into the realms of a manipulated body presentation; this is compelled by the changes of puberty, the opportunities of youth and the drive of adolescent culture and fashion
Adapted from Price (1993) (with permission)

Direct effects

Alopecia

One of the most distressing and noticeable effects of chemotherapy is the loss of hair. Preparing children for hair loss is extremely important and it is quite unfair to assume that it is a temporary price to pay when being treated for a life-threatening condition. Most children find the thought of losing their hair terrifying and so explaining fully what to expect may help to alleviate fears. Hair loss will be gradual, as the hair starts to thin first and (depending on the type of drugs received) there will be partial or total alopecia. If the hair loss is incomplete the remaining hair will be brittle and fine. It must also be explained that eyebrows, eyelashes and pubic hair may be lost, something which is particularly difficult for teenagers for whom this is an obvious sign of sexuality.

There are several measures that can be taken to reduce the effects of chemotherapy on the hair, in an effort to reduce the degree of anxiety and distress caused by this alteration to body image. Radical measures that can be used, such as scalp cooling and scalp tourniquets, are rarely offered to children. To reduce the stark visual alteration to body image more conservative methods are usually advised, for example, a haircut before total hair loss occurs. This allows children to gradually see themselves with a different and shorter hairstyle and it causes less distress when shorter hair strands fall out. Loose hair causes irritation when it gets into the mouth, eyes and on the clothes and acts as a constant reminder of the disease and altered body image.

Nursing note:

Although it may not look elegant, wearing a hairnet at night helps to reduce the irritation of hair on the pillow. Another remedy is to brush the hair well before bedtime to get rid of loose hairs.
Remember to tell young children that hair loss will be painless.

To delay hair loss, infrequent hair washing with a gentle shampoo and minimal brushing with a soft brush should be advocated. Teenagers should be made aware that hairdryers, heated brushes or strong chemical treatments, such as highlights or perms, are not advised. Very short hair or a shaved head may be accepted as fashionable especially to teenagers, but it may still not be their choice and choice has an important bearing on a person's self-esteem.

A wig may be offered as an option to the child, in an effort to maintain some normality to their appearance. Allowing the child this option helps to reduce the negative effect of the threat of hair loss, and the skills of a wig-fitter are of great importance if it is to be successful. Matching eyebrow colour, previous hair colour and style, and teaching the child how to manage the wig are extremely important. It is therefore preferable that children are seen early in their treatment whilst they still have their own hair. Teenage girls tend to take up this option, although once fitted, few wear their wig all the time. It appears that in hospital where the environment is safe and their condition is understood they do not feel the need to wear the wig, but outside it becomes their only means of controlling a normal outward appearance. Children who are normally very active and keen on sport may find wearing a wig problematic, posing a confusing threat to body image especially when such activities are important to them.

Hats, scarves and caps are often worn and can be seen as a fashionable clothes accessory. Care must be taken during hot weather to protect the head and a sun block cream or sun hat should be worn. During winter hats should be encouraged as a third of body heat can be lost though the top of the head. If the scalp becomes itchy or flaking skin develops then a simple mineral oil can be gently rubbed in. There may be some cultural or religious differences that may have to be considered with some families, as hair loss may be a very sensitive issue, possibly more so to the parents of young children than to the children themselves.

Nursing note:

Encouraging a positive appearance is extremely important, especially for teenagers, and suggestions such as wearing their own jewellery, make up and other accessories may improve their self-image. Encouraging the use of a beautician or hairdresser for teenage girls can help them to create a positive self-image. They may need help with managing wigs or tying scarves. Some teenagers are able to turn the experience into a positive one by experimenting with their appearance.

Haematological problems

These include thrombocytopenia (bruising, bleeding), anaemia (being pale, tired, listless), and leucopenia/neutropenia (infections, wounds, poor wound healing).

These haematological disorders are all well-recognised side effects of chemotherapy as a result of bone marrow suppression. Although they are temporary they still cause fluctuating influences on a person's body image because altered self-image or self-concept does not have to be a physical alteration to the body. Being aware that changes are occurring inside the body, such as a disruption to the normal number and function of blood cells, can be as emotionally upsetting to self-image and feelings towards the individual's own body as an outward physical change.

Young children usually have more bruises and falls than adults due to their more active and boisterous lifestyle or learning to walk or coordinate their actions, whereas for teenagers bruising may be a threat to their body image. Anaemia may have the same effect as it can create a visible change in appearance for all age-groups.

Gastrointestinal disturbances

These may lead to anorexia, nausea, vomiting, diarrhoea, weight loss, constipation or stomatitis leading to dysphagia.

Chemotherapy is commonly known for its unpleasant side effect of nausea and vomiting. Irritation of the bowel mucosa can cause diarrhoea, and certain cytotoxic agents can cause constipation. The effect of chemotherapy on the rapidly dividing cells of the mucous membranes may cause stomatitis which may lead to dysphagia, halitosis and infections such as candidiasis.

Any of these side effects may lead to anorexia and weight loss. Weight loss can sometimes be quite dramatic and particularly distressing for teenagers, as it may affect their normal activities due to loss of muscle bulk and body shape. This, in turn, may affect their ability or desire to participate in sports or their other activities and has a profound effect on body image. Relationships with their peers may be compromised affecting an already 'shaky' self-esteem, and may lead to a downward spiral when they begin to stop seeing their friends and stop taking part in activities.

All of these changes provoke an alteration to a person's normal bodily function and result in a feeling of loss of control over bodily activities (Blackmore, 1988). This loss of control affects the child's sense of normality because the concept of body image is based on the attitudes, values and feelings that the individual holds about their own body. Measures can be taken to reduce the side effects of chemotherapeutic agents, such as use of antiemetics and increased oral hygiene, and involving teenagers in their own care will help to increase their sense of control.

Nursing note:

Wearing a tracksuit helps to hide unwanted changes in appearance. Baggy clothes like big jumpers have the same effect and will hopefully remain trendy!

Impaired fertility / sexuality

Chambas (1991) found that teenagers with cancer had numerous sexually related concerns not identified by healthy teenagers, highlighting the importance of discussing these issues. Many chemotherapeutic drugs have an effect on fertility, although this is not always the case. The child's age and understanding of fertility and sometimes the parent's wishes will dictate whether this subject is discussed. In some cases it is necessary to suppress menstrual periods with norethisterone; in addition, some drugs may cause amenorrhoea. This is usually temporary, but the reasons for this should be explained to teenagers and their parents as this is a sensitive subject and teenagers are often embarrassed to talk about it themselves. This is a very critical developmental stage, when young people are discovering their personal feelings and their sexuality, and can be a very damaging time emotionally if normal developmental processes are disrupted. Not only has their external bodily appearance changed due to their cancer treatment, making them different from their peers and feeling less attractive, but their normal internal sexual development has also been affected.

> **Nursing note:**
>
> **It is important to make it clear to teenagers that they cannot assume that they are unable to conceive. Advice about contraception may therefore be required. In some instances religious and cultural issues may need to be borne in mind when discussing infertility.**

Practical issues, such as loss of pubic hair, can be very distressing for the sexually developing teenager as can stomatitis which may hinder kissing. Loss of muscle bulk and weight loss may alter the appearance, and fatigue may reduce the ability and desire for a physical relationship. Youngsters are often encouraged to have a central line inserted without recognition that this is likely to affect sexuality.

Teenagers who are sexually active may find this even more difficult to cope with than adults in a similar situation who may have more permanent and long-standing relationships. They may find that it is easier to talk to the nursing or medical staff than their parents about altered body image and sexuality and they should be given the opportunity to do so through open, leading questions. It is important to remember that teenagers should be given the opportunity to make their own decisions and choices as this affects their self-esteem and ultimately their body image. Burt (1995) identified that nurses are often reticent about approaching a young person to talk about sexuality as they are embarrassed themselves to approach the subject and this, too, may contribute to this age-group being ignored as potentially sexually active. It may be that the teenager identifies better with someone of their own age or a 'mother figure'. The support of family, peers and health care professionals are all needed to help teenagers to cope with so many difficult issues.

Skin changes

Skin discolouration, pigmentation, flushing, photosensitivity and dermatitis are all side effects of chemotherapy. The child should be made aware that these changes may occur, that they are a side effect of the treatment and that the changes are temporary and will return to normal over a period of time once the treatment has finished. These changes may be particularly distressing to teenagers and help should be offered to create a positive self-image.

Nursing note:

A creative outcome can be developed to make the changes a positive experience, such as the clever use of make up. It may also be possible to involve the skills of a beautician. Placing children's transfer tattoos over the discoloured skin is another idea.

Peripheral neuropathy

Certain chemotherapeutic agents cause temporary peripheral neuropathy with a reduced ability to control coordination, including clumsiness, reduced dexterity and drop foot. These side effects can cause embarrassment, frustration and avoidance of physical activity. Some children may find it difficult to write and this could cause all kinds of difficulties at school. When this side effect becomes so marked that it interferes with even simple daily activities a dose reduction or change to a different drug may be considered.

Other signs and symptoms, such as tingling in the fingers and toes, jaw ache and nerve pain, are a constant reminder of the disease and a loss of control over normal bodily functioning and thus a perceived alteration in body image.

Nail pigmentation and ridging

For the self-conscious teenager this is yet another insult to external body image. It should be emphasised that this condition is a temporary alteration which lasts only for the duration of chemotherapy treatment.

Nursing note:

This side effect can be turned into a positive and creative experience by the use of different coloured nail polish.

Stunting of growth

Chemotherapy has less of an effect than radiotherapy on normal growth and development but it has been found that growth does slow down whilst children are receiving it (Hawkins & Stevens, 1996). This is not a permanent side effect and children often have a growth spurt after completing treatment. It may become more of a problem in the teenager's eyes during puberty when growth spurts are more common and there develops a noticeable difference between the teenager who has had treatment for cancer and their peer group. Younger children may wonder about the disparity between themselves, their parents and their siblings if growth spurts are slowed down whilst receiving treatment.

Indirect effects

Reduced mobility

This leads to weight loss and loss of muscle bulk.

Fatigue, tiredness

Extreme tiredness is debilitating and the fact that the body is not functioning to full capacity has a negative effect on body image. During cancer treatment the body is coping with defence against infection, numerous drugs and the altered metabolism of tumour growth and it is not surprising that the child often feels exhausted. Anorexia and lack of sleep may add to the problem. As Price (1992) observed 'fatigue provides an all-encompassing filter through which we experience our body' (p. 644).

Pickard-Holley (1991), Nail and Winningham (1995) and Glaus et al. (1996) all found from studies that adult cancer patients did suffer from fatigue which involved decreased physical performance, extreme tiredness, weakness and an unusual need for rest, which is distinctly different to healthy people. There is no reason to believe that children do not suffer from similar symptoms but studies do need to be carried out to determine if this is the case. These are important and long-neglected symptoms and comparatively little effort has been invested in developing techniques to alleviate them. Anaemia also causes lethargy and fatigue and the child may feel that they cannot keep up with their peers. This affects the normal ability to participate, for example at school during lessons or in sports, which can easily lower self-esteem.

Liver dysfunction

Ascities, jaundice and oedema are all physically distressing symptoms which can cause noticeable changes to a child's appearance and have a strong effect on body image.

Weight gain, stretch marks

Caused by steroids; these can be noticeable and distressing side effects, especially to teenagers who may take great pride in their physical appearance. Darbyshire (1986) talked about the 'beautiful is good' phenomenon and this view certainly permeates our society, causing pressure on those who are unable to fulfil this expectation.

Interruption of skin integrity

Central venous access via long line or 'implantable port'

The safest, most direct and painless route for intravenous administration of cytotoxic drugs is through a central venous catheter or 'implantable port'. Daniels (1995) describes the placement of a central venous access device as a 'crisis experience' and outlines the psychosocial effect this has on body image. Its physical presence is a constant reminder of the diagnosis and the need for treatment. It causes an alteration to body appearance and is an invasion of a person's body integrity. The thought of a long term indwelling catheter emerging from the chest wall or metal port reservoir under the skin could be quite alarming. This information needs to be conveyed to the child in an age-appropriate and extremely sensitive manner.

The positioning of the central venous access device is particularly important for teenagers with respect to clothes, sports and girls who wear bras.

Implantable ports can be less unsightly than central lines and an advantage is that they are more acceptable in terms of body image and, in particular, sexuality. The port reservoir can protrude from under the skin, if the person is very thin, however, and still requires needle access.

To reduce some of the fears and anxieties and to assist with co-operation during this invasive procedure it must be explained to the child why it is necessary to have a central venous access device and the benefits it will offer by preventing peripheral cannulation and venepunctures for routine blood tests. The fact that it will remain in place for a period of time, including being at home, going to school, even going swimming, must be emphasised so that the child can see that a degree of normal life can be maintained.

Younger children often accept this procedure when it has to be undertaken. They understand that some of their 'medicines' can be given into the central line or port, and that it is an alternative to having painful peripheral venepunctures. Teenagers, however, may find it much more difficult to come to terms with having a central venous access device. Some feel so strongly about this issue that they choose not to have one, often against advice from professionals who think that they know better! In a study about teenagers with cancer 'getting on with life', subjects made the point that the way others responded to them influenced how they managed their illness. It was important for them to emphasise that they were exactly the same person and that if anything had changed, it was the attitude of others, which could be unhelpful (Rechner, 1990).

Nursing note:

Breast development may need to be considered when a port is an option. It may be helpful to put children in touch with others who have found a central line or port helpful. A point of debate — it is worth considering for whose convenience a line is inserted and whether the protocol dictates it in terms of intensity of treatment. The choice rests with the child and this is usually appropriate. In addition the child may want to change their mind as to whether to have it taken out or put in.

Peripheral cannulation

This can potentially lead to extravasation with some cytotoxic agents causing phlebitis, severe ulceration, necrosis, scarring.

Long Term Effects

Survivorship is an issue which has received attention in the literature over recent years (Norman & Brandeis, 1992; Bushkin, 1993) and is particularly relevant in childhood cancer where survival rates are increasing at a steady rate. Impaired body image has implications for survivors in the long term, because it can affect psychological well-being (Muzzin et al., 1994). Not only do survivors need to cope with physical disabilities but they may also have to face social stigma and difficulties with forming long term relationships. They may be unable to pursue the career they had dreamed about and planned for. Sadly, the attitude of society towards people with cancer is not always helpful and the media do little to help. Price (1996) discussed the implications of 'the chronic illness experience' and highlighted the fact that in the long term there may be disappointment about body function to deal with and worries about how to manage the body, as well as concern about presenting a plausible social image.

Conclusion

The issue of altered body image is one which nurses must consider during all stages of the child's illness and beyond, as it has implications long after treatment is complete. It also affects the whole family as the effects can be far-reaching. It is only through an understanding of the theoretical concepts underpinning this important area that nurses will be able to consider their practice and take appropriate steps to help children and young people to come to terms with such a complex problem.

Close collaboration with the multidisciplinary team, both in the hospital and in the community setting, must be established so that care is matched to the needs of the individual whether at home or in hospital, or whether practical or psychological help is needed.

WHAT'S IT LIKE FOR A 14-YEAR-OLD GIRL TO HAVE ACUTE MYELOID LEUKAEMIA!!!

When I first went into hospital 6th January 1996. I thought I'd only be there for the weekend, a month later I came out. Home was so far away I thought I would never see it, but I did. I fought to see it and it's made me a much stronger person, but sometimes things get you down, I thought I'd never reach the end. Every time I got ill it got worse, but then it got better, but then it would get worse again and then it would get better and in the end you recover completely, but it only happens if you stay positive because if you don't, where's it going to leave you.

I have always loved my hair, trying out different styles and different hair dyes, when I knew my hair was going to fall out I wanted to make the most of it, so I had it cut different lengths and sprayed silver and pink. When it did all fall out I had a few wispy bits and thought it was fine. But then all the magazines started going on about how to style your hair and what products to use and that really got me down.

I've got a big collection of hats now, 14 odd, sometimes I just want to get rid of them all, but I know if I'm patient I will never have to wear them again. Now the weather's warming up I get really hot wearing them and when my mates come round showing off their fancy hair do it really depresses me.

I have got a big collection of clothes, I bought skirts, shirts, every outrageous piece of clothing going and that kept me amused for a while until I noticed I was putting on weight. I went from 8 stone to 10 stone and developed stretch marks on my inner leg, outer leg, under my arms and around my chest and bottom. So I've spent most of my time in track suit bottoms and baggy t-shirts. I haven't seen my jeans and shirts and little tight skirts in months, so I've moved on to shoes.

I bought red shoes and black shoes with really big heels on them and expensive outrageous ones but then I got fluid on my feet and all my shoes became too tight, so I moved on to make-up.

I bought every new product going on the market. I enjoyed playing around with that, but then my treatment started blowing me up and the make-up didn't look as good any more so I moved on to jewellery.

I've always liked jewellery so I had plenty of it, I had four holes up each ear and loved changing earrings, but then I got infections, and the four holes were reduced to 2 holes in one ear and 3 in the other, and it looked really odd.

So now I have moved on to painting my nails, I would have blue one day and black the next day, then white the next, but then the chemotherapy started to make my nails chip, and the varnish didn't look so good so I didn't bother.

Now I've finished my treatment, I'm hoping to lose my weight, then my hair will start to grow back, then I will sort out my stretch marks. Everyone says they will fade, but I won't believe them, same about my weight too. I have lost 5 pounds in just over a week so it might come off pretty quickly. I'm going to try toning and trimming exercise videos and control my diet. My stretch marks I will try slapping lots of cream into them to build the moisture back up. I've also got to build the muscle back up that I've lost after lying in bed for so long. I walk up the stairs in the hospital instead of taking the lifts, also I'm going to do plenty of bike riding. I'm going off to America soon so I've got be to be in ship shape condition for that.

I'm looking forward to my wiggly coming out, then I will know I'm back to normal as I don't feel it at the moment. I don't feel as if I can do what I want to, next to my friends I feel like an Alien. I miss my social life and I miss me, but I will be back soon then there will be no stopping me!

Sometimes I cry over all these things like the hair, the hats, the clothes, the jewellery, the nails, but I know there's a light at the end of the tunnel, I might have to work hard to reach it, but I'm going to, because if you don't work hard you'll never get there. I've had my good days. I've had my bad and when I've been really ill and have stayed in bed and never thought I'd get out again, but I did, and it's such a relief to know I'm going to have a life again because now every day is so precious to me.

by Cathryn McGlone

Chapter 5
Late effects of chemotherapy

Philippa Chesterfield

Introduction

Due to improved multimodal treatment with chemotherapy, radiotherapy and surgery, 65% of children diagnosed with cancer will be long term survivors. This means that by the year 2000 one in 1000 adults will be survivors of childhood cancer (McCalla, 1985; DeLaat & Lampkin, 1992, Green & D'Angio, 1992; Hammond, 1992; Hobbie et al., 1993). Beyer (1990) calculated that by the year 2010 as many as one in 250 people may be survivors of childhood cancer. Improved long term survival has led to new challenges for health professionals in identifying, treating and reducing the long term implications of treatment for these survivors.

Interest in the long term effects of cancer treatment is evidenced by the volume of literature now available regarding the physical and psychosocial consequences of survival. The United Kingdom Children's Cancer Study Group (UKCCSG) has formed a specific working party to consider late effects of treatment. In 1995 they published guidelines for long term follow-up care. Long term follow-up clinics are now an established part of paediatric oncology practice. These clinics involve other specialists, including paediatric endocrinologists, cardiologists, respirologists and neurologists, in the follow-up of survivors. Nurses are now grasping the opportunity to take the lead in such clinics and are able to raise awareness about important psychosocial issues, such as the specific needs of teenagers or the optimum time to provide information about late effects to the child or young adult (Waterworth, 1992).

Knowledge gained from the long term follow-up of survivors informs current protocols, to decrease late effects for future generations (Pinkerton, 1992). In addition, there is continuing debate about the relative costs versus the benefits of treatment (Morris-Jones & Craft, 1990).

The effects of chemotherapy can be both short and long term. The long term effects will be related to the combination of drugs and the dose given. These effects can also be exacerbated by radiotherapy and surgery, such as the removal of lung metastases or radiotherapy following bleomycin.

Toxic Effects of Chemotherapy

Lungs

Pulmonary toxicity is a dose-limiting and potentially lethal toxicity of certain chemotherapeutic agents, generally manifested as pulmonary fibrosis (Barton Burke et al., 1991). Bleomycin is the most commonly known chemotherapeutic agent to cause lung toxicity. In children, significant pulmonary toxicity can be seen with as little as 60 mg/m^2 (DeLaat & Lampkin, 1992). Nitrosoureas (BCNU/CCNU), busulphan, cyclophosphamide and methotrexate can all cause pulmonary fibrosis and interstitial pneumonitis (DeLaat & Lampkin, 1992; Hammond, 1992; Hobbie et al., 1993; Galvin, 1994). These drugs used in combination with radiotherapy will cause pulmonary function abnormalities. Children receiving whole lung irradiation, such as in Hodgkin's disease, thoracic neuroblastoma and Wilms' tumour; or receiving a bone marrow transplant with total body irradiation and priming with busulphan, will all be at high risk of pulmonary toxicity. Lung function can be further compromised by thoracic surgery for the removal of lung metastases. Changes include abnormal lung function tests, breathlessness on exercise and cough. (NB High concentrations of oxygen (i.e. anaesthesia) may cause respiratory failure in patients previously treated with bleomycin.)

Nursing note:

Respiratory function should be assessed, including chest X-ray, lung function tests with carbon monoxide diffusion and oxygen saturation. Support and counselling should be provided related to career, exercise and the importance of not smoking. Any chest infections should be treated promptly. Awareness of the potential risks of anaesthesia and the need to inform health professionals of the risk, should be emphasised. In some circumstances, careful monitoring of fluid balance is needed to avoid pulmonary oedema, for example, after surgery where large volumes of i.v. fluids may be given.

Heart

Anthracyclines (doxorubicin and daunorubicin), high-dose cyclophosphamide and mitozantrone can all cause short and long term cardiac dysfunction (Kaszylk, 1986; DeLaat & Lampkin, 1992; Hobbie et al., 1993; Galvin, 1994). Total doses in children of >350 mg/m^2 can lead to cardiac abnormalities but damage has ocurred at much lower doses (Pinkerton, 1992). It is also suggested that the younger the age of the child when given anthracyclines, the greater the risk (Galvin, 1994). Anthracyclines affect cardiac myocytes, causing loss of muscle fibres and shifts in intracellular calcium leading to myocardial dysfunction (Hobbie et al., 1993). The risk of cardiac dysfunction is also linked to the dose and peak plasma levels of anthracyclines (Kaszylk, 1986). Research suggests that anthracyclines given as a bolus over 20 minutes are more toxic to the heart than if given over a longer period, or divided into smaller doses (Kaszylk, 1986). In many protocols now, anthracylines are given as infusions over 4–6 hours to reduce the risk of cardiac toxicity. Cardioprotective agents and analogues of anthracyclines, such as idarubicin and epirubicin, have been developed to reduce the risk of cardiomyopathy (Pinkerton, 1992). Cardiac myopathy may also be exacerbated if the chest has been irradiated, such as in Hodgkin's disease (DeLatt & Lampkin, 1992). Most patients may be symptomless and signs of cardiac failure only noticed at times of increased cardiovascular stress, such as exercise, pregnancy and anaesthesia (Hobbie et al., 1993). In severe cases of cardiomyopathy, congestive cardiac failure may necessitate drug treatment and a few survivors may require cardiac transplant (Adwani et al., 1995).

Nursing note:

Cardiac assessment should be carried out before each course of treatment that includes anthracyclines. Analogues such as epirubicin are sometimes used when a high cumulative dose of anthracyclines has been reached. Chest X-rays, echocardiogram, electrocardiogram, multiple gated acquisition (MUGA) scans, angiography and cardiac biopsy may all be required in the follow-up of these patients. All patients who have received anthracyclines require an echocardiogram 1–3 months after the final dose and five-yearly therafter (Kissen & Wallace, 1995).

The educative role of the nurse involves helping the patient to understand the implications of anthracycline therapy. Support and counselling may be required related to career, exercise and smoking.

Health care professionals need to be aware of the added strain anaesthesia or pregnancy may put on an already compromised cardiac function. Fluid overload may also compromise cardiac function causing cardiac failure; close monitoring of fluid balance will be required if large volumes of fluid are to be given, such as in operative procedures.

Renal system and urinary tract

Cisplatinum is known to cause acute renal toxicity in 50–75% of patients (Lydon, 1986; DeLaat & Lampkin, 1992; Hobbie et al., 1993; Galvin, 1994). Toxicity is related to dose and duration of treatment. However, doses of below $50/m^2$ per course are rarely noted to cause renal toxicity. Some reversibility has been noted over time but creatinine clearance may continue to be reduced as long as 2–4 years after treatment. High-dose methotrexate and other drugs, such as dactinomycin, anthracyclines and nitrosoureas, can all affect renal function (Lydon, 1986; DeLaat & Lampkin, 1992; Hobbie et al., 1993; Galvin, 1994). Renal function can be further compromised by the use of aminoglycosides, vancomycin, amphotericin and cyclosporin (DeLaat & Lampkin, 1992; Hobbie et al., 1993; Galvin, 1994).

Drugs such as cyclophosphamide and ifosfamide can cause haemorrhagic cystitis, atypical bladder epithelium and renal tubular necrosis (DeLaat & Lampkin, 1992; Hobbie et al., 1993; Skinner, 1993; Galvin 1994). Skinner et al. (1993) highlight the potential risk of rickets due to hypophosphataemia related to proximal tubular impairment caused by ifosfamide The risk of renal and bladder damage may also be exacerbated by abdominal radiation. Children with Wilms' tumour may receive dactinomycin and doxorubicin which are also radiosensitisors; this can add to the potential long term damage by exacerbating the effect of radiotherapy (DeLaat & Lampkin, 1992). In some severe cases of toxicity, dialysis or renal transplant may be required. Another cited potential complication of cyclophosphamide therapy is invasive carcinoma of the bladder (DeLaat & Lampkin, 1992).

Liver

The liver is an important site for the metabolism of chemotherapy agents; the slow growth of hepatocytes enables it to withstand significant damage from most of the drugs. Certain drugs, however, are hepatotoxic.

> **Nursing note:**
>
> Renal function should be assessed within 6 months of completing treatment. In most cases, if this is normal, no further action is needed (Kissen & Wallace, 1995). Assement may include creatinine clearance or glomerular filtration rate, urea and electrolyte analysis. Phosphate levels should also be checked in order to detect the potential risk of rickets and supplements given if required. Blood pressure should be checked routinely to detect signs of hypertension. Urinalysis for blood, protein and casts should be a routine test at follow-up of patients at risk of renal toxicity. Excretory urograms or voiding cystoscopy may also be required. Where the possibility of carcinoma of the bladder is considered, urine for cytology and cystoscopy should be carried out. The nurse should help to identify any problems, such as frequency of urination, painful urination and urinary tract infection, so that symptoms can be treated early.

Long term liver damage is most commonly associated with daily low-dose methotrexate and 6-mercaptopurine, such as in treatment for ALL, rather than high-dose intermittent treatment (DeLaat & Lampkin, 1992; Hobbie et al., 1993). Chronic liver damage is often insidious with patients being asymptomatic. Liver function tests and size of the liver can remain normal until liver fibrosis and cirrhosis develop.

> **Nursing note:**
>
> Liver function tests should be carried out at the end of treatment and further action taken if indicated (Kissen & Wallace, 1995). If necessary, imaging of the liver may be required. Alcohol and various drugs are known to be hepatotoxic, which may further compromise liver function. The nurse should give advice related to levels of alcohol consumption and avoidance of hepatotoxic drugs where posssible.

Gonads

It is widely documented that both radiotherapy and cytotoxic therapy can affect gonadal function (Clayton et al., 1988; Shalet, 1989; DeLaat & Lampkin, 1992; Pinkerton, 1992; Saunders, 1992; Shalet & Wallace, 1992; Hobbie et al., 1993; Galvin, 1994). This is related to the production of hormones and the viability of germ cells. Alkylating agents, such as cyclophosphamide and procarbazine, are the most likely to affect fertility. Factors such as age at diagnosis, nutritional status at time of treatment, and combination therapy affect the degree of dysfunction (Hobbie et al., 1993). It is difficult to assess gonadal dysfunction until puberty as abnormal gonadotrophin levels only become evident when puberty is reached (Shalet & Wallace, 1992).

Where appropriate, sperm saving for males before treatment should be considered. There have been recent advances in medical research into the possibility of growing human oocytes to maturity *in vitro* (Spears 1994), but as yet this is not common practice. Clearly there are many legal and ethical issues surrounding this subject and there exists a useful document related to the legal issues, published by the Human Fertilisation and Embryology Authority (HFEA). They have also identified guidelines for the storage of gametes and embryos for cancer patients within their code of practice (HFEA, 1995).

Males

The germinal epithelium in particular is the most vulnerable to cytotoxic agents causing azoospermia or oligospermia. Total doses of more than 11 g of cyclophosphamide can cause azoospermia. Combination chemotherapy that includes alkylating agents can cause permanent infertility, and the number of courses given will increase the risk of azoospermia (Hobbie et al., 1993). Males who have compromised germinal epithelium often have small testes.

Females

The ovary is relatively well protected from chemotherapy as oocytes are present from birth. However, a decreased number of ova are found after cancer treatment in prepubescent females (Hobbie et al., 1993). Doses of up to 20 g of cyclophosphamide do not appear to affect the onset of puberty in prepubescent females (Hobbie et al., 1993). These patients, however, may be at risk of an early onset of the menopause due to a reduction in the number of ova.

Growth

According to Hawkins and Stevens (1996) some studies have indicated that chemotherapy does not affect growth and yet clinical observations often demonstrate treatment-related growth impairment followed by 'catch-up' growth. They conclude that the intensity of chemotherapy may be what matters.

Nursing note:

Careful assessment of pubertal staging by use of the Tanner scale should be carried out at follow-up during puberty (Shalet, 1989; Shalet & Wallace, 1992). A history of a girl's menstrual cycle should be obtained, and for both males and females, baseline LH and FSH levels should be taken. More specifically, males will require testosterone levels to be taken, and females oestrogen levels, with referral to an endocrinologist if necessary. Advice about contraception is essential for this group of patients as not all patients will be infertile, even after bone marrow transplant (Senturia & Peckham, 1990; Nygaard et al., 1991; Murata et al., 1995). Females who wish to have children should be told about the possibility of early menopause. Referral to a fertility clinic for assessment and counselling should be made early rather than after the usual one-year wait. Many of the agents that are used to treat cancer interfere with DNA and cellular metabolism and also with cell division which may cause mutation and genetic disorders in humans. Although the data is limited Mulvihill and Byrne (1992), on reviewing the literature, did not find an excess of genetic defects except in the case of some hereditary cancers (Wilms' tumour, retinoblastoma). This is obviously of concern to cancer survivors wishing to have a family. Where appropriate, this should be addressed by the nurse, or referral made to a genetic counsellor.

Hearing

Auditory loss includes ototoxicity, the hearing loss induced by cisplatin as a single agent is high-frequency, bilaterally symmetrical and irreversible. The deficit is directly related to dose and inversely related to age (McHaney et al., 1992). This is of particular importance when treatment involves cranial radiotherapy X-ray, less is known of the synergistic effect with other chemotherapeutic agents. McHaney et al. (1992) found that cisplatin given before cranial radiotherapy was less ototoxic and this is of particular relevance to children treated for brain tumours. It was also suggested that ifosfamide given prior to cisplatin can potentiate the ototoxicity of cisplatin. Use of aminoglycosides may also exacerbate ototoxicity and where possible should be avoided when chemotherapy involves cisplatin. This has implications for future treatment regimes for children with brain tumours. Long term hearing loss may affect speech development and learning in these children.

> **Nursing note:**
>
> Poor hearing has an effect on both schooling and social interaction. Hearing assessment with audiograms for these children is essential, if necessary with a referral to the ear nose and throat department. Hearing aids should be fitted and help with speech development and education given if required.

Neuro/psychological

The effect of cranial radiation is well documented and discussed in the section on late effects of radiotherapy. Changes in white matter and calcification can be noted on computerised tomography (CT). Deficits in IQ, visual motor integration, memory, seizures and many others have all been noted after radiotherapy and intrathecal chemotherapy (Ochs et al., 1983; Mulhern et al., 1988; Chessells et al., 1990; Ochs & Mulhern, 1992; Hobbie et al., 1993; Stehbens et al., 1994).

Treatment for ALL has included cranial irradiation, intrathecal methotrexate, oral and intravenous methotrexate. It is therefore difficult to isolate the effect of methotrexate on neuro/psychological functioning because of the multimodal treatment to the central nervous system (CNS). Ochs and Mulhern (1992), however, found almost identical frequency of change in IQ and achievement scores when radiotherapy or both intrathecal and intravenous methotrexate were given as CNS prophylaxis. Balsom and colleagues (1991), using a small cohort of patients, in a retrospective study, found a protective effect with pre-irradiation intrathecal methotrexate. This has implications for treatment of ALL. The relative toxicities of cranial irradiaton, intrathecal and high-dose intravenous methotrexate continue to be investigated.

> **Nursing note:**
>
> Assessment of neuro/psychological functioning is essential so that any problems can be treated early. Referral to clinical psychologists for assessment and help with education may all be needed. The nurse has a role in asking about school and the child's ability to concentrate and memorise (Ferguson, 1981). Support and counselling can help these children and families understand, overcome and adapt to any disabilities due to treatment. Some children develop a phobia to school because of absenteeism or because they were made fun of. Paediatric oncology outreach nurse specialists and community children's nurses are often able to help by visiting the school and talking to teachers.

Second malignancy

The development of a second malignancy is probably the most feared consequence of therapy and is now becoming well documented in long term survivors (Hawkins et al., 1987; Frazier & Tucker, 1988; DeLaat & Lampkin, 1992; Hawkins et al., 1992; Hobbie et al., 1993; Robison & Mertens, 1993; Galvin, 1994). Robison and Mertens (1993), in their review of second malignancies, indicate that 68% of second malignancies are due to radiotherapy and are predominantly solid tumours. The issues of secondary malignancies related to radiotherapy is addressed in the radiotherapy section.

Alkylating agents (cyclophosphamide and busulphan) and epipodophyllotoxins are known potentially to cause non-lymphocytic leukaemia. This is well documented in patients who have Hodgkin's disease and have been treated with both alkylating agents and epipodophyllotoxins (Frazier & Tucker, 1988; Hawkins et al., 1992). These secondary leukaemias often develop between two and five years following treatment and have differing characteristics to spontaneous acute myeloid leukaemia. Treatment-related leukaemia is always preceded by a period of pancytopenia and appears to be part of a broader spectrum of myelodysplastic syndromes. These leukaemias also seem to be refractory to treatment and have a poor survival rate.

Nursing note:

The increased risks of malignancy should be discussed with the child and the family, and appropriate investigations undertaken as clinically indicated (Kissen & Wallace 1995). In the event of a second malignancy, it will be a shock for the family to receive the news and appropriate support will be required.

The Role of the Nurse in Long Term Follow-up

This is a developing area of paediatric oncology nursing and is addressed by authors such as McCalla (1985) and Hobbie et al. (1993). Although the physiological effects of chemotherapy have been examined, the psychosocial impact of treatment cannot be underestimated. Nurses need to be involved not only in identifying and treating late effects but also in ensuring that appropriate referrals are made. Research into this area continues to be needed both at a nursing level and at a collaborative level with other health care professionals. Nurses need to be actively involved in developing policies for follow-up of long term survivors and could be involved in setting up survivor groups so that experiences and problems can be shared. These long term survivors need health education and information related to their treatment and the likely late effects; thus helping them to develop an appropriate health locus of control.

Nurses have a responsibililty to facilitate support and counselling, to help survivors to adapt to any disabilities they may have. Everyone has expectations for their future and goals they wish to achieve. Nurses can help long term survivors re-assess and set realistic goals; helping to develop their self-esteem. Survivors may have problems gaining employment and insurance due to lack of understanding and may require information and letters for employers and other agencies (Evans & Radford, 1995). The dissemination of information via new technology, such as the Internet, would benefit not only long term survivors but also other health care professionals and the general public by raising awareness. With expanding practice boundaries, nurses have the opportunity to play a key role in the follow-up of these children and young adults. In the future nurses may specialise in late effects of cancer treatment with nurse-led long term follow-up clinics becoming common practice in paediatric oncology. The issue as to the ideal location for follow-up of survivors into adulthood is still under debate and requires urgent consideration.

Chapter 6
Future trends

Louise Hooker

Introduction

Developments in chemotherapy treatment have been matched by progress in nursing practice in response to the needs of children and their families. Intensive, multiple-drug chemotherapy schedules have drastically improved the prognosis of most childhood malignancies, but have increased the toxicities experienced by children receiving treatment. Knowledge of the potential side effects of chemotherapy regimes, both in the short and long term, has enabled the design of strategies aimed at prevention and monitoring, and the provision of appropriate treatment and support. This has meant that more children survive the potentially lethal effects of cytotoxic treatment and thereby have the best possible chance of surviving their cancer.

As new treatments are developed, paediatric oncology nurses face fresh demands upon their practice. If nurses are to be able to meet the needs of future patients they must be involved in discussions about the care those patients may require. All aspects of paediatric nursing practice, patient and family care, research, the management of services, and professional education, must meet the challenges presented by treatment innovations if the achievements of the past are to be sustained into the future.

Rapidly advancing scientific knowledge of specific tumour types, the genetic basis of cancers, the behaviour of normal and malignant cells and the exact mechanisms by which chemotherapy agents exert their cytotoxic effect are increasingly influencing treatment developments. As more is known about prognostic indicators of specific tumour types and presentations, drug treatments are becoming more 'tailored' to the needs of individuals.

154

New chemotherapy strategies are being developed with two inter-related aims:

- To increase tumour response
- To limit the toxicities of treatment.

The ideal cancer therapy would be one that was capable of eradicating all malignant cells whilst causing no harm to the patient. As yet this is not available, and treatment developments are attempting to improve the efficacy of existing drugs, alongside development of new agents and innovative approaches to therapy. This chapter explores future possibilities for progress in drug treatment for childhood cancer, based on current treatment trends and research activities, and discusses the possible implications of these for nursing practice.

Strategies Aimed at Increasing Response

For those children with poor-prognosis disease, the aim is to devise therapies which offer an improved chance of cure. Once the high-risk groups are identified, through analysis of the results of previous clinical trials, treatment protocols can be modified with the hope of greater success in the future. A number of the strategies described here have already had an effect upon childhood cancer treatment, and it is anticipated that many of these will continue to be used.

High-dose therapies

The relationship between the dose of chemotherapy agents and tumour response is well established (Bronchud, 1992). Administration of high doses of drugs is also thought to overwhelm some drug resistance mechanisms (Kaufman & Chabner, 1996). High-dose therapies are already a component of many paediatric chemotherapy protocols, and managing the toxic effects of these is a predominant feature of nursing care. Drug doses are limited by their toxicities; the benefits (increased response) must outweigh the harmful effects (potentially life-threatening organ failure). There is more scope for high-dose therapy with drugs in which the limiting toxicity is primarily myelosuppression than for drugs which cause irreversible damage, such as cardiomyopathy or nephropathy. This is because of the development of haematological rescue procedures following 'megatherapy' and the availability of colony stimulating factors (CSFs). CSFs will have an increasing role in supporting children receiving high-dose myelosuppressive therapies, with the application of new cytokines which stimulate various blood cell lineages, reducing not only the degree and duration of neutropenia but also thrombocytopenia and anaemia (Furman & Crist, 1992). Although the risk of infection may be reduced, the escalation of drug doses will inevitably increase the observed incidence of other side effects, which will become the new dose-limiting factors, and the focus for supportive care.

Dose-intensive therapies

Chemotherapy schedules involving intermittent 'pulsed' treatment blocks, are based upon the fractional cell-kill hypothesis and the ability of normal tissues to recover more rapidly than malignant cells. Such strategies have, however, been implicated in the development of subpopulations of resistant cell lines in solid tumours (Bertino & O'Keefe, 1992). This is thought to be related to repeated exposure of cells to the same drugs over a long period of time, the phenomenon of acquired drug resistance. Treatment intensity can be described as the dose of drug given over a period of time $(mg/m^2/week)$, and dose-intensive protocols are thought to reduce the potential for resistance to develop (Kaufman & Chabner, 1996). Dose-intensification can be achieved in two ways. By alternating myelotoxic drugs with non-myelotoxic drugs, given at the neutropenic nadir, it is possible to continue the cytotoxic onslaught on malignant cells, whilst permitting bone marrow recovery. Another approach is to reduce the duration of marrow aplasia by combining intensive chemotherapy with administration of CSFs, either as primary supportive care or to permit serial peripheral stem cell mobilisation, harvesting and rescue. If current randomised trials of dose-intensive protocols in osteogenic sarcoma and neuroblastoma improve survival, the development of more intensive therapies will follow. Currently, the limiting toxicity with administration of granulocyte-CSF, is thrombocytopenia, but the advent of thrombopoietic cytokines will reduce the transfusion requirement. Extra-medullary side effects will not be reduced, however, and supportive care will primarily require nursing input.

Schedule-dependent therapies

Greater understanding of the cytotoxic action of drugs and their pharmacokinetic profiles in children influences the design of administration schedules that exploit the behaviour of specific agents. Increasingly, there is scope for more refined approaches to therapy, based on cell-cycle kinetics.

Because CSFs initiate 'resting' cells into the cell cycle, their use in conjunction with chemotherapy agents is under scrutiny. Carefully timed sequential administration of CSFs and phase-specific drugs increases the proportion of a leukaemia cell population within the replication cycle and therefore vulnerable to cytotoxic action, and thereby increases cell-kill (Bassan et al., 1994). Schedule-dependent synergy between cytotoxic agents has been described. Administration of L-asparaginase following high-dose cytarabine in the treatment of acute leukaemia can overcome acquired resistance to cytarabine (Capizzi et al., 1984). Sub-cytotoxic doses of fludarabine, when given prior to cytarabine increase the cellular accumulation of the active form of cytarabine, with improved response (Gandi et al., 1993). The potential for increasing numbers of such schedule-dependent regimes is envisaged, as theoretical models of cell-cycle kinetics are applied in protocols where cycle- or phase-directed administration optimises the actions of existing drugs.

Administration schedules also affect drug metabolism and excretion profiles. Bolus injections or short infusions create high plasma concentrations over a short period of time, relative to the half-life of the drug. Cell-kill, particularly for phase-specific agents, can only take place in cells that cycle through that phase while therapeutic levels are maintained. Continuous, prolonged adminis-tration of these drugs, rather than bolus injection or short infusions theoretically offers response advantages. By sustaining plasma concentrations at therapeutic levels for longer periods of time, a higher proportion of the cancer cell population will pass through the proliferative cycle and be vulnerable to cytotoxic action (Collins, 1996). Whereas efficacy generally requires a minimum blood concentration to be achieved, toxicity is related to peak levels (Kerr, 1994). If the level sustained by continuous administration falls between these two values, in what is known as the 'therapeutic window' then optimum cell-kill may be combined with minimal adverse effect. The main disadvantages of prolonged administra-tion are practical, related to the inconvenience of lengthy infusions. This may be minimised by the use of ambulatory infusion pumps, with drugs being given via central venous access devices, or prolonged daily oral dosing.

Overcoming drug resistance

As the different mechanisms which mediate drug resistance are discovered, strategies are developed, aimed at overcoming them. Combinations of the non-specific strategies previously described will optimise effectiveness; high-dose, intensified protocols involving schedule-dependent dosing are already in use and may increase in prevalence. Another approach is the development of therapies which target the cellular mechanisms of drug resistance.

One area of current research is focused on the use of compounds that block the action of the P-glycoprotein pump. If the pump can be rendered ineffective, intracellular concentrations of chemotherapy drugs will reach cytotoxic levels. Drugs that inhibit P-glycoprotein activity include verapamil, nifedipine, the phenothiazines and cyclosporin. When given in conjunction with cytotoxic drugs to which tumours have previously shown resistance response has been demonstrated (Hardy & Pinkerton, 1992). If reversal agents prove effective, their use will increase, initially in the treatment of relapsed or refractory disease. The development of analyses that detect the presence of P-glycoprotein in tumour cell populations could serve to identify those tumours which are resistant (Beck et al., 1996) an indication for the administration of resistance modifiers in the tumours of individual children.

The effectiveness of such approaches, and the side effects of the resistance modifiers themselves are currently under investigation. For example, the cardiac effects (hypotension) caused by the dose of verapamil required to overcome multidrug resistance may limit its practical application, and the risk of increased chemotherapy-related toxicity to normal tissues has yet to be eliminated (Newell, 1992).

Strategies Aimed at Reducing Treatment Toxicity

Existing multi-modal treatment is successful in around two-thirds of children with cancer. However, the toxic effects of current therapies incur significant morbidity in many children, in the form of acute, prolonged or delayed side effects. These may have a substantial and life-long impact upon the quality of life of those who are cured. For those children who are judged to fall in favourable prognostic groups, increasing emphasis and research interest is being placed on evaluating strategies that may reduce these short and long term sequelae. Children receiving treatment are increasingly closely monitored; planned investigations for early signs of toxicity have become incorporated into standard treatment protocols. For example, routine monitoring of cardiac function during and after anthracycline treatment has become accepted practice, and treatment modified according to the degree of damage (Bu'Lock et al., 1996).

Reducing doses

High-dose therapies have been responsible for many of the improvements seen in the treatment of childhood cancers. Randomised studies are now being conducted which seek to evaluate whether some children can be treated at lower doses without reducing treatment efficacy. The main focus is to attempt to reduce the cumulative, dose-related cardiotoxic effects of the anthracyclines, and the infertility and/or risk of second malignancies associated with the alkylating agents. It is hoped that the optimum balance between effective treatment and low toxicity can be achieved by reducing the total doses given, by substituting less toxic analogues of effective drugs and, when possible, by avoiding anthracyclines or alkylating agents completely. Children who are involved in such studies will require particularly close monitoring for response, in order that treatment may be modified back to the standard therapy, if the dose-reduction strategy fails to control their disease.

Chemoprotective agents

Much interest has been generated by the development of drugs which may block the toxic effect of chemotherapy drugs while maintaining anti-tumour effectiveness, in particular agents which may protect the myocardium from damage by anthracyclines. Anthracycline-related cardiotoxicity is caused by the release of free radicals in the drug, which damage the heart muscle. This damage is dependent upon the presence of free iron ions which bind with the anthracyclines to produce the free radicals. By administering a drug which selectively binds with the iron ions immediately prior to chemotherapy, this process cannot take place, and the myocardium is protected (Chiron, 1995). It has been suggested that, by using a cardioprotective agent, the previous maximum dose limits may be safely exceeded in high-dose therapy for relapsed patients receiving intensive 'salvage' regimes (Steinherz et al., 1994). However, in children the focus of research is whether cardioprotective agents may enable standard doses to be given with less toxicity (Bu'Lock et al., 1993). Other chemotherapy protective agents, such as amifostine, have yet to be studied in children, but may offer similar protection to other organs, including bone marrow and kidneys, from a wide range of cytotoxic drugs (Schering-Plough, 1994). The development of liposomal drug technology also offers potential protective mechanisms, by trapping the cytotoxic drug within the lipid molecule structure (Nexstar, 1995).

Administration schedules

The potential response benefit of prolonged drug administration has been described above. For those drugs in which toxicity is related to peak serum levels, such as the anthracyclines, slow administration can also reduce toxicity. Some authors advocate very protracted (72-hour) infusions of anthracyclines, as the damage to the myocardium is related to the peak levels in the blood (Casper et al., 1991). However, the relative benefits of these regimes over shorter infusions have yet to be substantiated.

New Chemotherapy Agents

The development and investigation of new cancer drugs is a complex and often emotive issue. The implications for families and staff of involvement in trials of new therapies is discussed at the end of this chapter. The conduct of drug trials in the UK is closely regulated and monitored by a number of bodies, including the UKCCSG and the Association of the British Pharmaceutical Industry (ABPI), to ensure that all such research is undertaken scientifically and ethically. The design of the studies is carefully planned to ensure that scientific knowledge is advanced as quickly as is feasible, involving as few children as possible, whilst ensuring that the results gained are scientifically valid. However, the process of ensuring that a new drug is both safe and effective typically takes many years. There are three main stages of clinical investigation by which a new drug is tested; the basic structure of the studies will be described.

Phase I studies

Phase I studies are the first trials in humans. Prospective drugs will have undergone extensive pre-clinical laboratory testing on *in vitro* tumour cell populations and animal studies, to characterise their cytotoxic potential and preliminary toxic dose profile. The primary aim of phase I studies is to determine the maximum tolerated dose (MTD), and the dose-limiting toxicities (DLT). The first human studies are undertaken in adults, but as children often have different tolerance patterns for chemotherapy drugs, the paediatric dose cannot be accurately extrapolated from the results of adult trials. Paediatric studies often have as their starting dose 80% of the adult MTD. Children who have received all standard treatments, and who have relapsed or have refractory disease are eligible for entry into phase I studies. A mathematically defined progression of dose-escalation is undertaken (Blackledge & Lawton, 1992) whereby three children are given the drug at each dose level and are monitored closely for side effects. If they do not experience unacceptable toxicity (according to World Health Organization guidelines), a further three children are given the drug at the next dose. This step-by-step progression is continued until MTD and DLT are defined. In the absence of adverse side effects, or if disease response is apparent, children who enter the study at a specific dose level can usually continue to receive the drug at that dose, if they and their families wish it. Pharmacokinetic data are often collected, via serial blood and urine sampling, to determine the absorbtion, bioavailability, and excretion patterns for the new drug.

Phase II studies

These aim to determine the potential efficacy of the new drug in different types of cancer. The maximum tolerated dose is given to a statistically defined number of children with different relapsed or refractory cancers, and response is monitored. Once again, according to the wishes of the family, an individual child's 'treatment' can usually continue after evaluation for the trial, if the child is receiving some benefit. From the results of the phase II study, a picture should emerge concerning in which (if any) paediatric tumours further investigation is warranted. The final stage involves comparing the new drug with the best standard therapy for those tumours in which significant response was found.

Phase III studies

In childhood cancer, these phase III studies are the large-scale, multicentre national or international randomised trials into which the majority of children in the UK will be entered at the time of diagnosis. Large numbers of children will be given the new drug, usually in combination with standard therapy, to determine whether significant survival benefit is achieved by its addition to the previous 'best known' treatment.

Treatment Strategies Not Involving Chemotherapy

Historically, the major breakthroughs in cancer treatment occurred when the existing treatment modalities were, in their turn, introduced. By refining their use, alone and in combination, their effectiveness has increased. Two-thirds of children with cancer are now cured, and advances in the treatment of the still-incurable minority are likely to be on a smaller scale than previously. It is possible that the limits of existing modalities are being reached, and that further refinements in their application will make small steps, rather than giant leaps forward. Research into new chemotherapy agents and strategies to optimise the use of existing drugs continues, but for those malignancies that are proving largely incurable despite contemporary therapies, perhaps entirely different approaches are required, rather than new drugs. Increased scientific understanding of cellular biology and the genetic basis of malignant transformation pave the way for novel treatment approaches. Some exploit the natural control and defence mechanisms of the body, whereas others seek to alter the DNA within cancer cells to therapeutic advantage. These new modalities are, as far as childhood cancer is concerned, in the investigational stage; a brief overview of some of them is given here.

Differentiation therapies

The ability of some malignant cells to differentiate is well demonstrated by the example of neuroblastoma. Neuroblastoma can be viewed as one extreme of a spectrum of diseases, ranging from benign ganglioneuroma to the highly malignant childhood tumour, with the existence of an intermediate form, ganglioneuroblastoma (Brodeur & Castleberry, 1993). Stage 4S, usually found in infants, has the ability to regress spontaneously, and the continued presence of an apparently benign residual primary mass is well-documented. Some tumours are, at diagnosis, found to contain some mature elements: this is thought to be a favourable prognostic factor

(Ninane, 1992). An innovative approach to cancer therapy involves compounds that are capable of inducing cancer cells to differentiate. If cells can be influenced to mature they lose the invasive and metastatic characteristics of malignancies, developing into benign variants of the tumour.

Differentiation agents currently under investigation in cancer therapy include the retinoids and other fatty acids (Parkinson et al., 1996). Retinoids exist naturally as derivatives of vitamin A, and are known to influence normal cell growth and maturation via a number of biochemical mechanisms (Lupulescu, 1996). The ability of retinoids to influence cells relies upon the presence of appropriate receptor sites on the cell membrane. All-trans retinoic acid (ATRA) affects disease response in acute promyelocytic leukaemia because the chromosomal abnormality existing in this form of leukaemia involves a retinoic acid receptor site (Parkinson et al., 1996). Patients treated with ATRA may go into complete remission, although chemotherapy is required to consolidate the remission.

Retinoids are under investigation in the treatment of neuroblastoma. Retinoic acids have been shown to initiate a differentiation response in neuroblastoma cell lines *in vitro* (Hill, 1986) and clinical trials are under way to establish whether this can be achieved *in vivo*, with the aim that any residual malignant cells remaining after first-line treatment may be induced to undergo benign transformation, reducing the risk of relapse (Lie, 1990).

Nursing note:

Increasing public awareness of the potential cancer-protecting properties of some vitamins, including vitamin A, from which retinoids are derived, may encourage some parents to administer over-the-counter vitamin A preparations in large doses to their child. The fact that clinical trials are in progress may give this added credibility. As with any 'alternative' therapies, parents should be encouraged to discuss their ideas with staff in a non-judgemental atmosphere of mutual learning. With regard to discussions with parents, it should be remembered that vitamin A is also powerfully teratogenic, and women who are pregnant or planning a pregnancy should avoid 'cancer-protective' preparations containing vitamin A.

Immunotherapy

The healthy immune system has a cancer surveillance function. A number of immune mechanisms are involved in identifying and destroying abnormal cells (Graubert & Ley, 1996). The increased incidence of cancer in immunocompromised individuals is a clear demonstration of the role of the immune system in the development of malignancy. People receiving long term immunosuppressive treatment following organ transplant, or who have diseases affecting the immune system, such as HIV, are two such groups (Roitt, 1991).

Increased scientific understanding of the body's cellular defences has led to the development of strategies that exploit these mechanisms in the treatment of cancer. The role of immunotherapy has been explored to a greater extent in adults than in children. This is possibly because relative successes with cytotoxic chemotherapy in paediatric tumours make the exploration of alternatives less of a priority. There exists a potentially greater role for immunotherapy in paediatric oncology in the future as the limits of success with existing approaches are reached.

Advances in genetic engineering have made possible the mass production of the components required for immunologically mediated therapies. These components include cytokines, which are naturally occurring cellular messenger proteins which can be mass produced through recombinant DNA technology. Cytokines already established in paediatric oncology practice are those which stimulate haematopoietic stem cells along chosen maturation pathways; the colony stimulating factors. The CSFs most commonly employed are the granulocyte cell line cytokines, administered either to reduce the length of neutropenic episodes, treat bacterial infection or to enable harvesting of haematopoietic stem cells from the peripheral circulation. The clinical potential of other haematopoietic CSFs, such as erythropoietin and interleukin-3 (Furman & Crist, 1992), is yet to be explored fully. In the treatment of childhood cancer the principle cytokines under investigation are the interferons and the interleukins.

Interferons (IFNs) can suppress viral replication, regulate immune responses and exert a cytostatic effect on cells, inhibiting protein synthesis and slowing replication (Wujcik, 1993a). There are three distinct types: alpha, beta and gamma. IFN-alpha is the most widely used in cancer therapy, it has shown activity in a number of malignant tumours including myeloma, hairy-cell leukaemia, chronic myeloid leukaemia, non-Hodgkin's lymphoma and AIDS-related Kaposi's sarcoma (Witt et al., 1996).

Interleukins are a group of cytokines which have varied actions and include a number of haematopoietic CSFs. Interleukin-2 (IL-2) is naturally secreted by helper T-cells, stimulating peripheral lymphocytes to transform into cytotoxic lymphokine-activated killer

(LAK) cells, or the more active tumour-infiltrating lymphocytes (TILs). Administration of IL-2 may prove to have a role in mobilising immune surveillance of minimal residual disease cell populations following existing multimodal therapies (Favrot et al., 1990). In other strategies, known as adoptive therapies, IL-2 is administered to patients in order to mobilise LAK or TIL cell production. Macrophage populations (including the LAK/TIL cells) are then harvested from the peripheral circulation via leucopheresis, and further stimulated with IL-2 in the laboratory, before being returned to the patient. Response but not survival benefit has been demonstrated in some adult cancers (Cohen et al., 1996), and whether there is a future role for such therapy in paediatrics remains unclear.

Immunotoxins

Immunotoxin therapy represents a novel, theoretically cancer-cell specific therapy. It exploits another advance in biotechnology, the production of monoclonal antibodies, which are single-antibody molecules designed to target specific antigens. These are created by injecting human tumour antigens into mice to initiate an immune response, collecting the resultant antibody-producing B-cells and fusing the encoded B-cell DNA with immortal cancer cell DNA. This provides a hybridised cell population which produces a perpetual supply of specific tumour cell antibodies (Roitt, 1991), to which cytotoxic compounds, pro-drug-converting enzymes or radioactive particles may be attached (Junghans et al., 1996).

An immunotoxin consists of a bonding segment, known as a ligand, linked to a toxin. The ligands are, most commonly, monoclonal antibodies for the target cancer cell surface membrane antigens. The ligand transports the toxin to a cell-surface antigen or receptor. The toxin then enters the cell and destroys it through blocking essential metabolic processes (Wawrzynczak, 1991). The toxins used are highly potent, cell-cycle non-specific compounds, killing both resting and dividing cells. They are also unaffected by multidrug resistance mechanisms that limit the potential of traditional chemotherapy. By creating tumour-specific ligands, the toxin is directed only to those cells which express that antibody on the membrane, and normal cells are selectively spared. To offer effective therapy, the ligand must selectively target tumour cells, penetrate the cell wall and release the toxin (Wawrzynczak, 1991). By creating 'cocktails' of common tumour cell-membrane antigens attached to toxins, increased proportions of cell populations could be targeted

(Vitetta et al., 1991; Flavell et al., 1995). However, early studies suggest that immunotoxins may prove to be another therapy that is most effective in the removal of comparatively small numbers of cells, following massive cyto-reduction by traditional treatment methods (Rowe, 1994).

Limitations to immunotherapy include toxicity, specifically a dose-limiting capillary leak syndrome, the precise mechanism of which is as yet undefined. Intracellular fluids move out into extracel-luar compartments, characterised by a reduction in serum proteins and related oedema (Wawrzynczak, 1991). The production of anti-toxin or anti-mouse antibodies in the patient may also limit the effec-tiveness of repeated doses (Junghans et al., 1996) and produce unpleasant immunological response symptoms such as rashes, fever, hypotension and, potentially, anaphylaxis.

Gene-directed therapies

In paediatric medicine, gene therapies for children with inherited disorders such as severe combined immune deficiency syndrome or cystic fibrosis have triggered much interest. However, such treat-ments, if available, would only benefit the tiny minority of childhood cancers caused by single gene abnormalities, such as hereditary retinoblastoma. Of more widespread potential are therapies that are directed at the genetic material of tumour cells.

Cancer cells have undergone one or a series of chromosome mutations in order for cell populations to escape genetically programmed regulatory controls such as the rate of cell death, cell-cycle duration, and the proportion of cells undergoing proliferation. The ability to reliably identify those mutations specific to certain tumour types is influencing the development of cytogenetic analysis as an aid to diagnosis (Mertens & Heim, 1994), to determine prog-nostic indicators (Schaison, 1993) and to assess minimal residual disease (Kelly et al., 1996).

An understanding of the alteration in cellular biology brought about by these mutations, together with developments in biotechnol-ogy, have indicated possible future strategies for therapy by either directly altering the genes responsible for malignant transformation and proliferation, or targeting cytotoxic therapies. If the genetic error can be identified and corrected, the influence of oncogenes can be blocked, loss of tumour-suppressor gene activity reversed, or growth-factor receptors inhibited and the normal regulatory mecha-nisms could re-exert control. Gene-mediated strategies that would influence malignant cells to differentiate terminally have also been postulated (Clark, 1996).

As with other therapies that are designed to specifically target tumour cells, the problem of directing the therapeutic 'bullet' effectively must be overcome. Techniques have been developed, such as micro-injection, liposomes, and the use of vectors, or gene-delivery vehicles (Ho, 1994), but as yet effective transfer *in vivo* has to be perfected (Cohen et al., 1996). Viruses and retroviruses are of particular interest as vectors, as they are capable of inserting genetic material directly into cell DNA which is then replicated, passing the altered gene to daughter cells. The viruses are modified before use by removing the genes responsible for replication, to prevent infection (Wheeler, 1995).

Gene-transfer techniques can be combined with existing treatment modalities to target cancer cells with cytotoxic agents. Liposomes can transfer DNA, contained in the lipid structure, to tumour cells which then makes those cells produce enzymes capable of converting pro-drugs to their active cytotoxic counterpart, thus delivering localised chemotherapy (Clark, 1996). Another strategy is the transfer of 'suicide genes' into tumour cell populations, where the genetic material of tumour cells is manipulated to make them vulnerable to specific therapies. For example, by introducing viral DNA into tumour cells and then administering specific antiviral drugs, the cells which contain the virus/tumour DNA complex will be selectively killed. This has been investigated in adults with unresectable brain tumours (Cohen et al., 1996).

New Treatments for Cancer — the Nurse's Role

Research into new therapies is a prerequisite for advances in treatment, but presents many challenges. As previously described, participation in trials of investigational treatments may be offered when all known therapeutic options have been exhausted, when efforts are usually directed at symptom control and providing emotional support for families who are facing the death of their child. Conducting research within the context of palliative care is challenging (Ling & Penn, 1995), and can create tensions within the multidisciplinary team, as some people perceive any research involving dying patients as exploitative (Thorpe, 1992). Conflicts may also arise in relation to what course of action is considered to be in the best interests of the child if the parents make decisions that nurses disagree with (Akers & Bell, 1994). Nurses involved in trials of potential new treatments play a pivotal role in the ethical conduct of the research, and often bear the brunt of such conflicts (Cogliano-Shutta, 1986). Working with families participating in investigational drug trials requires knowledge, open communication, sensitivity and organisational skills in order to meet the needs of the terminally ill child and his family whilst fulfilling the rigorous requirements of clinical research.

Norville (1995) describes the multifaceted role of nurses working in clinical trials as patient and family education, direct caregiving, accurate implementation of study procedures and data collection. The research nurse is in a unique position, working with families, medical staff, trial coordinators (often from the pharmaceutical industry) and other nursing teams. The needs and perceptions of these groups may be disparate; the research nurse must maintain good working relationships with all parties whilst working effectively and ethically.

The families of terminally ill children are vulnerable, and their desire to avoid or delay their child's death may make them susceptible to suggestions that a new treatment strategy may hold a last hope of cure. It is vital, therefore, that full and frank discussion regarding what is offered by trial participation takes place, and that they are not pressured into making a decision. The role of the research nurse as advocate for families is critical (McEvoy et al., 1991) to ensure that, whatever decision is made, when the child eventually dies, it is not regretted.

Consent to trial participation must be freely given and informed, and families must be reassured that a decision not to participate, or to withdraw, may be made at any time without having to give a reason, and without fear of prejudice regarding their child's future care (British Paediatric Association, 1992). Clearly written information about the nature of the trial, the alternatives that exist, what participation will involve, and the possible benefits to the child and to society should be given in addition to verbal discussion (Hendrick, 1997). Booklets concerning the conduct of clinical trials have been produced for adult patients, and may prove useful for parents and teenage patients (Patient Education Group, 1994; BACUP, 1996). The consent of competent minors (Alderson & Montgomery, 1996) and the assent of younger children to undergo new therapies should be sought, and reconfirmed throughout the trial, based on information that is appropriate to their age, understanding, previous experience and concerns.

Withdrawal of children from new agent studies, due to deteriorating health, toxicity or the wishes of the family is a difficult and emotionally charged event. The family may have perceived, despite explicit and honest discussion prior to and during the trial, that the new drug offered a final hope, which has now faded. It is important to stress here that participation in research trials does not preclude excellent symptom management or the process of psychological support in preparation for the child's eventual death, and by ensuring that the child and family have enjoyed the continued support and input from the hospital and community nursing teams throughout the trial, the transition to palliative care may be eased.

SECTION TWO
BONE MARROW
TRANSPLANT

Chapter 7
Background to the bone marrow transplant procedure

Nikki Bennett-Rees and Louise Soanes

History

From 1891 bone marrow, in the form of an oral preparation, was given to treat patients with leukaemia and disorders where there was a known defective blood formation (Quine, 1896). This treatment appeared to have little effect on the patient. However, minimal changes in treatments were made over the following decades.

In 1937, Shretzenmayr (cited in Treleaven & Barrett, 1993) treated patients with intramuscular preparations of bone marrow. This was the first time the technique of transferring live cells into a patient was attempted, and with fair effect. However, two years later Osgood et al. (1939) infused bone marrow cells intravenously and, in 1940, there were reports of bone marrow being injected into the intramedullary space (Santos, 1983). Unfortunately, these first two attempts at the use of therapeutic doses of bone marrow in patients with aplastic anaemia were unsuccessful.

As a result of the discovery of atomic energy and the release of the atomic bomb in the mid-1940s there was a revival in research into the effects of an intensive dose of irradiation on the bone marrow of survivors in Hiroshima and Nagasaki. Pioneering work carried out by Jacobson et al. (1950) and Lorenz et al. (1952) was the forerunner of today's successful bone marrow transplants. In 1950 the work of Jacobson et al. demonstrated that mice whose spleens (a haematopoietic organ for a mouse) had been shielded from lethal doses of irradiation, could recover. Their work continued to demonstrate that infused bone marrow cells could also provide protection against death. Lorenz et al. (1952) went on to prove beyond doubt that normal bone marrow function could be restored to lethally irradiated mice and guinea-pigs by infusing bone marrow cells.

With the knowledge that engraftment of bone marrow cells was a possibility, clinicians made several attempts in the late 1950s and 1960s to treat a variety of human disorders. The clinicians were presented with numerous difficulties because most of these experimental transplants were carried out on patients with end-stage disease. Consequently, the patients died either before engraftment could be established or from a 'secondary disease' (Barnes et al., 1962). This is now recognised as 'graft versus host disease' (GVHD).

In addition to these problems there was the lack of treatment for life-threatening viral or fungal infections.

During the 1960s progress in developing effective treatments was slow and only approximately 10% of patients receiving allogeneic bone marrow transplant showed a clinical improvement (Pegg, 1966). However, the work of Thomas et al. (1957) on preventing GVHD, with that of Terasaki and McLelland (1964) on the human leukocyte antigens (HLA) system pushed the role of bone marrow transplant (BMT) into a new era. There was now increasing success in the treatment of patients with aplastic anaemia and leukaemia. Meanwhile work carried out in Holland by De Koning et al. (1969) led to the successful treatment of infants with severe combined immunodeficiency syndromes (SCID), until then a fatal disorder. In fact, as Morgan (1993) reports, the first successful HLA-matched sibling transplants were performed in 1968, on two children with primary immunodeficiency disorders.

By the end of the 1970s progress was such that BMT became a treatment modality which had a measurable success rate for diseases such as SCID, severe aplastic anaemia and leukaemia. The 1980s saw a vast increase in the number of BMT centres world-wide. Data banks were set up and the number and range of diseases treated by BMT expanded. In the paediatric setting, children with haemoglobinopathies, such as sickle cell disease and thalassaemia (Borgna-Pignatti, 1992), and a variety of ultimately lethal metabolic disorders (Vellodi et al., 1992) were able to undergo transplant successfully using HLA compatible siblings.

During the 1990s there continued to be further developments in the field of BMT:

- An improvement in the technology of HLA typing enabling more children in whom there is no matched sibling donor to receive bone marrow from a matched, or mismatched unrelated donor.
- The expanded use of prophylactic drug therapy both before and during the transplant period.
- The continued development of efficacious antiviral and anti-fungal therapy thus reducing both morbidity and mortality.
- The development and increased use of cytokines and growth factors therefore enhancing both haematological and immuno-logical reconstitution.
- The ability to successfully HLA type, harvest and cryo-preserve stem cells from the umbilical cord of newborn infants.
- The development of gene transfer in the autologous setting for the treatment of children with genetic disorders (Jenkins et al., 1994).
- The development of successful mobilisation, collection of allo-geneic and infusion of allogeneic and autologous peripheral blood stem cells (Gray & Shea, 1994; Walker et al., 1994; Vaux, 1996).

Types of Transplant

A bone marrow transplant involves harvesting bone marrow from a donor and then transfusing (or grafting) these cells into the recipient. There are three different types of transplant:

- Autologous marrow — these cells are harvested from the patient (i.e. self) prior to receiving dose escalating intensive myeloabla-tive therapy. Autologous marrow is used in gene therapy. Its use in children is, however, usually for those with a malignancy such as a solid tumour or acute myeloid leukaemia (AML). The advantage of an autologous transplant is the lack of GVHD. The disadvantage is the risk of tumour cells being present in the harvested marrow; also there will be no graft versus leukaemia (GvL) effect (discussed in detail later).
- Allogeneic marrow — bone marrow cells are harvested from another person who may be related or unrelated, matched or mismatched. Ideally, the donor will be an HLA-identical sibling.
- Syngeneic marrow — bone marrow cells are harvested from an identical twin. These transplants are ideal in children with an acquired bone marrow failure, such as aplastic anaemia, as both

the donor and the recipient are identical in every aspect and there will be no risk of the recipient developing GVHD.

The use of peripheral blood stem cells (PBSC) for transplant is increasing. Autologous PBSC is used more commonly. However, haploidentical (i.e. use of a child's parent who is a half-match) PBSC has been used successfully in conjunction with haploidentical marrow. An area which is open to future research and development is the use of allogeneic PBSC transplant. Furthermore, successful engraftment using umbilical cord stem cells from an identical HLA-matched sibling, is becoming more of a treatment option.

Diseases for which Bone Marrow Transplant is a Treatment Modality

For a child with a malignancy the aim of treatment is to eradicate the malignancy and then 'rescue' the child from the life-threatening effects of the myeloablative therapy. For the child with leukaemia there may be an additional GvL effect from allogeneic bone marrow transplant.

Cells used for transplant can be bone marrow or peripheral blood stem cells, and can be autologous, allogeneic, matched or mismatched (Table 7.1).

Table 7.1: Malignant diseases for which bone marrow transplant is a treatment modality

Leukaemias
  acute lymphoblastic leukaemia
  acute myeloid leukaemia
  chronic myeloid leukaemia
  juvenile chronic myeloid leukaemia
  myelodysplasia

Lymphomas
  non-Hodgkin's lymphoma
  Hodgkin's disease

Solid tumours*
  brain tumours
  Ewing's sarcoma
  primitive neuroectodermal tumour
  retinoblastoma
  rhabdomyosarcoma

*Cells used are usually autologous bone marrow or PBSC.

For a child with a non-malignant disorder, such as bone marrow failure or bone marrow dysfunction, or who requires replacement of a missing enzyme in an otherwise healthy bone marrow the aim is to remove the malfunctioning marrow and replace the system with healthy cells, thus restoring a normal functioning haematopoietic system.

Cells for transplant are used from bone marrow and are allogeneic, either matched or mismatched (Table 7.2).

Table 7.2: Non-malignant diseases for which bone marrow transplant is a treatment modality

Acquired marrow failure
   severe aplastic anaemia

Congenital marrow failure
   Fanconi's anaemia

Genetic/metabolic disorders
   Hunter's syndrome
   Hurler's syndrome
   Maroteaux–Lamy syndrome

Haemoglobinopathies
   thalassaemia major
   sickle cell disease

Immune disorders
   severe combined immune deficiency
   X-linked α gamma globulinaemia

The successful outcome of BMT depends on a variety of factors, such as:

- Ability of the underlying malignancy to go into remission pre-BMT
- Amount of previous therapy (such as chemotherapy and blood transfusions) the child has undergone
- Tissue-matching of donor
- Age and sex of donor and recipient.

As this field of medicine is continually evolving so the results of long term survival will change. Table 7.3 provides a current summary of long term survival.

Disease	Transplant	Long term survival (%)
Table 7.3: Survival outcomes for children undergoing bone marrow transplant		
Malignant disease		
ALL (1st CR)	allogeneic	60
ALL (2nd CR)	allogeneic	40
AML (1st CR)	allogeneic	50
AML (2nd CR)	allogeneic	20–50
AML (2nd CR)	autologous	40
Myelodysplasia	allogeneic	60–70
Neuroblastoma stage IV	autologous	30
Non-malignant disease		
Aplastic anaemia	allogeneic (non-transfused)	80
	(multiple transfusions)	70
SCIDS/CID	allogeneic (sibling)	90
	(haploidentical)	50
	(unrelated donor)	70
Thalassaemia major	allogeneic (sibling)	70–75
Inborn errors of metabolism	allogeneic	Early studies show good results for some hereditary metabolic diseases

ALL = acute lymphoblastic leukaemia; AML = acute myeloid leukaemia; SCIDS = severe combined immune deficiency syndrome; CID = combined immune deficiency; CR = complete remission.
Sources: Fischer et al., 1990; Lucarelli et al., 1990; Chessells et al., 1992; Barret et al., 1994; Nesbit et al., 1994.

Tissue Typing

Tissue typing is a key process in the pre-transplant phase. It is the basis by which the most suitable donor for transplant is chosen. Blood is taken from the patient, parents and siblings to establish HLA type and determine matches within the family group. Failure to find a match here will necessitate extending the search to the extended family members and/or unrelated donors on national and international registries.

Tissue type refers to a series of polymorphic proteins found on the surface of almost every cell in the body. These proteins are known as human leukocyte antigens (HLA) and are involved in the cell-to-cell interaction of the immune system.

Tissue type is, in simple terms, a list of these antigens carried on the surface of these cells (Ord, 1995). In BMT, the donor is chosen according to the similarity of their HLA in relation to the patient's HLA (Figure 7.1).

The HLA system is a major determinant in the success of BMT (Welte, 1994). Before its introduction in the 1960s, the results of allogeneic BMT were very poor. At the time of HLA introduction, enthusiasm for BMT was falling and the future of the speciality was in doubt. Today its impact and development in the field of BMT are well-known. It is, however, only 28 years since the first BMT using HLA matching was carried out (Treleaven & Barrett, 1993).

There are over 90 separate HLA antigens that can form 26 million combinations. Despite this, some tissue types are fairly common and yet others may occur only once in a million individuals. Individuals inherit their HLA antigens from their parents in a Mendelian inheritance in the same way that eye colour is inherited (Welte, 1994). Certain tissue types are found in certain ethnic and racial groups and a matched unrelated donor is more likely to be found in these groups for patients from these backgrounds.

HLA genes are found on the short arm of chromosome 6. Individuals inherit two sets of antigens: a paternal haplotype and a maternal haplotype (see Figure 7.1). There are two groups of antigens. Class I antigens (of which at least 17 have been identified) are expressed not only in leukocytes but in most nucleated cells in the body cells (HLA-A, HLA-B and HLA-C are the ones of prime concern in BMT). In contrast, Class II antigens are only expressed in a limited range of cells (B lymphocytes, macrophages, endothelial and dendritic cells except in the placenta and CNS). These are known as the HLA-D region and have been mapped into five distinct subregions: DN, DO, DP, DQ and DR. In BMT the HLA-DR is the most important of the Class II antigens (Roitt & Male, 1996).

The function of the HLA system

The most important role of the HLA system is reactivity with foreign antigens. The antigen is processed by being presented to macrophages and scrutinised by a T-cell receptor, which then initiates the appropriate T-cell response in order to rid the body of invading antigens. There are some T-cells, however, which are capable of responding directly to cells bearing foreign HLA, without prior

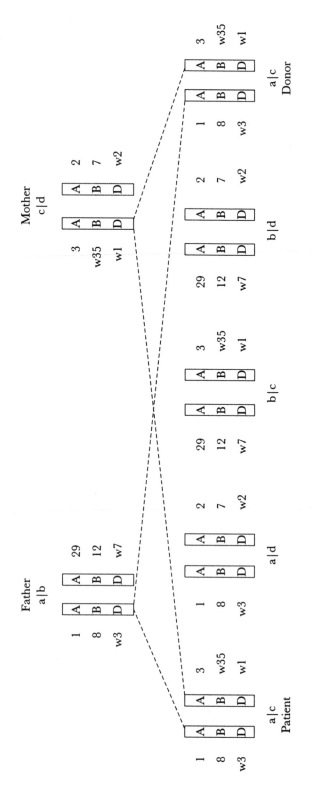

Figure 7.1: Possible combinations of human leukocyte antigens (HLA)

processing. Methods of identifying the number of these circulating T-cells, such as cytotoxic T-cell precursor assay (CTLP) and mixed lymphocyte culture (MLC), are a useful adjunct to choosing a suitable donor. A high CTLP frequency is an indicator that a donor may induce GVHD if used in transplant.

As well as the major histocompatibility antigens there are so-called minor histocompatibility (mH) loci that encode molecules in recognition and rejection. Despite their name these mH loci are strongly implicated in GVHD, particularly in the setting of HLA-matched related BMT (Reiser & Martelli, 1995). Minor histocompatible differences are not routinely assessed in BMT donor recipient pairs. In the future, matching mH may further reduce the incidence of GVHD, but in transplants for leukaemia such minor histocompatibility can be an advantage in the production of the GvL effect (Volelsgang & Hess, 1994).

ABO blood typing

ABO-incompatible marrow grafting can be accomplished with little of the haemolytic transfusion reactions seen in the past. This is due to improved techniques to remove red blood cells from the marrow, but if unmanipulated marrow is to be used then, as with normal blood transfusions, haemolytic transfusion reactions will occur. Appropriate blood products need to be compatible with both the donor and the recipient in the early stages of the transplant. The patient and the family should be informed that following BMT the patient's ABO blood type will convert to that of the donor. The time taken for this varies and therefore the recipient's blood group should be determined prior to a blood transfusion in the early stages post-transplant.

Adult unrelated donors

The birth rate in the industrialised world has been falling for many years. At present the average number of children in a family is 1.9. This has meant that only 30% of patients needing a BMT have a suitable donor within their immediate or extended family (Vowels et al., 1991). The failure to find a donor within the family group leads to the search for compatible marrow from an unrelated donor. Currently, the use of children as non-related donors does not occur, for the ethical and moral reasons discussed in a later chapter on sibling donors. Adult donors used for unrelated transplants volunteer to donate their marrow and are required to register with one of the bone marrow registries that exist throughout the world.

Donor panels

Donor panels arose as a result of the growing need for centralised unrelated bone marrow registry in the 1970s. This need was recognised following the failure to find suitable donors for individuals in a variety of countries at this time. In the UK the case of Anthony Nolan, a small boy with Wiskott Aldrich Syndrome, and the unsuccessful search for a donor in 1974 led to the formation of the Anthony Nolan Bone Marrow Registry now better known as the Anthony Nolan Bone Marrow Trust (ANBMT). Similar registries exist in many countries.

These registries provide information that may lead to the identification of a suitable donor for patients in both national and international bone marrow units. Through this collaboration, the pool of potential bone marrow for those patients for whom a suitable donor cannot be found on their national register, has widened.

The people on the registries are volunteers who have agreed to enter details of their HLA status to a central register. Initially, details of their relevant medical and social history are recorded and a sample of blood taken to determine their Class I antigens. Details of these are added to a database and held until required or the donor becomes too old to donate. A bone marrow transplant unit approaches the registry with details of patients requiring a donor. At this stage, further matching of Class II antigens identifies potential donors and further tissue typing is undertaken to elicit the most suitable donors.

Those identified as being the most likely potential donors are then screened for their suitability, using a lengthy selection process which can take months, and assesses both physical and mental suitability to donate marrow or stem cells.

Selection of adult unrelated donors

Due to the complexity of human major histocompatibility, approximately 10% of transplants are carried out as a result of volunteered matched unrelated donors.

Although the aim of HLA typing in BMT is to select the donor with the closest possible match this may not necessarily identify the most suitable donor. Other factors that come into play in donor selection are listed below:

- Donor age
- Donor/recipient sex
- Cytomegalovirus (CMV) status
- Ethnic group
- Physical and mental health.

The age at which volunteers can donate their marrow varies from country to country. At present the minimum age in the UK for joining a register is 18 years and the maximum is 40. The maxium age at which a potential donor can donate marrow recommended by the ANBMT is 56 years (this relatively young upper age limit is due to the increased risk of a general anaesthetic in older donors).

Ideally, the donor and recipient should be of the same sex, this is due to the risk of GVHD which is higher in female-to-male transplants. In contrast, male-to-female transplants increase the risk of rejection in aplastic anaemia.

The CMV and Epstein Barr Virus (EBV) status of donors is of paramount importance. The highest risk of infection is from CMV antibody-positive donors donating marrow to CMV antibody-negative recipients. This risk is reduced by the use of CMV negative blood products before, during and after transplant for those at risk. Donors are also screened for HIV and hepatitis B and C antibodies.

Ethnic group is of prime concern in BMT, as a matched donor is more likely to be found among the recipient's own ethnic group. The majority of unrelated donor volunteers are Caucasian and this has led to a shortage of potential donors from ethnic populations. Added to this, some ethnic groups have cultural and religious objections to the donation of marrow or stem cells.

There is also a shortage of male donors which may compound the above situation, as the incidence of many of the conditions requiring BMT in children is higher in males or has an X-linked inheritance; Wiskott Aldrich Syndrome being an example of this situation. Campaigns to recruit from ethnic groups and to encourage male donors to come forward are frequently undertaken by the registries in order to raise awareness and recruit more suitable candidates for donation.

Evaluation of the unrelated adult donor

Donors are required to complete a detailed medical questionnaire before entry to the registry. The physical criteria for donation includes stringent assessment of the donor as suitable for general anaesthetic. Exclusion includes previous medical history of respiratory disease, cerebrovascular disease, current pregnancy and back problems. Exclusion from donation on these grounds is due to the potential risk to the donor as a result of the anaesthetic or the process of marrow collection. Once admitted to the registry the potential donor waits to be called forward to donate their marrow (this may take many years). Each registry has its own limits as to how many times a person may donate their marrow. Adult unrelated donors may donate to two separate recipients with a gap of one year between donations. Agreement to donate more than twice is extremely rare due to the increased risk to the donor of repeated anaesthetics. However, a collection of T-cells from the donor may be collected in the case of pending rejection four to six weeks after the initial collection of marrow (Anthony Nolan Bone Marrow Trust, 1996).

Once called for donation the donor will not only be assessed physically but also psychologically for suitability to donate. During this early physical and psychological assessment written consent is sought from the donor to proceed with preparation to donate; though not legally binding, consent is sought on moral and ethical grounds.

Assessment of the donor's perceptions and attitudes towards transplant may uncover distortions in the donor's concepts of the procedure. Many donors have no previous experience of hospital and may have misconceptions of what the procedure entails. Education about the donation process and potential complications following donation and general anaesthetic are given (donors who are not fully confident in their decision to donate are encouraged to withdraw as soon as possible from the selection process). It is also explained that should the recipient of the marrow die or face serious complications as a result of the transplant, the donor is not responsible (Gordon-Box, 1996).

Personal information about the recipient is given only on request and disclosure of personal details is kept to a minimum (gender, age-group and country in which the transplant is to take place). Strict confidentiality between the two parties is maintained and contact discouraged throughout the pre- and immediate transplant period. This ensures that the privacy of both the donor and recipient is maintained (Cleaver, 1993).

Receiving a gift of such magnitude as bone marrow without thanking the donor is difficult for many families. In such cases cards and small gifts may be passed on through the registry to the donor at the time of the transplant. Sometimes the donor and recipient may meet or make contact, months after the transplant has taken place. Again, the registries offer support and advice in these situations, to protect both parties from over-involvement by the other and to offer support for the emotional response such a meeting may produce. The preparation of the related adult donor does not involve the support and services of the bone marrow registry and is coordinated by the BMT centre caring for the child. The physical preparation is similar to that already described.

Chapter 8
Preparation for transplant

Nikki Bennett-Rees and Louise Soanes

The Family

As BMT becomes the accepted form of treatment for an increasing range of childhood disorders, families who are referred for their first meeting with a BMT consultant fall into four categories:

- Those whose child has a malignant disorder
- Those whose child has a life-threatening non-malignant disorder
- Those whose child has a metabolic disorder
- Those whose child has a haemoglobinopathy.

For the family whose child has a malignancy the progression to a BMT may be the natural course of events or it may be the last hope for cure following either a relapse or a disease refractory to treatment. Such families have experienced chemotherapy and maybe even radiotherapy. There will be aspects of BMT which will be very new to them; however, if the oncology unit is attached to the BMT unit, the families will know their surroundings and staff. If the BMT unit is in a referral centre, these families will have to leave behind everything which has been familiar and supportive during previous treatments.

For the family whose child has SCID or severe aplastic anaemia (SAA), there may be either little or no hope of cure without a BMT. Such children may have had varying experiences ranging from long intensive hospitalisation to minimal inpatient treatment.

Children with metabolic disorders may also have had minimal hospital admissions, but without a BMT may suffer progressive deterioration, making their quality of life untenable (Vellodi et al., 1992).

The life expectancy for children with haemoglobinopathies has increased dramatically over the years. Thus, parents have a difficult decision to make when balancing the chance of potential cure versus acute and long term side effects of BMT (Borgna-Pignatti, 1993). No matter how much information and knowledge the family already has, there is still a great deal of information to be given and discussed at the first consultation. Specific information will include the child's need for a transplant; long term outlook with or without the transplant and the problems that might be faced during and after the transplant. At the first consultation, it is essential that a BMT nurse, as well as the unit psychologist, is present (Table 8.1). This serves to build up a relationship between the family and extended team as well as ensuring that continuity of information is given. In future, meetings with either the nurse or psychologist will be able to provide further answers to queries.

Table 8.1: Summary of the role of the nurse in giving information before bone marrow transplant
Be included in the initial family/consultant meeting Have the ability to assess the family's understanding Be consistent in giving information appropriate to the family's understanding Be able to discuss levels of family involvement in the care of their child Be available to answer questions in the coming weeks Be able to support the above with written information Maintain support of the family

The possibility of parents feeling confused, frightened and shocked is not uncommon (Haberman, 1988). It is therefore essential that, following this consultation, the BMT nurse has the time to go through what has been discussed, step by step with the parents. The nurse is in an ideal position to further this discussion with the family, as he or she will be caring for both children and families undergoing BMT, and thus will be able to answer a wide range of questions (Carney, 1981). It is the role of the BMT nurse to deliver information and support which is individualised for each family (Downs, 1994), ensuring that the information given is both accurate and paced appropriately.

In families for whom English is not the first language or whose 'medical' knowledge of English is limited, it is essential to make use of an interpreter at this meeting, preferably one who is attached to the hospital services. Experience has shown that using a family member as an interpreter (especially if a sibling) places too great a burden on that person; ultimately, it can become questionable whether all the information is relayed accurately. Whilst the interpreter is present, it is important to find out if the family follows any cultural routines or has special dietary needs to ensure that these can be met.

For families who are new to the area, a visit to the BMT unit following the meeting will help to allay some of their fears of the unknown. It is often a time where, to relieve the anxieties of the day, toys and activities for the child can be discussed. Ending the day by giving the parents a taped copy (Hogbin, 1989) of the first meeting will enable them to go through relevant information in the safety of their home. In addition, a specifically designed book about BMT, which includes the treatments, side effects, restrictions and daily routines of the unit, will enhance the family's knowledge and understanding. An added advantage of the book and/or tape is that the extended family can feel involved in what is going to happen.

Before admission the family and the child may have further appointments at the hospital. These visits offer an ideal opportunity to consolidate family knowledge, answer problems as they arise and give the family time to revisit the unit, thus making it more familiar. Some families may find it beneficial to meet another family going through the BMT process. If possible, this can be arranged in conjunction with the family meeting their primary nurse, play specialist and, if appropriate, school teacher.

On admission to the unit, usually the day prior to commencing conditioning therapy, most information is given by the nursing staff. It is essential to confirm what the family's and the child's knowledge of the forthcoming treatment is and to establish what their immediate needs are. Once the family has adjusted to the new environment, the forthcoming treatment can be discussed and the child's care planned. This time before transplant is enormously stressful for the parents. On top of the worry about the 'sick' child, there will be worry about the safety of their 'healthy' child donor. In the case of the donor being unrelated, the added worry concerns the donor's fitness or, indeed, whether he or she might change their mind. Keeping the parents well-informed through each day of conditioning helps to reduce their anxiety (Haberman, 1988). The length of the conditioning regime and the timing of moving the child into isolation will dictate how much additional information needs to be given in the first few days.

Parents should be given a copy of their child's conditioning protocol. This protocol can then be used to guide the parents' questions through each stage as well as explaining each of the individual drugs and their side effects. In addition, the parents will need to understand and learn about the isolation technique. This will vary between units but should range from the way to enter the room, to making a snack for their child.

Negotiation

Generally, once the bone marrow has been transfused the parents feel less stressed and are able to take in much more information. As soon as the time is right for the parents, discussion as to how much involvement they are either able or willing to offer, should be negotiated. Research provides overwhelming evidence of the benefit of parental involvement (Gibson, 1989; Taylor & O'Connor, 1989; Cleary, 1992). Thus, for the child to receive optimum care, he or she should be nursed in an environment which actively promotes the practice of parental involvement (Casey, 1988). Nurses need both to recognise and to value the expertise that the family brings to their sick child, yet it must be taken into account that not all families will either want, or indeed be able to participate in their child's care (Casey, 1988). However, whatever the level of parental involvement, for parents to be effective in their child's care, they need appropriate teaching and support. Furthermore, to create a truly effective partnership with nurses, care for the child's needs must be negotiated between the child, the parents and the nurse, and then evaluated. Some parents will be expert carers in terms of their child's 'medical' needs, able to perform tasks ranging from giving oral medicines to intravenous medications (Evans, 1994) and caring for the central line (Pike, 1989). Others will be novices in dealing with a hospitalised child. Whatever the contribution to the child's care, it must be valued and regarded positively. For the child, the parent's sheer presence acts both as a support and as a buffer against the unknown.

Thus, from admission through to discharge, the daily planning of the child's care will enable parents to be involved in the 'nursing care' in which they feel able to participate. Unless this negotiation occurs at each shift, staff may be unable to appreciate that parents may have days when they feel unable to give their child's care or, alternatively, wish to undertake additional roles.

Support

Both during the time leading up to BMT and during hospitalisation it is crucially important to provide support for parents. It can be given in many ways, but two of the most fundamental are staff providing detailed and accurate information and being freely available to parents. The sharing of care between staff and parents and acceptance by staff that parents have unique knowledge of their child's needs empowers parents who may find themselves in an alien environment. This acts as a support.

Support can also be offered at a very practical level. For example, some parents may find the financial burden extremely heavy while one or both is taking time off work, sometimes for an extended period. In addition to loss of earnings, extra expenses may be incurred, such as extra child care for siblings, travel costs and accommodation fees. Funds may be available through, for example, the Malcolm Sargeant Cancer Fund for families whose child has leukaemia or cancer. For other families, there are some charitable organisations which may help with travel expenses and holidays for siblings and families, especially at discharge. Access to information of this kind can act as an invaluable support. At another level, offering two simple stress-reducing thera-pies, such as massage and aromatherapy, on the unit allows parents some relaxation which again acts as a support.

Each person's need for support is unique, whether it is emotional, financial, practical or indeed a combination of all these things. The experienced BMT team should be able to recognise this and ensure that support is ongoing. If the parents are well-supported they, in turn, will be able to support their child. The overall effect of this will help ensure a good atmosphere in the ward, which has a direct result on the well-being of the child (Pot Mees, 1989).

Preparation of children

No matter what role a child plays in the transplant procedure (i.e. as donor, recipient or sibling) each will have individual needs and concerns. In order for these to be met, the preparation required should be both age- and developmentally appropriate to that child. This is particularly important for children where the recipient of bone marrow does not have a malignant disorder and consequently 'bone marrow' and 'bone marrow transplant' are entirely new words and/or concepts. Examples of misconceptions can vary from confusing bone marrow with the 'marrow bone' which comes in tins and is fed to dogs, to the child who thought his brother was having a 'bow and arrow' transplant! Another 'experienced' child, having undergone many surgical procedures for multiple abnormalities, none the less thought that his umbilical cord cell transplant meant that his 'belly button' was going to be cut open to give blood in. Words and procedures which are common everyday experiences to BMT staff are totally new and often bewildering to many adults, let alone children.

Ideally, preparation of children should be a shared family experience rather than an individual procedure, with family members being facilitated in the continuous process of information-giving, questioning and support. Research indicates that shared preparation enables family members to better understand the experiences and feelings each undergoes and they are therefore able to identify their role in supporting each other (Lwin, 1996). For some families, however, this may be neither practically nor emotionally possible. The need or desire for some individual preparation should be respected and provided in addition to family preparation.

Psychological preparation of a child undergoing transplant

The child who is to undergo a BMT may be a baby with no outside experiences; a child who has had a previously uneventful life and now needs a transplant to cure an acute illness; or a child who has had years of treatment. The needs of each child will be unique. The preparation will be based on their actual knowledge, and at a level appropriate and individualised to their needs.

The key to successful preparation is to reduce the anxiety that results from lack of knowledge. The play specialist will be able to discover the appropriate emphasis and extent of preparation the child will need pre-BMT. This preparation will be determined in the main by the child's age, development, knowledge and previous hospital experiences, but the child's need to know and consequent ability to cope with stress has to be balanced with the parents' wishes. For example, parents may not wish their child to be told about certain procedures or issues and staff must always respect this. Staff should indicate to parents, however, that if the child asks a direct or specific question an honest answer would have to be given. It is a delicate area, needing sensitive handling for all parties.

For the younger age group, preparation involving therapeutic play sessions using 'models' (e.g. teddy bears) with a variety of Hickman lines, peripheral lines, nasogastric tubes *in situ* proves very successful. The child is able to give medicines either by mouth or by one of the lines, take blood samples and change dressings, in the hope that new and possibly painful procedures will be learnt and coping strategies acquired. For the older child, preparation includes the use of prepared books showing what various treatments look like, and handling equipment such as Hickman lines, syringes or needles as well as giving accurate information. This should help the child to formulate questions, and encourage an understanding of why and how certain procedures will happen.

Essential for all children is the ability to build up a trusting relationship with the play specialist and nursing staff. Without this trust, it can be difficult for the child to believe that he or she is being told the truth and that there are no hidden surprises.

For the teenager undergoing BMT the whole procedure can become exceptionally stressful. In addition to the causes of stress described earlier, there may be additional ones linked particularly to adolescence:

- Awareness and resentment at loss of independence and control
- Consequent dependence on parents and nursing staff
- Concern about alteration in body image
- Concerns about changes to 'sexual' identity.

This last stress factor involves reactions to future loss of fertility and the repercussions not only of having someone else's blood in one's system but also possibly the blood of someone of the opposite sex (Wiley et al., 1984; Futerman & Wellisch, 1990). In the ideal setting teenagers should have their transplant in units which are able to provide adequate physical and emotional care to meet their special needs.

The general nursing preparation for the child receiving the transplant will need to take into account age, development, experience and need. Bearing this in mind, the methods and details of nursing will consequently vary for each child. The following general issues, however, will need full explanations of what to expect and how to cope with them (Table 8.2):

Table 8.2: General preparation of children for hospitalisation for bone marrow transplant

For previously non-hospitalised children
  Hickman line insertion
  Hickman line dressing
  nasogastric tube
  mouth care
  hair loss
  compliance with oral medication
  finger pricks
  isolation
  altered body image

For children with experience of hospitalisation
  new environment
  new staff
  new method of nursing
  nasogastric tube
  finger pricks
  isolation
  altered body image

Physical preparation of the child

Physical preparation of the child before BMT will show slight variations between units. The most frequent pre-BMT evaluations are highlighted. Much of the physical preparation is undertaken on an outpatient basis. Information is needed to assess the child's health and disease status before being deemed fit enough for the transplant to proceed. This also serves as a baseline for measurement of the child's future growth and development following the transplant. The process also monitors the effects of conditioning regimes and treatment in the long term.

The coordination of physical preparation is usually undertaken by a BMT coordinator and this is often a nursing role. The physical and psychological preparation, if coordinated by the same person, can allow a seamless preparation period for the child and the family. During this time, the BMT coordinator can introduce members of the multidisciplinary team with whom the child is likely to come into contact at a later date. The child and family can also familiarise themselves with the hospital, its routines and staff over this period of time. It offers an opportunity for questions and concerns to be raised and dealt with as they arise.

Information overload is a threat during this time, and support through open telephone access to the coordinator and clear written information will be needed to support the plethora of information given to the family. The presence of a third party, a primary nurse or BMT coordinator at interviews and new investigations can offer support to the family and can help in the later clarification of this information.

Physical preparation can be stressful and time-consuming. Fear that one of the many investigations will reveal an obstacle to the transplant or indicate disease recurrence or progression is reported by many parents at this time. Support for the family is vital in a period of intense physical and psychological activity.

In order to save time and reduce travelling for the family many of the physical investigations should take place on one day. Follow-up calls by the BMT coordinator to the family after such days can help the family to feel supported and allow the opportunity to discuss issues raised. The stress of such days should not be under-estimated. In response to this some units are now offering separate days on which to address issues of psychological preparation for the child, the family and, if applicable, sibling donors.

Physical preparation of the child for bone marrow transplant includes:

- *Medical history and physical examination*
  previous treatment history
  diagnosis treatment history
  identification of other medical problems
  transfusion history
  allergy and immunisation history
  psychological and neurophysiological assessment
- *Histocompatibility*
  confirmation of HLA and MLC testing and selection of donor
  transfusion support planning
  determination of markers for engraftment (allogeneic patients)
- *Major organ assessment*
  full blood count, differential and platelets
  electrolyte assessment
  hepatitis screening
  viral assessment (CMV, *Herpes simplex*, *Varicella zoster*, Epstein Barr)
  pulmonary function
  cardiac evaluation (ECG, echocardiogram)
  glomerular filtration rate (GFR)
  chest X-ray
  nutritional evaluation
  dental evaluation (teeth with evidence of caries should be extracted before the insertion of new central lines and should not be undertaken at the same time; this is due to the release of pathogens from the affected teeth which may be released into the peripheral circulation and may colonise the newly inserted line)
- *Tumour/disease evaluation*
- *Central line insertion*
- *Sperm banking*
- *Back-up bone marrow harvest* from child (this is collected and stored in case the donated marrow in allogeneic bone marrow transplant fails to engraft and the child needs 'rescuing' from the ablative therapy of conditioning regimes).

Conditioning Regimes

Prior to the bone marrow being transfused, the child will undergo a preparative conditioning regime. Conditioning regimes vary according to the child's diagnosis, age, type of transplant and any additional research therapies which may be introduced. The rationale behind conditioning therapy is:

- To treat any residual disease
- To produce 'space' for the donor marrow to grow
- In the allogeneic setting, to immunosuppress the child in order to decrease the risk of graft rejection.

To achieve these three goals the regimes may be:

- A single high dose of chemotherapy
- A combination of high-dose oral and high-dose i.v. chemotherapy
- A combination of high-dose i.v. chemotherapy and total body irradiation (TBI).

Depending on the match of the donor, further immuno-suppression may be used, such as antithymic globulin (ATG) or campath (a monoclonal antibody). Table 8.2 outlines the most common combinations of therapies used.

Table 8.2: The most common combinations of therapy used in conditioning regimes		
Drug therapy	Type of bone marrow transplant	Disease
High-dose melphalan	autograft	solid tumours
Oral busulphan and i.v. cyclophosphamide	allogeneic	children less than 2 years old and/or with a non-malignant disease
i.v. cyclophosphamide and TBI	allogeneic	children more than 2 years old with a malignant disease

Due to the large doses of treatment used, any combination of the tabled therapies will result in the child having some degree of nausea and vomiting. Vomiting can range from mild to severe, but over the years, antiemetic therapy has brought about great improvements. By using a combination of ondansetron (i.v.) and dexamethazone (i.v.) the antiemetic effect can be enhanced. On a few occasions, a third antiemetic may need to be considered, such as cyclizine, given as a slow i.v. bolus. Although there is little docu-mented research, experience has shown that babies and young children appear to tolerate conditioning very well and are less likely to vomit, but the degree of nausea they experience is unknown. It would therefore be reasonable to give a single-agent antiemetic, such as 7–8-hourly i.v. ondansetron. If the child's nausea and vomiting are well controlled, both the parents and the child will feel more in control and better able to cope. This, in turn, will have a direct effect on staff morale.

In addition to the nausea and vomiting and the well-documented general side effects of chemotherapy, the conditioning drugs have specific side effects. Cyclophosphamide when given in high doses can cause haemorrhagic cystitis. To counteract this, the child is given hyperhydration containing mesna. Nursing staff need to measure the child's in/output accurately to ensure that fluid retention is not occurring. Urinary output must be tested for blood.

Nursing note:

For children wearing nappies, the safest way of testing for blood is to place a cotton wool ball into each nappy. The wet cotton wool can then be squeezed on to the multistix.

It must be noted that occasionally a late-onset haemorrhagic cystitis may occur after engraftment, therefore it is important that urine output is always observed and tested. Treatment for haemorrhagic cystitis may include hyperhydration, bladder irrigation and maintaining a high platelet count.

Busulphan is a drug which is only available as an oral preparation. It has been shown to be as effective as TBI when combined with high-dose cyclophosphamide (Lucarelli et al., 1985) in children without a malignancy or those under two years of age who are undergoing rapid development and are therefore saved from the additional side effects of radiotherapy. It is essential that the child is able to take and absorb the busulphan tablets and if there is any doubt about the child's ability to take the dose, a nasogastric tube must be passed for the duration of the drug. For some parents, this can be extremely distressing. If the issue of passing the tube is approached appropriately and the safety measures for the child, parents and staff are discussed the night before commencing the busulphan, stress levels can be reduced.

Research studies have shown that busulphan is significantly better absorbed if given on an empty stomach. The best regime is for the child to be nil by mouth one hour pre- and two hours post-dose. To achieve this, negotiation of dosing times, within a 12-hourly schedule, which suit the child and the parents is essential to ensure compliance. It appears that busulphan is of a low emetogenicity. None the less, because it is an oral medication it is preferable to give i.v. ondansetron with each dose to avoid having to calculate the amount of busulphan lost in vomit.

The main side effect of busulphan is that some children may suffer seizures. On account of the small chance of seizures occurring it is advisable for the child to remain in the unit for the duration of the course of busulphan. Again, experience shows that seizures are more likely to occur in older children who are verging on adult weights, or in children who have had CNS problems. On account of this, it may be a good policy to give anticonvulsants for a period of time surrounding the busulphan course. Busulphan also causes alteration in skin colour. This is particularly noticeable in non-Caucasian children, and on the scrotum of Caucasian boys. For some parents this causes concern, but the skin colouring should return to normal several months post-BMT.

A later side effect associated with high busulphan levels is the occurrence of veno-occlusive disease (VOD) (Bearman, 1995). Nurses play a significant role in the early detection of VOD by commencing twice-daily weight and girth measurements at the start of the busulphan therapy (discussed later).

TBI is the most effective treatment in reaching sanctuary sites (i.e. the CNS and testes) in children with a haematological malignancy. It is also the single most effective immunosuppressant therapy. The unpleasant side effects seen when TBI was given as a single dose have been greatly decreased since the introduction of fractionated TBI over 6–8 doses. Most children tolerate the treatment well and an oral dose of ondansetron before treatment is usually sufficient. When there is no 'on site' radiotherapy facility, children and parents appear to enjoy the trips out to the radiotherapy unit, taking in a few toy shops after the treatment!

Campath is a drug which may be used in units where children receive unrelated donor marrow. A monoclonal antibody, campath is used to irradicate lymphocytes. Generally given over 5 days, the most toxic effects occur on day 1, when there is greatest activity following breakdown of the lymphocytes. The main side effects are hyperpyrexia, tachycardia, headache and nausea.

Nursing note:

If a pre-medication of i.v. pethidine, chlorpheniramine, methylpred-nisolone and ondansetron as well as paracetamol is given 1.5 hours pre-campath, the toxic effects are reduced. The paracetamol must be continued 4-hourly during the infusion to ensure maximum comfort is achieved. On day 1, the campath should be infused slowly over 8 hours. If this regime of pre-medication and infusion is well-tolerated, on the subsequent days the campath can be infused as fast as tolerated, but no faster than over 2 hours. In addition, if the drug is well-tolerated the pre-medication can be weaned down so that by day 3–4, the child may not need any pre-medication.

At the start of the conditioning regime, it is the nurse's responsibility to both teach and explain to the parents the safety aspects of caring for a child receiving chemotherapy. This will include the wearing of vinyl gloves when changing nappies, helping with bedpans and urine bottles or vomit bowls. The length of time recommended for the use of gloves is 7 days following the last dose of chemotherapy. However, universal precautions would include the wearing of gloves when in contact with any body fluids at any time.

No matter which regime is used the two most important aspects for nurses are:

- To be aware of actual and potential side effects and thus be able to act effectively on that knowledge
- To be able to support both the child and parents.

For parents whose child is undergoing chemotherapy for the first time, this is a new and frightening experience. Similarly, for parents whose child is receiving radiotherapy for the first time, the fear of TBI may be overwhelming and a point of no return, where they need to continue with the transplant.

Fertility issues

The issue of fertility has been discussed in the chemotherapy section of this book. However, it warrants further discussion in this section as children who have undergone previous chemotherapy may regain some fertility, with boys retaining spermatogenesis and girls possibly retaining a small degree of functioning ova (Sanders et al., 1996).

Before the start of the conditioning regime it may be possible to collect semen from older boys and thus retain the hope of fatherhood for them; sadly, at the time of writing the successful collection and storage of ova remains elusive in clinical practice.

It is the use of conditioning regimes in BMT that will render the child sterile. The most likely causes of such sterility are total body irradiation (TBI) and the use of cyclophosphamide. It has been shown that 90% of males who received TBI are permanently azoospermatic (Sanders et al., 1987).

In adult patients it has been suggested that sperm may be collected up to 30 days after the commencement of conditioning chemotherapy. The rationale for this time being that the life expectancy of mature sperm in the epididymis is 30 days so, in theory, these sperm will have matured before the onset of chemotherapy. This extra time may be vital in adolescent boys in the preparation time for the collection of sperm. In girls, the damage to ova is more devastating as females are born with a finite number of ova and once damaged there is no opportunity for regeneration (Sanders et al., 1996).

For most of the children who undergo BMT the issue of sperm banking does not arise due to their age. However, parents should be informed of their child's future infertility and the effect this may have on the family should not be under-estimated. Although at the time of preparation for BMT the prime concern of the parents is the potential cure of their child, issues such as loss of future grandchildren may have future implications for some families (Heiney, 1989).

By the age of 14 most boys have entered puberty and may be able to masturbate and ejaculate. Raising this subject will require great tact and diplomacy at a time of family stress (Williams & Wilson, 1989). Discussion of sperm banking will need the following areas to be taken into consideration: information, privacy, confidentiality, support and follow-up (Hopkins, 1991).

Discussion with the young man will need to include why sperm collection is necessary and this may be difficult for the family to instigate. Discussion of a young son's sexuality at any time is difficult for families; during preparation for BMT with stress already at a high level it may be impossible.

After discussion with the parents and the young man a male nurse or doctor may be chosen to talk in private about the issue of sperm donation. This includes concerns about masturbation (which in some religions is seen as a sin, for example, the Roman Catholic and Jewish faiths). Masturbation still has a stigma attached to it in western society (Hopkins, 1991). Information as to how the sperm is collected and stored should be discussed, with attention being paid to the amount of information given. The ability and comfort of the young man to comprehend what is discussed should be clues as to the length of such sessions.

Centres vary in their time limits of sperm storage. Ten years is the average time and this means that although provision for fatherhood has been made, even this has a limit. This will have implications for the future for the young man involved in deciding when to have a family. Arrangements for longer storage will need to be considered according to age at donation and will require negotiation with the local sperm bank.

Following preparation and the decision about sperm donation by the young man, even with guidance and support the collection of the sperm may still be difficult to achieve. Masturbation, even in a secluded room within the hospital with sexual stimuli from magazines, may be impossible (Hopkins, 1991). The specimen can be collected at home, but needs to be stored within four hours, making this option difficult. In the event of failure to obtain a specimen, psychological support and information on other options available will be needed by the young man. If collection is successful he will need information as to how to recover the sperm at a later stage, and details should be given about the length of storage time (Kaempfer et al., 1983).

For girls this situation is further complicated by the lack of technology with which to collect and preserve ova successfully. Experimental advances in the collection of ova or sections of ovaries have yet to prove successful in the clinical setting; in the future this situation may improve. But, for those young women faced with infertility as a result of conditioning regimes of BMT, counselling and advice, by trained infertility counsellors, in order to make clear future options should be offered prior to the preparation for transplant. Recent research (Sanders et al., 1996) indicated that 5% of prepubertal girls receiving TBI or high-dose chemotherapy prior to transplant developed normal gonadal function.

Preparation of a Sibling Donor

Sibling donor preparation begins once the choice of donor has been established. It may be that informed consent from the child has not yet been dealt with because up until this point the parents will have given consent on behalf of the donor (Lwin, 1996). In the first instance the parents, with the help if necessary of the unit staff, will need to discuss with the child, or children, the need to have a blood sample taken. Preparation should include practical issues such as blood taking and understanding the need for repeated blood tests if a child is a donor. The donor is a 'well' child and may have no understanding of the need to be in hospital having needles and medicine. There may be children who fear the truth has not been told. At the same time the donor should be prepared (if old enough and with parental consent) for wider issues, such as the patient developing severe GVHD, rejecting the marrow or dying. These negative aspects can have a huge impact on the donor and may result in the need for ongoing support, possibly from outside the family. The unit psychologist may well be the best person to provide continuity of support and long term follow-up of the donor. Preparation of the donor prior to admission must aim to allow them to accept that whatever the outcome is it is not their responsibility. None the less, this must be balanced with the hope that the healthy marrow will enable the sibling to undergo BMT safely with a positive outcome.

Once the admission date of the donor is established, being able to address any other worries is essential. These may range from physical concerns to emotional fears, depending upon the age and development of the child. Physical worries may arise from repeated blood tests, anaesthesia and the anticipation of post-procedural pain from the aspiration sites. The emotional fears in the young child may include those of separation from family and home even though only for a short time, to the fear of having a Hickman line or becoming bald like the other children on the unit. For the older child the fear of the bone marrow not being good enough may be a huge burden. In addition, the donor may not want to go through with the procedure and may be feeling guilty and frustrated (Freund & Siegel, 1986). Some of these fears may be lessened by being made to feel special and important during the period of the donor admission. As the donor is generally an inpatient for only 48 hours, good preparation is clearly essential. The donor should have a clear understanding of what bone marrow is, where it comes from and how they are likely to feel and look on return to the ward from the harvest. Being able to address some of the deeper issues surrounding the fears of the older donor may be difficult to achieve in such a short time span.

During the inpatient time the donor is often made to feel very special and receives a good deal of attention from the parents. Once discharged, however, both the parents may become deeply involved in the care of the child receiving the BMT. If the donor is the only sibling, the feelings of isolation will increase as he or she is shut out of the sibling's room and away from the attentions of their parents. The sibling donor needs to be given a gentle and tactful explanation as to why it is not possible to go into the isolation room. If this child is to remain a frequent visitor to the unit, continued work and involvement with the play specialist will be beneficial (Rollins, 1990).

Ethical use of sibling donors

Thirty per cent of donated marrow used in BMT comes from family members. Of this, a large proportion comes from siblings. In adult transplants the sibling donor is often an adult too, and is, therefore, able to understand what is required, give informed consent and understand the implications of donating marrow. However, when the sibling donor is a child the situation is different and becomes more complex. Ethics is a branch of moral philosophy which aims to enquire into the good/bad and rights/wrongs of human actions. It calls us to consider our everyday actions and judgements but is not an examination of what is 'legal'. Ethical theories, as with other theories, describe the world as it ought to be rather than as it is. This is not to say that ethics is purely an academic ideal for those in ivory towers. Ethical theories offer nurses a framework to guide the principles of clinical activity. The use of such a framework can give nurses a basis on which to examine and clarify values and beliefs in practice and begin to understand the reasons behind them (Richardson & Webber, 1995). The use of ethics in conjunction with moral theory can offer the experience of examining what has gone on before, evaluating events and aiding decision-making processes for the future (Brykczynska, 1990).

An awareness of these issues is important in an area of medicine such as bone marrow transplant where new and experimental treatment is undertaken in an effort to prevent a child from dying. Of all the members of the multidisciplinary team, nurses often have the greatest contact with families. They spend longer periods of time with them and intense relationships with the child and immediate family can form. Indeed, it may be the nurse who first identifies and confronts the ethical and moral dilemmas related to bone marrow transplant. How they then deal with these issues in support of the family will in many cases have an effect on the final outcome of the situation. If nurses wish to have a voice that is heard in the growing debate surrounding paediatric BMT, and hope to be part of the decision-making process in the future, they need first to examine and be comfortable with their own beliefs and values.

Two of the most common ethical issues that confront nurses in paediatric BMT are informed consent and the rights of donors, particularly donors that are children.

Informed consent has been discussed in the chemotherapy section of this book. Briefly, informed consent involves a two-part process. First, the patient (or parent on behalf of their child) consenting to treatment should be fully informed and understand the benefits and risks of treatment. This information also needs to include the identification and discussion of the alternatives available to this proposed treatment. The second part of the process involves the explicit giving of consent; this should not be assumed through the lack of dissent. The health care professional giving this information should not use their power or influence to coerce the potential patient in this decision-making process.

What, though, if the person to whom the treatment is directed is below the legal age of adulthood, as is often the case in the use of sibling donors? Do they have the right to informed consent and, if so, is it afforded to them by adults acting on their behalf? Do they also have the right of dissent, that is do they have the right to say 'No' at any point during the time before the marrow is collected if they feel they have not been fully informed?

Despite the legal precedents concerning when children are deemed competent to give consent to medical treatment they may be able to give informed consent at a much earlier age than thought (Nitschke et al., 1982). Kubler-Ross (1982), as cited in Brykczynska (1990), worked with children facing terminal cancer and showed that children can take part in complicated decision-making and are able to make appropriate treatment decisions.

In legal terms 'child' refers to individuals from birth to 18 years of age. These 18 years encompass the mental development of the child from infant to adulthood. The level at which a child understands information given to them and the cognition to cope with the implications of making decisions develop throughout this same period. Both are affected by the child's life experiences and may differ greatly from child to child. This diversity faces nurses and other health care professionals in paediatric BMT both with patients and with donors in the process of gaining truly informed consent from paediatric donors.

Through the use of play therapy and psychological support, young children can be supported in their decision to become a donor (Kinrade, 1987), although the final decision as to whether the child is competent to give informed consent is still held in the power of the adults involved (Ellis, 1992). Issues such as these have been raised in the case of a mother of half-siblings to a child needing a transplant being taken to court in an attempt to tissue-type the children. The court upheld her decision to refuse the testing. The opinions of the children involved were not stated in the reporting of this case (Gibbs, 1990; Morrow, 1990).

When it is discovered that a child within the family is a match for the sick child requiring a BMT the news is greeted with relief and joy. A potential life saver has been found close at hand and often the transplant procedure commences without further ado. But what of the rights of the sibling donor?

Brykczynska (1990) states that society expects organs and tissue to be donated without concern for the donor. The cost of such a gift can be high and has been identified as a process that is not without psychological and emotional implications (Kinrade, 1987; Pot Mees, 1989). The giving of a gift is not as simple as it may seem. It involves three stages: giving, receiving and repaying (Mauss (1967), as cited in Brykczynska (1990)).

In donating marrow there is no exchange of gifts but just one person giving to another. In receiving bone marrow from a sibling a child can never adequately repay such a gift; the child may feel indebted to their sibling for such a gift yet how do they know when the debt has been repaid? For the child who donates, more than a donation of marrow is involved, indeed, the survival and future functioning of a family is included. Giving such a gift accompanies feelings of responsibility for both the recipient's life and possibly death (Fox & Swanley, 1974). This may be a burden to the donor and again, the question arises as to when the responsibility stops (Lwin, 1996, personal communication). A young child is rarely in the position to refuse offering such a gift to the sick sibling and the above issues often go unrecognised.

Delaney (1996) argues that it is not clear whether harvesting bone marrow from a well sibling is legal and states that the Children Act (Department of Health, 1989; Scottish Office, 1995; Department of Health and Social Services, 1995) permits a medical procedure to occur only if it is in the best interests of the child. She goes on to state that the donation of marrow involving a painful procedure necessitating a general anaesthetic may not be in the child's best interests and may be carried out under pressure from parents and health care professionals and without the child's informed consent.

Delaney (1996) advocates the use of an independent panel to assess the regulation of sibling donors in order to judge whether the donation of the marrow to a sibling is in the best interests of the child. Month (1996) argues that this approach is to ignore the benefits to the family as a whole in preventing the child donating bone marrow to a sibling. He argues that the child is, in effect, saving the family from the trauma of losing one of its members, stating that the loss of a sibling is potentially more harmful than the physical risks of donation even when the sibling is too young to have formed an emotional bond with the recipient. His evidence is based upon psychological research relating to children whose siblings have died rather than the sibling donors of bone marrow transplants, so can parallels be drawn?

The siblings of children who are chronically ill are known to be a population at psychological risk and many experience both positive and negative effects (Dunn, 1988; Eiser, 1989, 1993). Siblings who donate marrow may similarly be at risk and a five-year longitudinal study is currently being funded by the Bone Marrow Research Fund to investigate the impact and psychological cost and benefits to children donating bone marrow to their siblings.

The role of the nurse in the ethical debate surrounding sibling donors is complex. Appropriate education regarding the issues involved in marrow donation is a key factor in informed consent (Downs, 1994). The nurse can be seen as the family's advocate in providing for, assessing and supporting the family and the child in their decision to donate marrow.

The sibling donor will for a short while be a patient afforded the same rights as their sick sibling in accordance with the Children Act (Department of Health, 1989; Scottish Office, 1995; Department of

Health and Social Services, 1995). If a sibling donor should disclose doubts about donating marrow to their sibling, the ethical and moral duty of the nurse is to the sibling donor. Should the child receiving the marrow die, the nurse has a duty to understand the needs of the donor and the family by coordinating care and identifying families at risk.

Cord blood transplants raise many ethical issues in their own right. These sibling donors can be seen as an agent in achieving a goal. Cases exist of children being conceived in the search for a source of suitable stem cells to save a family member (McBride, 1990). This is not a situation unique to BMT; children are conceived for many reasons other than the desire for children. Jecker (1990) argues that the conception of a child to save a life of another is an event not likely to harm a family as it is an individual decision, made on behalf of the family as a whole. The question may be asked, 'What if the outcome of the transplant is not successful?' Will the child grow up in the knowledge that he or she failed the family before being conscious of their existence? Questions such as this will remain unanswered until those involved are at an age where they can reflect.

Who ultimately owns the cord blood is another question raised but not yet answered in cord blood donation. Does it belong to the child or the parent?

At present in the UK cord blood is collected and stored centrally for use as needed. This treatment modality is in its infancy and as yet the situation has not arisen where a child, or sibling, whose cord blood has been collected and saved has needed a source of stem cells at a later stage. What rights do those children have over the saved cord blood and what right of redress do they have if that cord blood has been used? These transplants are not suitable for all types of the conditions requiring BMT and the use of siblings as sources of stem cells from bone marrow is likely to continue for some time.

In conclusion, nurses need to be aware of the current ethical decisions concerning paediatric BMT if they are to support the family in their time of stress and reach a decision regarding the use of one child to help another. Further ethical implications are raised in the light of NHS reforms and the case of Jaymee Bowen (*R.* v *Cambridge Health Authority, The Times,* 1995) as to the allocation of resources and BMT. The growing inverse relationship between resources and treatment options, so-called 'health care rationing', is likely to increase in areas such as BMT. Nurses need to be involved in the discussions on such issues. If the nurse is to act as an advocate for the child and the family, his or her communication and assertion skills in dealing with members of the multidisciplinary team will need to be backed with the value of allowing the child to be supported and helped in reaching an informed consent to their donation. Nurses should formulate and be comfortable with their own ethical opinions and be happy to act on them (Ellis, 1992). The support offered to the sibling donor incorporates the guidance of child psychologists and skilled play specialists, in sessions both as a family and as an individual; to ensure the child is fully informed of what donation entails, and that as an individual rather than as a child, they are happy with the decision to proceed.

Preparation of Non-donor Siblings

Initially, all the children in a family will have undergone blood tests to determine their tissue type and suitability to act as a donor. For the child who is not a 'match' various feelings may emerge. On the one hand, there may be great relief in not having to undergo any further tests. On the other, there may be feelings of guilt and anger at not being able to be included in the transplant process (Patenaude et al., 1979; Eiser, 1993). Furthermore, exclusion from the physical process means the exclusion of the 'healthy' children from their parents. In cases where both parents wish to be with their sick child, siblings are often sent to other family members. Visiting may then only occur at weekends when the children may only have minimal access to their parents. In the two different environments of hospital and alternative 'home', siblings may well feel a loss of control over what they can do, and restrictions not previously experienced may be placed upon them. The joy at being with their parents at the weekend may be lost if they are too worried or tired to provide the attention that is needed (Eiser, 1993).

With these issues in mind, the setting up of a weekend sibling support group can prove enormously beneficial for all the siblings of children undergoing BMT (Kramer & Moore, 1983). This special time given to siblings allows them to mix with other children in the same position, thus enabling them to share their feelings and act as a support to each other. In addition, it provides an outlet for possible feelings of frustration, guilt and anger (Patenaude et al., 1979; Kramer & Moore, 1983; Freund & Siegel, 1986).

Although the play specialist has a key role in the preparation and ongoing emotional support of all the children it is by no means exclusively his or her role. When the psychologist, ward nurses and the play specialist combine their skills and time to work together the emotional needs of both the child undergoing BMT and the siblings will be met (Harding, 1996).

Chapter 9
Collection and
infusion of bone
marrow

Nikki Bennett-Rees and Louise Soanes

Collection of Marrow

The method of collecting the marrow from the donor is an individual procedure that varies from unit to unit. However, the principles remain the same for both adult and child donors and these are described below.

The donor is admitted to hospital the day before the bone marrow is collected. A routine pre-operative physical evaluation is carried out in preparation for an anaesthetic and consent for the procedure obtained.

The collection of bone marrow is undertaken in an operating theatre using a sterile technique and lasts 30–90 minutes. The donor is laid in the prone position to allow aspiration from the posterior iliac crests; in cases of poor collection from this site the patient may be turned and the anterior iliac crests and possibly the sternum used. Epidural anaesthetics have been used in bone marrow collections, though not in situations where marrow collection from the iliac crests is likely to be insufficient and the sternum used.

Two or three skin punctures are made at the chosen site of collection. The marrow is then aspirated in 5 ml aliquots using multiple penetrations with the aspiration needle being redirected to a new area of bone as needed. The aim of using only two or three skin incisions and stretching the skin across is to minimise scarring.

The collected marrow is then injected into a blood transfusion pack containing anticoagulant. The total amount of bone marrow aspirated varies in each case and is calculated during the procedure by measuring the number of nucleated cells in a sample of marrow and estimating the required amount of bone marrow needed to supply an adequate number of stem cells to ensure engraftment.

The marrow is then filtered through a series of fine mesh filters in order to remove fat, bone and fibrin clots. If required within the next 72 hours the marrow will be stored at 4°C. Longer periods of storage at this temperature result in stem cell death. If the marrow is to be transfused after this time (as in the case of autologous marrow and cord blood) then it will be cryopreserved (marrow from unrelated adult donors should not be cyropreserved except in extreme circumstances). For effective cryopreservation the cryopreservative, dimethylsulphoxide (DMSO), is introduced; this involves DMSO being added to the marrow which is then frozen in either liquid nitrogen, liquid nitrogen vapour or mechanical deep freezers.

The freezing process can have an adverse effect on the marrow. If frozen too quickly damage to the stem cells may occur, ice crystals may form in the bags and the freezing process acting on different metabolic processes in the cell may cause disruption to the cell and result in cell-toxic metabolites forming. Large quantities of marrow may be divided into smaller bags in order to allow uniform freezing at a controlled rate; this is also valuable if one bag is rendered unusable in the freezing or thawing process as some marrow is still available for re-infusion. Marrow preserved in this way can be used up to five years following donation but the use of DMSO carries some risk for the patient; this is discussed in the section on transfusion of the marrow.

On completion of the harvest, up to a litre of bone marrow may have been aspirated from the adult donor (less from children). In preparation for this the donor will have given some of their own blood to replace that lost in the collection, autologous blood is used as it reduces the risk of transfusing white cell antibodies. Haemoglobin levels are assessed prior to discharge and the need for further transfusions or oral iron preparations made on an individual basis.

Nursing note:

Care of the donor (both adult or child) involves educating the donor, using appropriate techniques for age and cognitive level, in order to fully inform them of the donation procedure.

On return to the ward from the operating theatre the donor will require the same post-operative care as any patient after a general anaesthetic. Other specific post-operative care involves assessing the puncture sites for haemorrhage. If haemorrhage occurs it is usually slight and can be controlled with the application of pressure dressings to the puncture sites. Donors should be made aware that the skin incisions will result in scarring, although small and not visible during everyday life. The dressings covering the puncture sites can be removed after a few days and left exposed if the wound is clean and dry.

Discomfort is the most commonly reported side effect of donating marrow. Following donation, physical discomfort from the puncture sites may require oral analgesia for a few days and slight stiffness may be experienced on walking up stairs and, for adults, driving is reported to be difficult. Donors are advised to mobilise as soon as possible following donation, to prevent severe stiffness. For young children this is rarely a problem, though older patients whose bones are more dense than children may find mobilising quite difficult initially.

The donor is often fit enough to leave hospital the following day and rarely requires any further medical or nursing intervention. He or she may, however, feel a little lethargic as a result of the anaesthetic and should not return to work or school for a few days following the bone marrow collection.

On discharge from hospital, advice should be given on recognising the symptoms of complications that may need medical attention. Such problems may include persistent pain and signs of infection (discharge, pain and fever). Written documentation of the expected recovery time, signs and symptoms of complications and the telephone number of the person to contact, are useful and reinforce the verbal information given on discharge.

Complications of donation

The long term sequelae of unrelated adult donors are not well-documented. Most registries maintain contact and offer support to unrelated adult donors for a period of time after donation, this may be up to a year. Details of the welfare of the bone marrow recipient may be passed on in brief. In exceptional circumstances, the donor and the recipient may meet. In such cases both parties receive counselling to prepare for the emotional effects this may have. Complications following donation are very rare but reports exist of physical complications ranging from haematomas, to persistent back problems and continuing pain from the aspiration sites. In a study of 1270 donors, six life-threatening complications were reported, three of which were related to anaesthesia (Buckner et al., 1984).

Bone Marrow/Stem Cell Infusion

Harvested bone marrow will remain 'fresh' at room temperature for at least 72 hours but it should be infused as soon as both the marrow and the recipient are ready. Delays from time of harvest to infusion occur if the donor is much older and larger than the recipient or has a different blood group. In either of these cases the marrow will be plasma-depleted and the red cells removed. Alternatively, bone marrow from an unrelated donor may undergo a degree of T-cell depletion which may take several hours.

The aim of T-cell depletion of bone marrow is to remove the cells responsible for causing transplant-related complications, especially GVHD. In removing all the T-cells, however, the risk of graft rejection, or indeed the risk of leukaemic relapse is increased. It is for this reason that some transplant units either leave a residual amount of T-cells in the bag of bone marrow or remove a specific amount of T-cells and give them as an 'add back' prior to infusing a fully T-cell-depleted bone marrow.

Inevitably, the day on which the harvested bone marrow is infused is one of mixed emotions for all the family. There may be a sense of relief that the marrow has been safely harvested whether from a sibling or an unrelated donor, while there can be feelings of both optimism and trepidation about the actual infusion. If the marrow has been freshly harvested from a sibling, parents will want to spend time with both the donor and the recipient and may experience a swing of emotions relating to the situation of each child. Although the harvested marrow needs to be infused as soon as possible, if it is from a sibling donor both parents and the donor may need to be given some time to gather themselves and prepare for the next stage of the infusion itself.

Once the bone marrow arrives on the unit the recipient, donor and parents appreciate being able to see the bag of marrow before it is attached to the 'giving set'. However, seeing the bone marrow can be something of an anticlimax as it looks like a normal bag of blood, or in the case where the red cells are removed, the marrow is yellow and looks like platelets. None the less, it is not uncommon for the parents to take a photo of the donor holding the bag of bone marrow, to record this achievement. In a recent case a mother had difficulty in pinpointing exactly why she took photographs, but felt that it marked 'a new beginning'.

If the marrow has not undergone processing the child will not require any pre-medication. If there is an ABO incompatibility or a large volume of marrow, the marrow will have been red cell and/or plasma-depleted. A pre-medication of i.v. hydrocortisone and i.v. chlorpheniramine may be given to ensure any risk of reaction due to the processing is reduced. Depending upon the volume of the marrow to be infused, or the child's ability to cope with intravenous fluids, a diuretic may be necessary. If the child is to receive a T-cell 'add back' the cells can be given as a bolus followed by a 5–10 ml flush of 0.9% sodium chloride, ensuring none of the cells remains in the line. Following this the bag of marrow can be infused. The bag of marrow can be attached to a standard blood giving set and either set at a free-flow rate or infused via a pump to regulate the rate. Generally, the child will be 'specialled'. This will enable the nurse to record half-hourly readings of temperature, pulse, respiration and blood pressure. In addition, the nurse will be able to both support and act as a resource for the child and the parents during this emotional time. On completion of the infusion the marrow bag should be washed through with 0.9% i.v sodium chloride to ensure that all the cells have been infused through the bag and central line. If the infusion has occurred uneventfully the recordings of vital signs can return to four-hourly.

For patients who are to have bone marrow or stem cells (peripheral or umbilical cord) which have been harvested some time ago, both the procedure on the unit and the nursing implications are different. The bone marrow or stem cells will have been cryo-preserved in DMSO and prior to infusion the preserved bags of marrow or stem cells need to be thawed at 40° C in a large water bath. Ideally, this process should take place on the unit in order that time is not wasted in transportation after the preserved bags have been thawed. Once the bags are thawed, each bag should be infused over 15 minutes.

Before thawing the marrow or stem cells the child and parents must be prepared. Although cases of anaphylaxis, cardiac failure and arrythmias have been documented these are extremely rare (Davis et al., 1990b, cited in Patterson, 1993). Most of the side effects or reactions occur as a result of the DMSO. These may include nausea, vomiting, abdominal cramps, headache, hypo- or hypertension. These side effects can be minimised by ensuring the child has a pre-medication of i.v. hydrocortisone, chlorphrenamine, buscopan and ondansetron, 30 minutes prior to the infusion. In addition, some units recommend a regime of hyperhydration for several hours post-infusion.

Nursing note:

As the DMSO is broken down and excreted via the lungs an over-whelming smell of 'garlicky-sweetcorn' soon becomes apparent to everyone except the child who, instead, will have an extremely unpleasant taste in their mouth.Eating strong flavoured sweets, such as mints or cherry drops, will help to lessen this taste and it is worth having a good supply ready, out of the wrapper, before infusing the marrow.

On completion of the infusion the parents and the child need to be aware of the haemoglobinuria which can last up to 24 hours follow-ing the infusion so that they do not become worried about blood-stained urine. This is caused simply by the breakdown of old red blood cells. If the child feels well enough to drink, hyperhydration can be continued orally to prevent small-clot retention blocking the renal tubules.

The marrow infusion is generally a quick procedure and the record-ing of observations during the procedure is half-hourly. The child's general condition will alert the nurse as to how they are coping with the DMSO in the marrow.

Regardless of whether the bone marrow or stem cells are fresh or preserved, allogeneic or autologous, the family will generally have mixed feelings after the infusion, as they may have done prior to it. Although they may experience relief that the marrow has been infused safely and uneventfully, and the donor child, if there is one, is well, none the less they may turn their thoughts to the future and be concerned about what will happen next. Will, for example, the new marrow engraft successfully or will there be added complications? Might the disease return despite the BMT? Such concerns may well be at the forefront of their minds and the nurse has a vitally impor-tant role at this stage in providing both emotional and physical support.

Once the bone marrow has been infused it begins to migrate to the empty marrow spaces. From the day of the infusion, i.e. day 0 to approximately 14 days post-infusion, the child is most vulnerable to infection. From day 14 onwards, circulating neutrophils start appearing and generally, by day 28, engraftment has occurred with a neutrophil count greater than $1.0 \times 10^9/l$. Thus, during the first two weeks post-infusion the child has no functioning immunity and the expert assessment and care given by the BMT nurse, with medical interventions, should prevent overwhelming complications.

Chapter 10
The neutropenic phase

Nikki Bennett-Rees and Louise Soanes

Introduction

The consequences of life-threatening infections remain the major cause of morbidity and mortality in patients undergoing BMT. There are three distinct phases, depending upon the child's immune recovery, where they are at risk from the wide range of microbiological pathogens (Barnes, 1992a, b):

- The neutropenic phase (days 0–28)
- The post-engraftment phase (days 28–100)
- The late phase (day 100 onwards).

The main sources of infection are either environmental or from staff/parents (exogenous), or from the child's own skin and gut flora (endogenous).

The child will be at most risk during the neutropenic phase, when a period of physical isolation is required. In order to prevent exposure to exogenous sources of infection many BMT units advocate the use of laminar air flow (LAF) with or without the use of high-efficiency particulate air (HEPA) filtration. The use of these two systems should remove most bacterial and fungal spores from the air. For units in cities and where building work is ongoing, the use of LAF and HEPA filtration will have an effect on reducing the risk of infection with *Aspergillus* (Fenelon, 1995). It could be argued therefore that for children undergoing BMT who will have a prolonged episode of neutropenia (such as SCID or unrelated donor transplants) use of LAF and HEPA filtration is essential during the neutropenic phase. There is no evidence to show that LAF and HEPA filtration decreases the incidence of fever post-transplant or, indeed, the occurrence of acute GVHD. However, in units that combine LAF/HEPA filtration with skin and gut decontamination regimes, there appears to be a 'lower incidence of early infectious' problems (Skinh et al., 1987) (Figure 10.1).

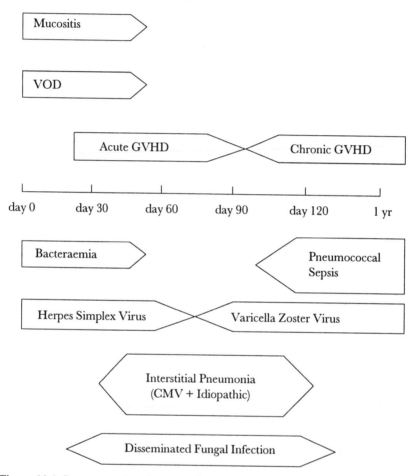

Figure 10.1: Sequence of major complications after allogeneic bone marrow transplant from day 0 (Source: Press, Schaller & Thomas, 1986, cited by Groenwald et al., 1992)

Infection Prophylaxis

The assessment and care needed to prevent infections during the neutropenic phase is a major concern for nurses. Infection prophylaxis is aimed at the prevention of fungal, viral and bacterial infections. Measures taken to prevent these three common types of infection in the child undergoing BMT include:

- Use of an air filtration system such as LAF or HEPA
- Restricting the number of people allowed into the isolation room
- Encouraging the child to cooperate and comply with oral medication, diet restrictions, mouth and skin care.

Although the environment may be protected by one or both of the filtration systems there is a need for additional environmental measures. These will include a daily cleaning programme, though it is sufficient to both 'damp dust' the surfaces and clean the floors using a new cloth and hot water with an appropriate detergent. Terminal cleaning need only be carried out on discharge or pre-admission of a child. Fresh flowers and plants must be avoided as both are sources of fungal and bacterial spores and their water is likely to harbour *Pseudomonas* (Barnes, 1992a, b).

Protective isolation

The issue of what constitutes protective precautions varies widely between units, not only throughout the UK but also throughout 91 BMT centres in the USA (Poe et al., 1994; Dunleavy, 1996). The type of precautions carried out will depend upon the physical ameni-ties available and whether the unit is a dedicated BMT unit, as opposed to one which is integrated with another speciality.

Exogenous infections come not only from airborne bacterial and fungal spores but are also transmitted on the hands and clothes of staff and parents (Barnes, 1992a, b). There are therefore some fundamental principles of protective precautions which must be adhered to regardless of unit specifications:

- Scrupulous hand washing and drying (Laison & Lusk, 1985; Gould, 1991; Fenelon, 1995).
- Use of a clean plastic apron on entering an isolation room; the apron must be changed when soiled (Pinkerton et al., 1994; Fenelon, 1995).

These two simple but essential precautions lay down the basis for good practice in nursing the child undergoing BMT. In addition, water (which is a common carrier of *Pseudomonas*) and food can trans-mit a multitude of infections with potentially serious implications for the child post-BMT (Barnes, 1992a, b; Fenelon, 1995).

Certain foods have high microbial loads, such as uncooked foods:

soft or raw eggs carry salmonella; soft cheeses carry listeria; pepper and spices carry bacteria and fungi; unpeeled fruit and salad carry *Pseudomonas*. Perhaps the most effective way to protect the child is the use of oral antibiotics to ensure gut sterilisation and by offering a sterile diet. Unfortunately, once the food has been irradiated to render it sterile, it often tastes unpleasant. Attempts to make children eat such unappetising food can lead to increasing stress for parents and the child. In a situation where the child is already reluctant to take oral medications, especially when they have severe mucositis, the pressure to take additional oral antibiotics is too great. Added to this is the risk of the child developing resistance to antibiotics. It is therefore recommended that it is sufficient for food to be freshly prepared and for the child to finish eating it before it has become cold. As water is a known carrier of *Pseudomonas*, it is good practice to provide the child with bottled sterile water both for drinking and teeth-cleaning.

Nursing note:

Although bottled sterile water has a 'plastic' taste, if it is cold and squash is added it will taste like 'normal' squash.

The more difficult infections to eliminate are the endogenous ones from the child's own skin and gut flora. As all children have a central line *in situ*, both the entrance site and the handling of the line present an ideal source for infection. In addition, with young children who explore with their fingers, the transference of infection from toys and scratched 'bottoms' to the mouth is a problem that appears to be unresolvable.

The restrictions necessary to care for the child under protective precautions must be both manageable and adhere to safe practice. It would be of great interest for a national working party to research this area and produce guidelines on the amount of protection needed by children undergoing allogeneic BMT. Thus, the implications for nursing children both pre- and during BMT will concern anticipating, reducing and treating infections before they become overwhelming.

Excessive numbers of toys, games and videos in the room should be discouraged, as they often sit on the floor/surfaces and collect dust. It helps the child to have a system whereby toys and games can be rotated to lessen the boredom. Generally, toys and games should either be washable, such as Lego® and Duplo®, or nearly new, as with books and games. Soft toys that the child may need should also be new or (in the case of the favourite teddy) should be washed and tumble-dried.

Nursing note:

If the soft toy is placed inside a pillow case when being tumble-dried, the rubber nose and glass eyes will remain intact.

Restrictions on visitors and staff will depend upon unit policy. Restrictions on the number of visitors allowed to enter the room or, indeed, the unit may be in place, but also taken into account will be the age and health of visitors. It should be mandatory that no one enters the isolation room if they have a cold, sore throat, are coughing, have diarrhoea and/or vomiting, have a cold sore or conjunctivitis. It may be argued that wearing a mask will give protection to the child from the infected person, but greater safety is provided if people with such afflictions do not enter the room. None the less, there are units where the wearing of masks as part of the isolation precautions is the norm. Again, it may be argued that the benefit of wearing a mask is heavily outweighed by the detrimental effect on the well-being of the child. In one unit the wearing of masks was abolished when a deaf child who could only lipread was admitted for BMT.

There does not appear to be adequate data to determine absolutely whether siblings should be allowed to visit. It is believed that school-aged children are more likely to bring a variety of viral infections, including chickenpox, and refusing school-age visitors entry to the isolation room appears to be a sound precaution. However, allowing children, especially the patient's siblings, into the unit to speak through an intercom link will both reduce the mystery of the BMT procedure and help to maintain the sibling relationship. The balance between the child's psychological needs and the increased risk of infection from a variety of people entering the room (or indeed the unit) needs to be carefully assessed in the formulation of the unit policy.

Finally, whatever the unit policy, it should be adhered to in order to prevent inter-family friction if different 'rules' apply to different families.

To continue to protect the child there are a number of prophylactic medications now used both pre-, during and post-BMT (Table 10.1).

Table 10.1: Drug therapy related to infection prophylaxis	
Drug therapy	Prophylaxis against
Antimicrobials	
cotrimoxazole (oral)	*Pneumocystis carinii* pneumonitis
ciprofloxacin (oral)	Gram-negative bacterial infections
Antiviral	
acyclovir (i.v./oral)	cytomegalovirus (CMV)
	varicella zoster virus (VZV)
Antifungals	
itraconazole (oral)	Aspergillus
fluconazole (oral)	Candida
amphotericin (oral/inhalation)	Candida, Aspergillus
nystatin (oral)	Candida
Others	
immunoglobulin (i.v.)	to improve post-transplant immunity
granulocyte colony stimulating factor (G-CSF) (i.v.)	reduces the length of the neutropenic phase

The effectiveness of prophylactic therapies depends upon the compliance of the child. Often, pre-transplant the child is able to comply, but unfortunately, as nausea and vomiting followed by mucositis occurs, compliance weakens. Not only is the child feeling miserable and ill but non-compliance may be the only form of control they have.

Nursing note:

To help the child continue with as many oral drugs as possible in a stress free manner, the use of a sticker chart is often recommended. It is also helpful to award a sticker for each painful procedure, such as mouth care, peripheral blood sampling, or taking oral medications. Once an agreed amount of stickers has been achieved, the child has a 'dip' in a treasure chest which is filled with amusing novelty toys and games.

The teenager will require a different approach to younger children and there is nothing to be achieved by using the seriousness of their condition to frighten them into compliance (Blotcky et al., 1985). If treated in a mature way, and explanations are provided with patience and clarity at the commencement of treatment and maintained throughout treatment, compliance should be more realistically achieved. Hopefully, if the child's pain is well-controlled and he or she feels well-supported by both parents and staff, the days when oral medications are missed will be minimal.

Dietary restrictions

Most children undergoing BMT stop eating as a result of nausea and/or vomiting following conditioning therapy, mucositis, feeling generally unwell, or because eating can become an issue over which they can exercise control in a situation where otherwise they have little or none. In addition, alterations in taste and smell (McDonnell-Keenan, 1989; Hanigan & Walter, 1992) or the onset of GVHD can cause further nutritional problems. During the BMT period both pre- and post-transplant, adequate nutritional support is vital to maintain target weight and, indeed, prevent weight loss. There is a belief that good nutrition may help to lessen the occurrence of severe acute GVHD (Gauvreau et al., 1981). As discussed earlier, the type of oral diet, whether sterile or low microbial, will depend on the unit policy. The child who is unable to maintain an adequate oral intake will require nutritional support. Nutritional support can be achieved either via enteral tube feeding or through total parenteral nutrition (TPN) via a central line. Enteral feeding has a vital role to play in nutritional support, both pre- and post-transplant and in the recovery of the child post-engraftment. During the first three to four weeks post-transplant, when the child is at greatest risk of infection, bleeding, oesophageal/oral mucositis as well as nausea, vomiting and diarrhoea, the passing and use of a nasogastric tube may exacerbate these problems. Therefore nutritional support is best achieved with the use of TPN. It has been noted that this method is particularly beneficial for children under the age of ten years (Souchon, 1992). Nevertheless TPN is not without potential problems, the two most common being an increased risk of infection and fluid overload.

Nursing note:

Maintain asepsis when handling the TPN lines. Avoid breaking the line for infusing blood products or blood sampling. Adjust TPN flow rates if additional fluids, such as drugs or blood products, are given via a second lumen so to avoid fluid overload. Daily urine testing for glycosuria. Daily monitoring for blood sugar levels.

The aim should be for the TPN to be concentrated and infused over 20 hours to enable the child, if well, to have a few hours 'off the lines'. As the child recovers and the mucositis resolves so their appetite will slowly recover. Equally, as the child's oral intake improves, the TPN rates and length of infusion can be decreased, allowing the child more time 'off the lines'. Following consultation with the dietician, food and drinks can be fortified if necessary thus enabling a high calorie intake. By approximately six weeks post-BMT, most children will have recovered their sense of taste and, in addition, when the child is discharged home and resumes a family life and home cooking, diet and fluid intake appear to return to normal.

For the very young child or baby who may have had long periods of reduced oral intake, the use of enteral tube feeding is beneficial to ensure that the child's nutritional and fluid requirements are met.

For the child who wants to eat there are some dietary restrictions which will have been decided upon by the unit staff in conjunction with the microbiologist and dietician. Foods that are excluded are those with high microbial loads, as mentioned previously. For children who are able to continue to eat portions of food, they should be of the right size to enable them to finish what they are given. Sometimes this might mean very small portions served on a small plate. The advantage of having a diet-cook employed to prepare meals for children undergoing BMT is that it allows the children to have some choice and therefore control over their diet. The cook will be able to discuss with the children and the parents the type of food and size of portion that will tempt them to eat. Many children appear to have an increased appetite in the evening and, in order to boost their calorie intake and satisfy their needs, it should be possible to make snacks for the child on the unit. Whatever the meal or snack the child, especially if young, will often want to eat with their fingers. There is no harm in this as long as the hands are thoroughly washed and dried before eating.

Mouth care

To ensure that the mouth, skin and especially the perineum, is kept at its healthiest, frequent mouth and skin care regimes need to be commenced on admission. Before admission for BMT, at one of the outpatient sessions, the child will have had a full dental assessment to identify and correct any problems such as dental caries or teeth which may need extracting. If treatment is needed, antibiotic cover is given to prevent colonisation of the central line with dental organisms and treatment given as far from the transplant day as possible. During the inpatient period the aim of mouth care is prophylaxis.

Mucositis, however (discussed further in Chapter 11), is almost a universal problem in patients undergoing BMT; mucositis appears to be more severe in patients who have been given methotrexate as part of GVHD prophylaxis.

To help prevent, or at least lessen, the impact of mucositis, the nurse's role is to ensure that thorough mouth care is carried out. Whilst the child's gums remain healthy and the platelet count is adequate, the following regime can be used. Teeth-cleaning using a 'favourite' brand of toothpaste with a soft-headed baby toothbrush followed by a chlorhexidine-based mouthwash with or without an oral antifungal agent to follow (Beck, 1992). For babies with no teeth the use of specially made foam sticks soaked in chlorhexidine replaces the toothbrush. The use of chlorhexidine mouth wash as an agent which can reduce the severity of mucositis (Ferreti et al., 1987) is debatable. Some researchers have found side effects, such as gingival bleeding and epithelial desquamation, to limit patient tolerance (Ainamo et al., 1982). To help prevent dental caries a once-daily dose of fluoride has been found to be beneficial (Gordon, 1983; Beck, 1992).

Skin care

A daily bath or shower promotes skin care. Damp flannels and sponges encourage the growth of *Pseudomonas* so the child must be given a new disposable washcloth at each bathtime. The use of commercial bars or liquid soaps should be avoided as they can cause further drying of the skin which is already affected by the chemoradiotherapy used during conditioning. The use of antimicrobial soaps or lotions on the skin followed by the use of antibacterial creams to various parts of the body may be standard practice. However, it is sufficient to ensure that the skin is bathed daily and kept supple to prevent drying. To prevent the skin from becoming dry, an oil such as oilatum should be used in the bath, followed by the application of an unperfumed moisturiser, such as diprobase, once the skin is dry. Whilst drying and then applying the cream, the parent and/or nurse will be able to observe the child for bruises, spots/rashes, scratches and the general healthiness of the skin. Particular attention must be given to children who still wear nappies to prevent breakdown of the skin in the nappy area. Nappies must be changed 1–2-hourly (especially during conditioning) to prevent excreted chemotherapy damaging the skin. With each nappy change the perineum can be cleaned using cotton wool and water, but if the area looks red and painful the use of an oil (instead of water) for cleaning is more soothing. Once clean, an effective barrier cream, such as a mixture of metanium and white soft paraffin, must be applied. The use of sucralfate to any broken areas of skin on the perineum has been shown to be effective in preventing further damage to the skin.

Nursing note:

The use of urine bags on children who have delicate or broken patches of skin should be avoided to prevent breakdown of the area. To collect a specimen of urine either place sterile cotton wool balls in the nappy or leave the nappy off and sit the child over a potty on the parent's or the nurse's lap and entertain the child until successful!

Specific skin care needs to be applied to the Hickman line exit/entry site. This care generally comprises cleaning the site with an antiseptic solution, drying it and then re-dressing with a transparent permeable dressing, such as Opsite 3000. This care should be maintained weekly unless the dressing is wet, is falling off or there is a problem with the entry/exit site looking infected (Maki, 1991).

Screening of stools and urine should be carried out once or twice per week. Swabs from the nose, throat and Hickman line exit site as well as any lesions on the lips, mouth or skin, should also be taken as indicated. Most children dislike having their nose and throat swabbed. If the child is taught how to carry out the sampling, he or she can do their own at a time when they are ready. Alternatively, if the parents wish to take on this 'nursing' role for their child they too can be taught and can undertake this procedure for as long as they wish to do so.

The Effects of Isolation

The protective precautions required to care for a child undergoing BMT result in the parents and child being isolated from other members of their family. In addition, the separation from previous support networks, including school friends, as well as the loss of freedom places a heavy burden on the whole family. It is therefore essential to work out strategies by which to lessen the impact of isolation.

To achieve a semblance of normal life the isolation room should be furnished with a television, video player, radio/cassette player and telephone. These items alone will help the family and friends to keep in contact with what is happening. Home-made videos and tapes from family and friends can often be a great source of support and amusement. Personal effects, such as photos, books and hobbies, for both the child and the parents are essential items which must go into the isolation room. Precisely which items may be taken into the isolation room will depend on individual unit policy. Items such as letters and cards can be taken out of their envelopes and taken into the room, postcards can also be taken in and used to brighten up the walls. Both cards and postcards can brighten up the clinical room, and more importantly, help maintain contact with home. However, it is not uncommon for staff to misinterpret which items may potentially be seen as an infection risk to the child. If staff are unsure, the parents may be misinformed or, worse, may receive conflicting information.

Nursing note:

In order to help staff to provide accurate information, the use of a short quiz covering areas such as isolation technique, diet restrictions, 'step down' precautions and psychosocial issues, can help to keep the changing workforce up to date with current practice on the unit.

For children of school age a daily visit from the unit school teacher will become routine. School sessions are planned around the child's ability to participate in a session. For babies, similar sessions with a physiotherapist may be appropriate. This is particularly important in infants with SCID who may have had long periods of hospitalisation prior to BMT. The work of the physiotherapist will help the infant to reach the normal developmental milestones.

The play specialist plays a major role in ensuring that a 'normal' atmosphere is maintained for all children in isolation and provides play to achieve developmental goals by ensuring that the physical, intellectual, language, emotional and social development of the child in isolation is maintained or enhanced. Physical development may be the most difficult to achieve due to the confines of space. Any activity which combines exercise and play, such as skittles, mini-snooker and basketball, gives both stimulation and enjoyment thus helping to lessen the feelings of boredom and isolation. It is crucial for play specialists and nursing staff to work well together and for nurses and doctors to avoid interrupting play sessions with medical/nursing activities.

Children who are old enough can be encouraged to write letters to school friends thus starting up a communication link which keeps friends and family in touch. Parents, especially if one parent is the main resident carer, can also be encouraged to keep a diary of life in isolation. This will help them, when discharged, to re-live their feelings and describe to the family at home what happened each day.

Some families also encourage siblings and other family members 'at home' to keep a similar concurrent diary. The respective experiences can then be joined and shared after discharge. For parents caring for their child in isolation life can become a round of 'nursing', entertaining and washing clothes. To relieve this stress they should be encouraged to have 'time out', especially when the teacher, play therapist or nurse is with their child. Families who are able to take turns at being resident often appear less overwhelmed by the isolation. Although initially relieved from the restrictions of isolation and having to manage their sick child's day the parents may remain anxious about their child when not with them (Darbyshire, 1994). None the less, one of the main feelings for both children and parents in isolation is the loss of control. By negotiating the daily schedule for nursing, play, and education with the parent and child, and encouraging participation in care and planning, the family will be able to regain a degree of control. This, it is hoped, will at least lessen the feeling of helplessness in such a restrictive environment (Abramovitz & Senner, 1995).

Chapter 11
Complications of bone marrow transplant

Nikki Bennett-Rees and Louise Soanes

Introduction

The complications described here are those that most commonly occur in the transplant period, days 0–100, and therefore include the neutropenic and post-engraftment phases. Most occur as a direct result of the ablative chemotherapy and radiotherapy used in conditioning the child for transplant. Complications rarely occur in isolation and signs and symptoms often overlap. The nurse's role in the prevention, early detection and management of these complications is discussed as they are often called upon to coordinate the care of these acutely sick children while offering support and education to the child and family. Good management of these complications has a direct impact on the successful outcome of BMT.

Mucositis

One of the predictable side effects of BMT is mucositis. The use of high-dose chemotherapy agents, such as cyclophosphamide, melphalan and TBI, gives rise to widespread gastrointestinal mucosal damage. This damage may be further compounded by the use of methotrexate in the prevention of GVHD.

Stomatitis first occurs within 7–10 days of conditioning and may last for 14 days (Kanfer, 1993). It can cause pain, ulcerations leading to bleeding and infection, taste alterations, and xerostomia which inevitably result in poor nutritional intake. This can have physical and psychological implications for the child.

A quantitative assessment of the oral mucosa is necessary and provides documentation of the onset, severity and resolution of mucositis (Zerbe, 1992). An established oral assessment guide to ensure uniformity of assessment within the unit should be used. Many of these exist (Eilers et al., 1988; Beck, 1979). These assessment guides use numerical and descriptive data to assess the level of stomatitis and the effect on the patient. In order to be successful the chosen model should be user friendly and staff should be educated to ensure compliance and reliable use.

Nursing note:

Xerostomia is often due to TBI, older children may find relief in sucking chips of ice or sucking ice lollies or hard sweets. Small frequent warm drinks are easier to swallow than ice-cold ones if stomatitis extends to the oesophagus, as will frequently be the case.

The loss of mucosal integrity can lead to infections both locally and systemically. Most units initiate prophylactic antifungal and antiviral agents; with the loss of the ability to swallow, these may temporarily need to be administered intravenously until the mucosa recovers, along with the establishment of white cell recovery approximately two weeks following bone marrow infusion.

The treatment of mucositis aims to offer physical support to the patient and prevention of complications.

The physical risks of stomatitis due to immunosuppression and infection account for some of the morbidity associated with BMT patients (Ezzone et al.,1993) as the loss of the epitheal lining of the mucosa provides a portal of entry for microorganisms into the systemic circulation and may result in life-threatening infections (Zerbe, 1992).

Psychologically, the loss of comfort from thumb and dummy sucking can be distressing for small children and alternative methods of comfort may be sought by the child, such as holding the dummy, or alternative comfort measures found (attachment to soft toys). It is often the case that once the mucositis subsides the child reverts to the previous use of dummies and thumbs. Loss of verbal communication as the mouth becomes too sore to speak can be distressing for the school-aged child. Although alternative measures such as writing may be successful at first, as the child becomes weaker, these may be abandoned and the use of nods and shakes of the head for simple questions may be all that is tolerated. Loss of self-image due to inability to swallow saliva can distress the older child who may perceive dribbling and spitting into tissues embarrassing. The maintenance of privacy for the child in this instance is paramount.

For the child, pain is likely to be the worst symptom associated with an ulcerated mucosa of the gastrointestinal tract and this is often the first symptom reported by the child before the visible signs of mucosal damage appear. At first pain is often associated with swallowing, sleeping (due to mouth breathing) and speaking, progressing to continuous pain, often requiring the use of opiates to provide adequate analgesia.

As the mucositis progresses gastrointestinal manifestations emerge. Again, pain is often the first indicator of mucosal ulceration and nausea, vomiting and diarrhoea commonly occur. Due to the severity and frequency of diarrhoea, peri-anal excoriation and ulceration can occur, especially in small children and babies who wear nappies. The older child will find frequent diarrhoea and the dependence on others for toileting embarrassing and involving altered perceptions of body image. The recently toilet trained child may return to nappy-wearing in protest.

Treatment and nursing implications

Oral hygiene

Oral hygiene, although unable to prevent stomatitis, can help lessen its severity and prevent infection. The method, frequency and evaluation of oral hygiene will vary from unit to unit. Oral hygiene should be initiated during the first few days of hospital admission for the transplant. This allows the child and the family to become familiar with the unit's chosen methods and allows the child time to adapt to new ways of cleaning teeth. The use of play specialists to familiarise the child with toothbrushes, foam sticks and mouth inspections should be assessed on an individual basis. The child's developmental stage will be crucial to the success of this process.

Nursing note:

The use of chlorhexedine-based mouthwashes reduces oral soft tissue disease and decreases the Candida and microbial burden (Ferretti et al., 1987). Avoid commercial mouthwashes as they may dry and irritate the mucosa. Chlorhexedine mouthwashes can be painful and, as stomatitis and ulceration progress, encourage compliance and positive reinforcement of oral hygiene with the use of sticker charts, etc. Allow parents to opt out of this role as it becomes more difficult for the child so as to reduce stress for them. Toothbrushes remove plaque and food debris from the gum line. Soft-headed baby toothbrushes are best used by children whose platelet and white cell counts are suppressed. The toothbrush may be kept for a 24-hour period and then disposed of to prevent the risk of infection. The care of lips and the products used to prevent drying and cracking, again, varies from unit to unit, though petroleum jelly is still the most common lubricant (Ezzone et al., 1993).

Diarrhoea

Diarrhoea is a common early symptom of mucosal ulceration of the lower gastrointestinal tract. The greatest risk to the child is infection due to loss of mucosal integrity and damage to the peri-anal skin area as a result of frequent diarrhoea. Routine stool specimens will isolate pathogens and allow the early instigation of treatment. The collection of these stool specimens is often combined in the surveillance screening undertaken during the pancytopenic phase following BMT and reports of abdominal pain, fever and abdominal tenderness should be investigated rigorously.

Alterations in nutritional status

As mucositis progresses and the child's oral intake diminishes, reduction in nutritional status leading to weight loss will occur. The recognition of this has led some units to instigate prophylactic TPN at an early stage in the transplant (Graham et al., 1993). On recovery of the child's white cell count and the resolution of mucositis poor nutritional intake may persist; the involvement and support of a dietician will be needed to ensure adequate calorie intake following BMT. This may involve continuing supportive measures, such as nasogastric tube feeds or high energy sip feeds, after discharge from the BMT unit.

Nursing note:

Prepare the family and the child for the loss of appetite and slow recovery following BMT. Educate the family of the need for TPN. Monitor blood glucose and fluid overload on instigation of TPN. Involve the dietician to maintain maximum oral intake before mucositis prevents oral intake and on recovery. Weigh the child daily during acute phase, scales being kept in the child's room prevents cross-infection. On discharge, encourage parents to weigh the child no more than twice a week to reduce parental anxiety. Prepare the family and child for taste alterations. Provide oral hygiene as unit policy.

Pain

Pain is experienced by the child during BMT for a variety of reasons. Veno-occlusive disease, mucositis, procedures and GVHD can all be a cause of pain. Adequate evaluation is vital to ensure a successful outcome with a child in pain; evaluation not only of the level of the child's pain but also of the interventions and assessment applied to treating the pain.

A variety of assessment tools are available for measuring children's pain: CHEOPS (McGarth et al., 1985); the *Faces Scale* (Wong & Baker, 1988) and *The Eland Color Scale* (Eland, 1988). Whichever tool is used it must be reliable, provide consistent information, be user friendly and be appropriate for the child's cognitive level.

The choice of appropriate pain control often follows the World Health Organization (WHO) ladder approach to cancer pain (Patterson, 1992). However, individual unit guidelines vary and the initial use of analgesics such as paracetamol may be avoided as their antipyretic effect may be perceived as masking the signs of infection. Often, as the cause of the child's pain progresses and the pain worsens a step-up approach to analgesia is needed leading to the use of opiates as effective control of the child's pain.

The use of opiates for pain control in BMT is often necessary, particularly for controlling the pain associated with mucositis. These drugs may be administered intravenously or subcutaneously according to unit policy. The use of patient-controlled analgesia pumps (PCA) in older children provides both adequate pain relief and some degree of patient control (Gureno & Reisinger, 1991), an important factor for older children during BMT when so much surrounding this procedure is beyond their control.

Nursing note:

Prepare the family and child that pain may occur. Educate them about the unit's methods for assessing and treating pain. Anticipate and prepare for pain; early intervention. Adequate staff education is essential, as is the use of paediatric self-report pain assessment tools. Monitor pain relief measures accurately. Liaise with pain control teams. Produce a written evaluation of pain control. Offer local as well as systemic pain relief. Apply age and distraction therapy. Support the child and the family whilst the child is in pain.

Nausea and Vomiting

Nausea and vomiting in the transplant child is often the result of the chemotherapy and radiotherapy used in the conditioning of the child. This is often expected and prophylactic antiemetics should be given in accordance with the unit's policy. Following the expected nausea and vomiting associated with the use of radiotherapy or chemotherapy these symptoms frequently persist in the

BMT child. This can be for a variety of reasons, namely infection, pain due to mucositis, GVHD, veno-occlusive disease, TPN and swallowing of oral secretions. Multiple-drug therapy used to control these other symptoms includes antibiotics, and morphine can also give rise to nausea and vomiting.

Nursing note:

Vomiting
Initially this may be well-controlled with 5HT antagonists such as ondansetron. This may continue to be useful in controlling vomiting, although other agents may need to be added. Metoclopramide (both oral and i.v.) and cyclizine have been beneficial. Support for the child and family is vital. Vomiting is distressing for both the child and family. It can cause further damage to already fragile oral mucosa and, if the platelet count is low, bleeding can occur from the mucus membranes and petechial bleeds may occur especially around the eyes. The parents and child should be informed that this may occur. Monitor input/output and fluid balance accurately. Monitor electrolyte balance.

Nausea
This is a subjective feeling which is difficult for the child to describe and thus difficult to relieve. Avoid exposing the child to the smell of known causes of nausea (e.g. food, perfume). Intravenous antibiotics are a common cause of nausea due to the heightened sense of smell following chemotherapy and the powerful odour that these drugs exude. Inform the child of when such drugs are to be given and allow time for distraction to take place, some children find smelling soap or comforters help. Sucking sweets or infusing rather than injecting antibiotics can prevent the taste distortion that some children experience.

Pancytopenia

Following infusion of bone marrow or stem cells the child will be at considerable risk from both infectious and haemorrhagic complications. These two complications are as a result of the myelo-ablative therapy used in the conditioning regimes of either chemotherapy alone or chemoradiotherapy with, in the allogeneic setting, the use of further immunosuppressive therapy such as cyclosporin. Furthermore the occurrence of GVHD and its treatment will cause increased immunosuppression for the child.

Infection

The risk from the wide range of infections occurs at three distinct phases and coincides with the child's haematological and immunological recovery post-transplant (Wujcik et al., 1994; Veys & Hann 1997). The three phases for infection are:

- Neutropenic phase
- Post-engraftment phase
- Late phase.

The neutropenic phase lasts approximately 21 days post-BMT and occurs with the worst of the mucosal lining of the entire gastrointestinal tract. The post-engraftment phase lasts from approximately days 30 to 100 post-BMT.

Late-phase infections occur from day 100 and may last until immune recovery occurs at 1–2 years post-BMT. However, if the child is treated for chronic GVHD, recovery of T-cell function will be further delayed so the risk of infection may become a long term problem.

During the neutropenic phase the child is at risk from a wide spectrum of infections (Table 11.1). Prophylactic treatment varies between units, however the treatment for febrile neutropenia or proven infection appears to be universally very similar. Once the child's axillary temperature reaches the level for antibiotic commencement (as decided upon by the unit but generally 38–38.5°C) a first-line broad spectrum antibiotic regime is commenced which will cover both Gram-negative and Gram-positive bacteria. Additional antibiotic, antiviral or antifungal therapy will be commenced according to:

- The child's clinical condition
- The child's response to first-line antibiotics
- The results of various cultures and X-rays
- The results of the C-reactive protein level (CRP) (Barnes, 1992a, b).

The addition of recombinant G-CSF, which is a naturally occurring hormone, has been included in the drug regime post-BMT (Singer, 1992), although clear benefit to the use of growth factors following allogeneic BMT has yet to be demonstrated. G-CSF is given intravenously once a day (commencing between day 1 and day 8 post-transplant, depending upon the unit) to boost early bone marrow engraftment. An early marrow engraftment reduces the length of time the child is neutropenic, therefore reducing the risk of neutropenic fever and infections. There is a direct correlation between the length of time the child is neutropenic and the acquisition of a fungal infection such as Aspergillus (Barnes, 1992a, b).

Table 11.1: Infectious complications post-bone marrow transplant		
Phase	Infection	Organism
Neutropenic (days 0–21)	Gram-positive bacteria	*Staphylococcus epidermidis*, *Staphylococcus aureus*
	Gram-negative bacteria	*Pseudomonas aeruginosa*, *Escherichia coli*
	Fungal	*Candida albicans*, Aspergillus
	Viral	*Herpes simplex* (HSV), Rota virus
Post-engraftment (days 30–100)	Viral	Cytomegalovirus (CMV), Adenovirus, *Pneumoncystis carinii*
Late (day 100+)	Viral	*Varicella zoster* (VZV)
	Encapsulated bacterial organisms	*Streptococcus pneumoniae*, *Haemophilus influenzae*

Sources: Barnes (1992a, b), Wujick et al. (1994), Veys & Hann (1997).

Haematological complications

Haemorrhagic problems can initially occur during conditioning therapy pre-transplant as a result of the use of high-dose i.v. cyclophosphamide. Acrolein, a harmful metabolite of cyclophosphamide, causes bladder toxicity which may result in haemorrhagic cystitis. The resulting haematuria can range from microscopic, demonstrated on multistix testing, to the child having frank blood loss with clots, urinary retention and pain. Therefore, the goal is to prevent haemorrhagic cystitis and this is achieved by infusing mesna with the cyclophosphamide. Mesna is a drug which is activated by urine and works by binding to the acrolein thus helping to inactivate its toxicity. In addition, the child will need a regime of i.v. hyperhydration and be encouraged to pass urine frequently. At ward level, each urine sample must be tested for blood. If the sample is positive, measures such as increasing the amount of mesna and/or the rate of the hydration can be taken. In the event of severe haemorrhagic cystitis occurring, treatment measures may include the continuation of hydration fluids and bladder irrigation. In conjunction with this, the child's haemoglobin and platelet counts must be maintained at an adequate level. As haemorrhagic cystitis can also be a late occurring problem a daily urinalysis should be performed.

Transfusions of both blood and platelets will be necessary until the donor marrow becomes fully engrafted and functional. The level at which the child will need transfusing will depend on both the BMT unit's policy and the child's condition. For example, a haemoglobin of 8 g/dl or a platelet count of $20 \times 10^9/l$ or less should be transfused. However, a child with an infection, fever or an existing clotting problem may need to have a platelet count maintained at $50 \times 10^9/l$ or higher.

Whatever the unit's policy regarding the level at which the child must be transfused, it is essential that both the blood and platelets are irradiated and CMV-negative. By irradiating these two products the lymphocytes within them will be destroyed and therefore unable to cause an immune response in the child, thus preventing the child developing transfusional GVHD.

Nursing note:

Ensure the safety of connections of i.v. lines. Monitor daily full blood counts and twice-weekly clotting screen. Monitor the child's temperature. Perform daily urinalysis for blood. Observe all stools for gastrointestinal bleeding. Observe the child for any petechiae or bleeding. Observe the mouth for bleeding gums. Use a soft-headed toothbrush or foam sticks to lessen trauma to gums. Assess blood loss during nosebleeds. Administer blood and platelets according to unit policy. Assess the child for reactions to either product and administer i.v. chlorpheniramine and i.v. hydrocortisone if indicated.

CMV which can be transmitted in blood products is the main cause of morbidity and death in patients treated with allogeneic bone marrow. In the UK approximately 40–50% of the adult population is CMV-positive. For the CMV-negative child who receives marrow from a CMV-negative donor, it is essential that CMV-negative products are given. For a child who is CMV-positive or whose donor is CMV-positive, the ideal situation would also be to transfuse CMV-negative products although no additional benefit has been shown in this situation. If there is a shortage of CMV-negative products the use of a leukocyte filter for blood or platelet transfusions (the virus is transmitted through leukocytes) will greatly reduce the risk of transmitting CMV.

Graft Versus Host Disease

GVHD is a reaction of donor cells to histocompatible differences between the donor and the host (Witherspoon & Storb, 1993). GVHD was a major complication in the early days of BMT (Barrett, 1993) and today it continues to be a complication of allogeneic transplants. This situation is likely to continue with the increasing use of unrelated and mismatched donors.

Originally, GVHD was seen as a T-cell-mediated disease, brought about by infiltration of effector cells into target tissues with their resultant destruction (Treleaven & Barrett, 1993). It has now been shown that the situation is far more complex with involvement of natural killer (NK) cells, macrophages and cytokines (Witherspoon & Storb, 1993).

Cytokines are produced in response to the conditioning regime prior to marrow re-infusion. The release of inflammatory cytokines such as tumour necrosis factor (TNF) and interleukin 1 (IL-1) increases the HLA expression and upregulates the immune response. This enhances the recognition of donor histocompatibility by the donor T-cells. The activated T-cells proliferate and secrete cytokines, mainly interleukin 2 (IL-2), which in turn activates more donor T-cells and mononuclear cells. This is the afferent pathway of GVHD. The mononuclear cells are induced to produce IL-2 and TNF which again stimulates further T-cell activity. In this way a positive feed-back loop is initiated amplifying the immune response and increasing tissue damage. The individual contribution of lymphocytes, macrophages and cytokines in mediating tissue damage during the efferent phase of GVHD remains unknown (Veys & Hann, 1997). The resulting damage is focused on the rapidly dividing cells of the epithelium, gastrointestinal tract and liver.

The diagnosis of GVHD is usually clinical, however skin, gut or liver biopsy may be used to confirm diagnosis. Individual organ grading and overall GVHD grading is used (Figure 11.1). Patients with grades III and IV GVHD have a reduced chance of survival.

Two forms of GVHD are described: acute and chronic. Acute GVHD (aGVHD) occurs in the first 100 days following transplant and may be a mild and self-limiting or a fatal disorder (Veys & Hann, 1997). In its mild form, treatment may be symptomatic, with control of itching and monitoring of the condition. If the child becomes systemically unwell or the GVHD progresses, oral steroids may be added and increased or reduced as necessary. With progressive GVHD which has failed to respond to steroids, other treatment approaches, including the use of monoclonal antibodies, thalidomide and IL-2 receptor antagonists have been used.

Individual organ system grading:			

SKIN Rash		GASTROINTESTINAL TRACT Diarrhoea		LIVER Bilirubin μmol/l		GRADE
◔	<25%	▭	8–15 ml/kg	▨	12–20	1
◑	25–50%	☐	16–25 ml/kg	▦	20–50	2
◕	>50%	▯	>25 ml/kg	▨	>50	3
●	Desquamation	○	Pain/Ileus	◍	Raised AST/ALT	4

Overall grading			
SKIN	GIT	LIVER	GRADE
1–2	–	–	I
1–3	1	1	II
2–3	2–3	2–3	III
2–4	2–4	2–4	IV

Figure 11.1: Grading systems of GVHD (adapted from Barrett, 1993)

Chronic GVHD (cGVHD) occurs beyond day 100 of the transplant. It may occur earlier, in isolation or as a progession of aGVHD. cGVHD affects more organ systems than aGVHD and the effects on the child appear to be similiar to autoimmune diseases such as scleroderma. The nursing implications for both forms will be described separately (see Chapter 13).

Acute GVHD

There are recognised risk factors used to predict GVHD severity and occurrence. These are shown below:

- Mismatched or unrelated donor (increasing level of HLA mismatch, the greater the risk of GVHD)
- Racial mismatch
- Intense conditioning regimes

- Donor–recipient sex mismatch (increased GVHD in female donor to male recipient)
- Increasing age of donor and recipient
- Infections with DNA viruses (CMV and HSV)
- Cytokine administration
- Sunlight (can excerbate skin GVHD).

Prevention of GVHD is undertaken according to the perceived risk. At present, a variety of methods are used to achieve this, involving either T-cell depletion of the donor marrow prior to infusion or the use of cyclosporin plus or minus methotrexate in the patient post-marrow infusion. The chosen method of GVHD prevention is a matter of choice for individual units and the chosen methods applied in response to the specific requirements of that transplant.

Skin GVHD

Onset 7–10 days following transplant. Acute skin GVHD varies in intensity from a mild to a severe form with desquamation of large areas of the body. Frequently, the first sign is a rash or increased redness of the face, neck, palms and soles. This can progress to a maculopapular rash on the upper and lower body causing itching and discomfort to the child. Severe GVHD of the skin can progress to generalised erythroderma and desquamation (taking on the manifestation of second-degree burns).

Nursing note:

Daily skin care in an emollient bath oil to maintain skin integrity. Encourage the use of skin moisturisers. Assess the skin daily for rash. Educate the parents in the prevention and early detection of skin GVHD. Symptom control of itching with antihistamines (small babies may need to wear cotton gloves to prevent secondary infection). Loose cotton clothing can help to reduce skin irritation. Ensure the child has adequate sun protection; the education of parents on discharge is vital. Sunblock, long-sleeved shirts and trousers should be worn when outside even on cloudy days.

Gastrointestinal GVHD

Onset 10–21 days following transplant. Gastrointestinal GVHD often, but not always, follows skin GVHD. Presenting signs include diarrhoea with abdominal cramps, nausea and loss of appetite. Further gastrointestinal involvement can lead to increasing amounts of diarrhoea (stools are often green with mucous to begin with, becoming increasingly watery with strands of epithelial lining). As the involvement of the gut progresses, severe fluid loss, blood loss and bowel perforation may occur, requiring intensive medical and nursing care. Severe gut GVHD carries a high incidence of morbidity and mortality.

Nursing note:

Assess the amount, colour and consistency of the stools. Awareness of the gut signs of GVHD is needed to differentiate mucositis and GVHD (GVHD stools are green and watery with strands of gut lining present). Maintain an accurate intake/output and fluid balance. Observe the child for dehydration, blood loss and signs of infection. Monitor the electrolyte balance. Ensure the peri-anal area is cleaned following episodes of diarrhoea. Maintain skin integrity as per unit policy. Assess the peri-anal area for redness, fistulae and early signs of abscess (in the neutropenic child this may be difficult). Rest the gut; provide nutrition with TPN.

Liver GVHD

Onset 30+ days following transplant. Liver involvement in GVHD occurs as a result of the destruction of the hepatic bile ducts and mucosa (Wujcik et al., 1994). Elevated liver enzymes, enlarged liver, jaundice and right upper quadrant pain can be an early indication of liver GVHD but may be due to cyclosporin, other drug toxicity or liver infection.

Nursing note:

Provide comfort measures for itching as a result of jaundice. Provide analgesia and monitor its effectiveness. Position the child on the left side to decrease liver pressure. Provide support and comfort to the parents and the child.

The treatment and prevention of aGVHD frequently involves the use of cyclosporin, possibly combined with other drugs. The side effects of cyclosporin may compound those already apparent with aGVHD and these are listed below:

- Increased hirsutism (especially facial hair).
  This may be upsetting for the child and the parents. Information that this is likely should be given to the parents prior to the commencement of cyclosporin therapy. Reassurance that this hair will disappear as the drug is withdrawn should be given.
- Hypertension.
  Monitoring of the child's blood pressure should continue on discharge even if this has not been a problem as an inpatient. It

should be ensured that the community team is aware of the need to monitor blood pressure. Antihypertensive drugs may be needed to control this symptom.
- Cushingoid appearence
  The child and the family should be supported during this time. Reassurance should be given that this alteration in body image is temporary and the child's appearence will return to normal once cyclosporin is discontinued.

Graft versus Leukaemia

One of the specific advantages of BMT concerns the phenomenon of the Graft versus Leukaemia (GvL) effect.

Following BMT there is a high rise in cytokines, including interleukin-2 (IL-2), natural killer (NK) interferons and tumour necrosis factor (TNF). This 'cytokine storm' is thought to be responsible for unrestricted cytotoxicity towards leukaemia cells. On activation, T-cells demonstrate a wide range of cytotoxicity towards tumour cells. The use of IL-2 to amplify this response is currently the subject of clinical trials (Reiser & Martelli, 1995).

GvL is thought to be the result of minor donor T-cell recognition and elimination of host leukaemic cells' histocompatibility antigen differences on the surface of cells. This phenomenon is most readily seen in adults with chronic myeloid leukaemia (CML) both from donor T-cells infused at the time of transplant and with donor T-cell infusions following relapse of CML post-transplant. It may have a role to play in BMT for childhood leukaemia but the full implications and appropriate use in the clinical setting will be the subject of further medical research (Caudell & Adams, 1990; Magarth, 1994; Veys et al., 1994).

Veno-occlusive Disease

Hepatic veno-occlusive disease (VOD) is a major complication which can occur in up to 20% of children undergoing BMT (McDonald et al., 1984). VOD occurs as a result of the conditioning regimes pre-transplant, particularly in therapy regimes where busulphan is given (Ringden et al., 1994, cited in Bearman, 1995). It occurs as the result of damage to the endothelial lining of both the sinusoids and terminal hepatic venules, leading to necrosis of the hepatocytes (Bearman, 1995). The hepatic veins become increasingly occluded by cellular debris causing the blood flow from the liver to back up and the protein-rich fluid content of the blood to leak out into the peritoneal cavity, resulting in ascites (Grandt, 1989; Baglin, 1994).

As with GVHD there are some recognised factors to predict which children may develop VOD, such as those receiving:

- Allogeneic BMT
- Mismatch or unrelated donor marrow
- High doses of busulphan
- Second transplant following on from a failed first transplant
- Pre-existing infection during conditioning therapy
- Pre-existing chemical or viral hepatitis.

The diagnosis of VOD can range from mild to moderate or severe. The child may not develop all the symptoms but the more severe the symptoms are, the more severe the form of VOD. It usually occurs within the first three weeks post-transplant and lasts for approximately 10–14 days from the onset of the liver dysfunction (McDonald et al., 1985).

Signs and symptoms include:

- Unexplained weight gain
- Ascites
- Hepatomegaly
- Increase in bilirubin
- Refractory thrombocytopenia
- Increase in almine amino-transferase (ALT)
- Hypoalbuminaemia
- Clotting abnormalities.

Jaundice and encephalopathy are both late signs and symptoms. The diagnosis of VOD is usually made on clinical grounds and the differential diagnosis includes infectious or chemical hepatitis or GVHD of the liver. However, it is only in VOD that there is an unexplained weight gain and fluid retention (Bearman, 1995). There are two techniques available to confirm the diagnosis of VOD. The first is a non-invasive procedure using Doppler ultrasound, which shows reversal of hepatic portal venous flow. Alternatively, a liver biopsy can be performed. However, as these children are usually thrombocytopenic and may also have clotting abnormalities due to liver dysfunction a liver biopsy is not recommended.

The management of the child with VOD is the joint responsibility of nursing and medical staff. Early detection and support measures by both teams may help to decrease the damage to the liver, the aim being to reverse the liver disease rather than allowing it to prove fatal (Bearman, 1995). In children who are at high risk of developing VOD there may be an indication for treatment with continuous i.v. heparin (Bearman, 1995).

Treatment is usually supportive. Both intravenous fluid volumes and sodium content must be restricted. To reduce symptomatic ascites diuretics such as i.v. frusemide and i.v. spironalactone can be given. However, to maintain intravascular volume i.v. albumin may need to be given concurrently. In the event of gross ascites which are not responding to albumin, diuretics and fluid restriction, careful paracentesis with intravascular colloid replacement may need to be performed. This will remove the peritoneal fluid, thus improving the child's respiratory function and ensuring the child's comfort (Bearman, 1995).

In the case of severe VOD in a child whose condition continues to deteriorate, studies have shown that the use of recombinant tissue plasminogen activator (rtPA) has been successful in a number of cases (Baglin et al., 1990). Both the continuous heparin infusion or use of rtPA can cause significant and overwhelming bleeding, therefore the child will need careful monitoring and observation. The outcome for the child with VOD can range from full recovery to fulminant hepatic failure and death. Markers for a better prognosis are peak bilirubin levels <105 μmols/l and ALT levels <286 U/l.

Nursing note:

Ensure twice-daily weight recording and girth measurement. Make an accurate recording of the fluid balance chart. Restrict intravenous and oral fluids. Restrict i.v. sodium chloride. Give diuretics, e.g. i.v. frusemide and i.v. spironalactone. Administer pain relief, e.g. subcutaneous or i.v. morphine. Assess the child for petechiae and bleeding. Give platelets, albumin and Fresh Frozen Plasma. Maintain adequate respiratory function for the child. Assist with paracentesis. Provide support for the child and the parents.

Chapter 12
The post-engraftment phase

Nikki Bennett-Rees and Louise Soanes

Infections

During the post-engraftment phase (days 29–100 post-BMT) the child's new bone marrow will start functioning and producing neutrophils, thus decreasing the risk of bacterial and fungal infections which cause major problems. However, both cell-mediated and humoral functions take several months to recover and full immunity may take at least one year to recover post-BMT. Furthermore, if the child is receiving steroids as part of treatment for GVHD, his immunity will be further compromised, resulting in an increased risk of developing a viral illness. The most common viral infection at this stage is CMV causing an interstitial pneumonia, which carries a greater than 50% mortality rate.

CMV may occur as a result of:

- Primary infection
- Reactivation of infection if the child was CMV-positive prior to BMT
- Reactivation, if the child was CMV-negative and received CMV-positive donor marrow or blood products.

The following may all lead to an increased chance of developing CMV:

- Receiving allogeneic bone marrow
- Increased intensity of conditioning regimes
- The child being CMV-positive prior to BMT

- The donor being CMV-positive
- The child being treated for GVHD.

In children the incidence of CMV is lower than in adults. This may be due in part to children and their sibling donors being younger and therefore more likely to be CMV-negative. Secondly, the incidence of acute GVHD in children, which increases the risk of CMV infection, is far less than in adults.

The signs and symptoms of CMV pneumonitis include:

- Fever
- Dyspnoea
- Dry cough
- Respiratory failure.

The diagnosis of CMV pneumonitis needs to be confirmed to rule out other chest problems such as *Pneumocystis carinii* pneumonia. This is done by the child undergoing a bronchoalveolar lavage (BAL) and/or lung biopsy to confirm the diagnosis. A diagnosis of CMV in the child's blood and/or urine can be detected on cultures.

In addition to CMV pneumonitis the child may also develop a CMV gastroenteritis, hepatitis, colitis, retinitis and pancytopenia.

Treatment for high-risk children who received CMV-positive marrow or who are themselves CMV-positive is with high-dose i.v. acyclovir eight-hourly with or without weekly i.v. immunoglobulin to prevent reactivation of the virus (Schmidt, 1992). The treatment of choice for children who are excreting CMV in their urine, have positive blood cultures or who develop CMV pneumonitis is i.v. ganciclovir and i.v. immunoglobulin (Wingard, 1990).

In general the incidence of CMV infection post-BMT is dropping. This may be the result of improved blood product screening and the use of leukocyte filters, alongside the improved antiviral drug therapies.

Discharge Planning

The experience of a BMT, for both the child and the family, takes place over a long period. The experience begins with the search for a donor and this may take many months and be emotionally exhausting for the child and the family. Hopes and expectations are raised and dashed in the search for and identification of a suitable donor.

With the success of finding a donor comes the transplant. This often takes place at a regional BMT centre which may be a distance from the home and away from the support of family and friends. The extensive medical and nursing support needed following transfusion of the marrow and in the wait for engraftment requires weeks, possibly months, of hospitalisation. At last the child and the family reach the physical criteria required by the unit to be allowed to go home. This is the day everyone has been waiting for.

However, on discharge from a BMT unit parents may face a myriad of concerns and anxieties related to treatment, prognosis and the changes in their lives resulting from the transplant experience.

Once home the practicalities of family life need to be resumed. The financial cost of the transplant often becomes apparent on discharge, even in countries with free medical care the cost implications for families undergoing bone marrow transplant are vast. Usually one parent (often the mother) gives up a wage or takes a career break during the transplant period. This loss of income can have major implications for the family; the financial costs of a home and family carry on and although put on hold during the hospitalisation of the child they reappear once the family is home. This may lead to a change to the previous lifestyle of the family, affecting all its members, particulary the healthy siblings who may lose out on previously granted treats or pastimes.

On discharge there is a transition from an acute to a chronic phase of care, requiring an alteration in the coping mechanisms demanded of the family and the child. White (1994) has identified six major themes of concern to parents on discharge from a BMT unit:

- The return home
- Working with this
- Changing relationships
- Learning the rules
- The new norms
- The uncertain future.

Returning home

The return home is often seen by families as a mixed blessing. Reporting 'it's good to be home, to be a family again in familiar surroundings and in charge of our lives again' but also expressing concerns about leaving the safety and security of the unit with the 'experts on tap'.

Changing relationships

If the transplant has occurred far from home the follow-up care may be coordinated at a local paediatric unit. In some cases this might be the original referring hospital in which the child has been cared for in the past. If this is the case, relationships with staff will have been formed and the routines and environment of the hospital will be familiar to the child and the family. However, for those children with little or no previous experience of hospital, for example, children with metabolic disease or children for whom the follow-up hospital is not their referring hospital, the involvement of another hospital can be an added stress. New relationships will need to be formed with the staff of this hospital and a new philosophy of care learned. Parents can be helped in this with the support of paediatric community nurses from the shared care or tertiary hospital.

In such cases the family becomes a teacher, explaining the past experiences of the child and the practicalities of BMT to the new staff. The inexperience of the staff in the follow-up hospital in relation to the field of BMT can lead to further stress and anxiety for the family.

Learning the rules

Learning the rules of discharge can be a major component of the discharge experience for parents. The vulnerability of parents leaving the safety of the hospital, often perceived as clean and germ free, to enter the outside world again can be a time of fear. Physical care of the child is now their sole responsibility; monitoring vital signs and the symptoms of GVHD and choosing when to act on them is now their responsibility.

New norms

The skills parents have previously learned and once undertaken in order to care for their child whilst sick may need to be relearned prior to discharge, for instance the timing and safe administration of the many oral drugs required after a transplant and caring for central venous lines. Skills such as these may have once been second nature, but now physically and emotionally exhausted following the transplant, parents may have forgotten how to carry them out; or tasks may have been performed by staff on the BMT unit, so leading to loss of confidence. The assumption that because parents have successfully carried out such tasks before, they are capable or confident about resuming them on discharge, should not be made by staff. New skills need to be learned, such as nasogastric feeds. The monitoring of adequate calorie intake and other supportive care also needs to be learned by the parents prior to discharge.

The uncertain future

This sense of responsibility for the physical well-being of the child can lead to unrealistic expectations by parents as to how safe they can make their home in order to prevent complications and infections occurring. The extended use of hospital-based infection precautions, such as methods of washing clothes, and the adoption of hospital-type cleaning routines have been reported and in one case a child's bedroom was rebuilt as the the old wood was seen by the parents as a potential infection risk. Reluctance to return the child to school and the prolonged use of restrictions to the child's activities may prevent the child's reintegration into 'normal life'.

To help these families make sense of the transplant experience and to help in the child's reintegration to normal life careful discharge planning is required.

Although a significant event, BMT is a temporary period in a family's life. Helping a family to make sense of this period and return to society post-transplant begins before the transplant and requires a multidisciplinary approach which is often coordinated by a nurse. Hare et al. (1989) suggest that the period and quality of preparation can have a significant effect on the the family's attitude towards treatment and recovery.

Discharge interviews are recommended by some authors (Heiney et al., 1994; Sormati et al., 1994); these interviews can act as debriefing sessions for the family and help them to begin to make sense of the transplant experience. Acknowledgement that the transition from the acute to the chronic phase of the bone marrow transplant and the return to the new norm may not be smooth is needed by the staff leading the discharge planning. The nurse leading these sessions needs to be someone the family already knows and with whom they have a working relationship. This may be their primary nurse, social worker or transplant coordinator. This person will need to be confident in their ability to coordinate the care of the child and the family's reintegration to home life. Skilled communication is called for, as is understanding of the role of the resources and functions of the multidisciplinary team.

Each family will require careful assessment, planning and implementation of a care plan as discharge approaches. The family's involvement is paramount to the success of discharge planning, the use of interpreters for both oral and written information should be considered in advance. For those families for whom English is not the first language, the use of interpreters and cultural advocates may be necessary to provide coordinated discharge from hospital.

The child whose care post-transplant is to be shared with other hospitals and agencies may require multidisciplinary discharge planning meetings, in which the anticipated transition can be discussed openly and supportive measures implemented. Prior to discharge, professionals within the multidisciplinary team for whom BMT is not the norm may be apprehensive about receiving the child into their care. This should be recognised as a cause of stress to staff and support mechanisms should be identified for them. Staff in such areas will need input from the discharging unit about the precautions and possible complications of BMT. Such information should include practical advice, for example restrictions on diet, immunisation and sun protection, as well as general advice on physical and psychological responses to BMT.

At the discharge meetings acceptance of each other's areas of responsibility and limitations should be recognised and respected. In both areas a named link person would be beneficial, and effective communication systems should be established before discharge of the family from the unit. As early discharge from units may be a feature of the future, due to pressure on resources and the expansion of transplants in paediatrics, this situation may become more frequent. The link person coordinating the discharge should be easily contactable by parents and staff and have a named associate to cover in their absence. Effective communication within the unit will help in the continuity of care and reduce confusion and stress for all those involved.

The first year after transplant has been shown to be the most stressful in emotional, physical and psychological terms (Pot Mees, 1989); support during this period is likely to be the most intense. As the family adjusts to the new norms, the intensity of involvement by the supportive agencies can be reduced; naturally there will be some families for whom longer term intervention is needed due to the physical results of treatment, such as the side effects of TBI and GVHD, or the psychological trauma of a difficult or complicated transplant. Long term support groups for parents have been used in some centres with beneficial results (Andrykowski et al., 1995).

For parents the need is for concrete information to help them cope with the physical and psychological care of their child and the knowledge that their fears and concerns will be acknowledged and acted upon (White, 1994). As discharge approaches and the child's physical health improves, care by parents can be increased and nursing intervention slowly withdrawn. 'Step down' units or transfer to a quieter more distant area of the unit can aid in the transition to home with less nursing intervention. Responsibility for drug administration by parents can be implemented with help and support from staff and the learning (or relearning) of skills, such as caring for central venous lines and nasogastric feeds, undertaken by parents (with negotiation and planning undertaken by parents and staff together).

Confidence is needed by both sides that the recognition of complications post-BMT, such as GVHD, and the required action, is understood and that other carers the child may have, for example grandparents, are aware of the need for precautions such as adequate sun protection and skin care. Support and reinforcement is once again vital if parents are to be confident in their child's care after discharge. Written information is needed to support the verbal information given, with a named person to contact if necessary. This may be included in a parent information folder or booklet. Again, consideration for families for whom English is not the first language needs to be taken into account.

The use of multidisciplinary outpatient clinics can be of benefit to both families and staff alike in providing a cohesive transition to home and the opportunity for parents to talk over their fears and concerns with the 'experts'. For successful transition from hospital to home awareness is needed by both the family and the staff. The family will require information that the transition from hospital to home may not be as smooth as they expect. Information about what to expect, both from their own and the child's reaction to returning home, will need to be discussed with them. Speaking to a family recently discharged from the unit may help to highlight areas only apparent to those who have experienced transplant at first-hand. Coping mechanisms and strategies for coping with setbacks (both physical and psychological) will need to be identified.

The transition from hospital to home can be managed well, allowing the family to reintegrate with support and education from the multidisciplinary team with the minimum of trauma.

Finally, as the day for discharge approaches and the isolation precautions have been reduced, the parents must be given sound discharge advice, balancing the continued need for the child's protection against infection with the need to resume a 'normal' life.

Chapter 13
Long term effects

Nikki Bennett-Rees and Louise Soanes

Introduction

For many children BMT offers a chance for a future. However, it is associated with a significant degree of acute toxicity and long term sequelae. Many of the late effects are comparable to those seen in children undergoing high-dose chemotherapy using anthracyclines and radiotherapy. In addition, these children will have had infections treated with amphotericin and the aminoglycoside antibiotics (Liesner et al., 1994). Nevertheless the late effects of BMT will be intensified as a result of:

- Higher doses of chemotherapy, particularly cyclophosphamide
- Higher doses of radiation
- Treatment for chronic GVHD.

The long term effects particularly associated with BMT are chronic GVHD, endocrine failure, secondary malignancy and cataracts (particularly found in those children who have had TBI).

Chronic GVHD

Chronic GVHD (cGVHD) is unusual in children, however, the risk of occurrence increases with age. For children under the age of 10 years receiving a sibling transplant and receiving GVHD prophylaxis of methotrexate and cyclosporin, the incidence is as low as 13% rising to 28% in adolescents (Sullivan et al., 1991). Chronic GVHD is defined as GVHD occurring 100 days post-transplant. However, the clinical and histological features may occur 30 days post-BMT (Barrett, 1993). It may occur alone or in conjunction with aGVHD

(Atkinson, 1990). Risk factors include increased age of donor, degree of HLA mismatch and previous aGVHD (Veys & Hann, 1997).

The primary feature of cGVHD is an increase in collagen deposits causing sclerosis and atrophy of the dermis. More organs are affected than in aGVHD and clinical signs reflect the organ affected. These may include joint and muscle contracture, skin colour changes, malabsorption and liver damage due to bile duct destruction (Frederick & Hanigan, 1993) (Table 13.1).

Treatment is both specific and symptomatic. Alternating oral steroids and cyclosporin is an effective regime and aims to minimise drug-related side effects (Sullivan et al., 1991). For those with a poor response to this regime, thalidomide has been used due to its immunosuppresive effects (Volelsgang & Hess, 1994). Symptom control is neccessary to maintain the child's comfort and quality of life. This includes a multidisciplinary team approach from occupational therapists and physiotherapists in order to maintain mobility and prevent contractures.

Table 13.1: Signs and presenting symptoms of cGVHD	
Skin	
scleroderma	red discolouration of the skin, stiffness of connective tissue, joint contracture
lichen planus	dry white patches on the skin
skin colour	can be increased or decreased
alopecia	sparse, uneven hair — both head and body
Sicca syndrome	dry eyes and mouth
lichenoid lesions	white, dry patches on oral mucosa, often mistaken for oral candida
premature dental decay	
mucositis	painful friable mucous membranes (this may also affect the vagina, oesophagus, external auditory canal)
xerostomia	dry mouth, difficulty in swallowing, reduction in saliva
Gastrointestinal tract	
malabsorption	weight loss, diarrhoea
anorexia	
dysphagia	difficulty in swallowing may be due to narrowing of the oesophagus
Musculoskeletal	
	muscular atrophy, weakness and wasting painful joints, knees and hips
Lungs	
obliterative pulmonary bronchitis	decreased activity tolerance
Sources: Frederick & Hanigan, 1993; Barrett, 1993.	

Due to the low levels of circulating antibodies which are a feature of cGVHD and the immunosuppressive nature of treatment, the risk of viral, bacterial and fungal infections is increased. Prophylaxis against pneumocystis and encapsulated organisms is also needed (Barrett, 1993). Response to treatment and the long term outlook depends upon the number of organs involved; thrombocytopenia less than $50 \times 10^9/l$ is also an indication of poor prognosis (Veys & Hann, 1997).

The occurrence of cGVHD can have emotional as well as physical effects. The child never becomes well after transplant, leading to depression and low self-esteem. This can affect all the family members as the affected child remains dependent on the parents for both physical and psychological support. For the sibling donor, extended feelings of guilt may be shown at having a part to play in the debilitation of their sibling through donation.

Nursing intervention includes recognising the family at risk of stress due to caring for a child with cGVHD and the implementation of support mechanisms.

Endocrine Failure

Growth

Children who receive i.v. cyclophosphamide and oral busulphan as their conditioning regime have far fewer growth problems than those who receive TBI as part of their therapy (Sanders et al., 1986, 1989). The dose of radiation used in TBI is the main cause of problems leading to growth failure. The younger the child, the greater the potential growth defect, with the greatest damage to facial, dental and spinal growth being seen in children who received TBI when younger than 6 years old (Sanders et al., 1989; Leiper et al., 1987). It is possible, however, that the long term growth problems may be reduced since TBI is now given as fractionated therapy over 6–8 doses as opposed to single-dose therapy (Sanders et al., 1986). Replacement growth hormone treatment may be indicated and may improve growth velocity. Unfortunately, the growth hormone supplementation will only maintain growth and does not allow the child to catch up with his peers.

Fertility

When cyclophosphamide alone is given as a preparative conditioning drug the return of normal sexual function will occur in most boys and girls (Sanders et al., 1996). A recent study in Seattle (Sanders et al., 1996) provides evidence that adult patients who receive TBI are not inevitably infertile, but that women are at high risk of spontaneous miscarriage, premature labour and giving birth to low birthweight babies. The pre-pubertal child who receives TBI may not have the same outcome; indeed, in the study by Sanders and colleagues (1996) the pregnancies of the five women who were pre-pubertal at the time of TBI all ended in spontaneous miscarriage.

Children who have delayed pubertal development should be given sex steroid supplementation. This serves both to maximise growth velocity and to lessen psychological problems in the developing child (Leiper, 1995).

Cataracts

Posterior subcapsular cataracts, which are easily removed, occur in approximately 20% of children receiving fractionated TBI. This is a great improvement on the 90% of cases seen when TBI was given as a single dose (Deeg et al., 1984).

Secondary Malignancy

There is a higher incidence of developing a second malignancy in children who have been treated for childhood cancer (Miké, 1982). Witherspoon et al. (1989) found that the incidence of secondary malignancy post-BMT was 6.69 times greater than a primary malignancy in the general population. Furthermore, in children whose conditioning regimes included TBI there was an increased risk of developing a secondary malignancy compared to children receiving 'chemotherapy only' regimes.

Some families find the risk of their child developing a secondary malignancy overwhelming. However, this risk needs to be balanced with the greater risk of the child dying from his original disease whether it is a malignancy, a haemoglobinopathy, a metabolic disorder or an immune deficiency syndrome.

A combination of ongoing refinements to the conditioning regimes, with an increased knowledge of the HLA system and tissue-typing may result in children developing less long term sequelae post-BMT. As the number of children who undergo successful BMTs and become long term survivors increases, so the late effects must be constantly monitored, treated and evaluated, thus allowing these children to develop into healthy adults.

Psychosocial Effects of Bone Marrow Transplant on the Family

The emotional cost of transplant has been discussed throughout this chapter. However, it is on discharge from the BMT unit that families often realise the full impact that the transplant has had on their lives.

A change in perspective occurs. The trivia of life that once seemed important, such as cars breaking down and delayed trains, no longer seem as crucial; one mother described it thus, 'the small things don't matter anymore, after this [the transplant] the rest is just not important.'

This change in philosophy can be accompanied with an alteration in spirituality. This may not take the form of religion but may be expressed as a growth in inner strength, conviction and life goals (Ferrell et al., 1992a, b). If faith was important to the family before it may be reinforced by the experience of transplant. In some cases belief in a greater being and prayer may have been used during the transplant and their use be afforded some responsibility for its success; these coping mechanisms may or may not be continued after discharge (Brack et al., 1988).

The spiritual issues of BMT can also lead to the question of 'Why did our child survive and others die?', so-called 'survivor guilt' (Whendon & Ferrell, 1994). Being aware that other families on the unit are not so lucky as to be discharged with a well child may lead parents and children to ask why they were chosen to survive instead of others. Survivor guilt has been reported to lead to feelings of despair in some survivors of BMT (Ferrell et al., 1992b). The discussion of survivor guilt is included in the following section looking at a potentially negative response to BMT, post-traumatic stress disorder (PTSD).

The perception (by both nurses and the family) that the transition from hospital to home will always be smooth is unrealistic and in some cases may be so difficult as to result in PTSD (Heiney et al., 1994). PTSD is defined as a 'psychological traumatic event that is outside the normal range of usual human experience'.

Often used to describe reactions to man-made or natural disasters it can also be used to describe any overwhelming life-threatening event. The presentation of PTSD is the development of a set of characteristic symptoms which include re-experiencing the event, avoidance, detachment, physiological arousal and feelings such as anger, guilt, depression and grief. Factors contributing to PTSD include decreased social support, the extent to which the sufferer played a part in the event and the origin of the stressor.

Heiney et al. (1994) used PTSD to examine the aftermath of BMT in paediatric patients and their families. In this work she found that seven factors in the transplant period affected the development of PTSD:

1. Degree of life threat
2. Duration of trauma
3. Degree of bereavement and loss
4. Displacement from home and family
5. Potential for recurrence
6. Role of the parent in the trauma
7. Exposure to death and destruction.

These issues are discussed briefly below and in detail in other sections of this chapter.

The transplant, an attempt to prevent death or improve quality of life, carries a risk of mortality and morbidity that continues throughout life with the occurrence of complications, rejection and the fear of relapse. Parents report lying awake at night worrying what to do if a relapse occurs, the graft is lost due to infection or the uncertain response to transplant.

Parents are involved in their child's care during transplant and give consent to the procedure. This involvement and the witnessing of complications and trauma for the child can lead to stress and feelings of helplessness by parents. The displacement from home and support networks can lead to feelings of isolation and detachment. In the place of usual support networks friendships are formed with other families on the unit. Some of the children in these families may die during their transplant. This, in turn, leads parents to face not only the possibility that their own child may die but also the death of children who they know well, an experience rarely faced by families in late twentieth century western society.

The relationships formed with other families on the unit are especially significant during the transplant period. On discharge, relationships with old friends and neighbours are resumed and this is taken to be a sign of returning to normal by others. Families report that the loss of contact with people with whom they have shared a common experience is difficult to adjust to, 'People who are in the same boat as you are lost', is how one mother described this loss of support.

Relationships within the family may also have altered during the child's admission. The parent who stayed in hospital and the sick child may have almost become a single family. A relationship can be formed in which each party knows the other more intensely than before or than other members of the family know them. The readjustment to their previous roles within the family can take both time and energy.

In their parent's absence, older siblings may have taken on the role of parent to younger siblings, and fathers may have taken on roles previously carried out by the mother.

In effect, the parent and child may return to a household in which the roles they once occupied have been filled. One mother, after a prolonged transplant admission, commented that on her return 'it was almost as if they didn't need me anymore'.

The transplant period of separation has also been described as having a negative effect on marital relationships and the personality of the parents (Freund & Seigel, 1986). The transplanted child has to readjust to being one of the family again and no longer the centre of attention. Relationships with and between siblings will also require adjustment. Siblings who have been sent to stay with relatives will need to adjust to the family rules again and a period of conflict may occur as old roles and domains are regained or adjustments made to permanent changes to family dynamics. In addition, for the mother, adjustment to the changed home environment may be compounded with her return to work. This can be additionally stressful, as leaving the child previously in her care can give rise to feelings of fear and guilt (Pot Mees, 1989).

Once home, many families do adjust to the new norm and rapidly gain confidence in their child's care, instigating changes and moving on from the hospital. The reintegration to school is one area that may be a significant event for the family. The point at which the child is allowed to return to school will vary from unit to unit. Often, once immunosuppressive drugs have stopped and the immune system is re-established school can be restarted. The fear of infection is one of the main reasons cited for the delay in restarting school and outbreaks of infections such as chickenpox may cause the child to be withdrawn from school again.

For the child, adaption to his peer group can be stressful. Old friendships will have moved on, the rules and culture of school, as with the family, will once again have to be relearned and the school work interrupted by the transplant will need to be regained. The provision of home tuition while the child is well but still immunosuppressed can help to reintroduce academic work. Once this hurdle has been overcome, confidence in reintroducing other activities usually grows, 'once he started school it seemed silly not to allow him to do the other things, we just slowly started them up again things like football and Cubs so far there's been no problem'.

Following BMT it can often take a year for the family to readjust to the experience (Pot Mees, 1989). This experience that has not been shared by the family as a whole, will mean that each member child, the parent who stayed in hospital, the parent who stayed at home, the sibling donor, and the sibling who was not a donor, will all have their own private feelings about the transplant. The year following the transplant will be a time of upheaval and resettlement for the family as they reform. This year can be likened to the 'golden hour' in emergency medicine, in that what happens during that time is vital for the long term implications for the family's health, both as individuals and as a whole. Planning for the family's discharge is a key area of responsibility for the BMT nurse.

Chapter 14
Peripheral blood stem cell transplant

Hilary Brocklehurst and Louise Soanes

Peripheral blood stem cell transplants (PBSCT) are increasingly used in the treatment of many of the conditions described in this section. Primarily, they are a treatment option for children with solid tumours as a rescue following so-called 'megatherapy'. This involves a large dose of cytotoxic drug(s) to induce increased cytotoxicity. The main side effect of this is profound and potentially permanent myleosuppression (Pinkerton, 1993). The transfused stem cells given following this chemotherapy act as a rescue from this potentially fatal side effect. Previously, autologous bone marrow was used as a rescue from 'megatherapy', however, in the last five years the rapid expansion of PBSCT has almost replaced autologous BMT as a source of stem cells. Table 14.1 provides a brief history of PBSCT.

Table 14.1: PBSCT — a brief history

1909	Documented existence of haematopoietic stem cells by Alexander Maximow (cited by Korbling & Fleidner, 1996)
1962	Stem cells identified in circulating blood
1965	Flow cell separator introduced (Freireich et al., 1965)
1980s	Autologous blood stem cell transplants used for adult patients with CML (Goldman et al., 1988)
1985	Peripheral stem cells shown to reconstitute haematopoietic function in humans (Kessinger et al., 1986)
1988	Use of cytokines to mobilise stem cells into peripheral circulation
1996	Peripheral stem cells mobilised with growth factors have widely replaced autologous BMT

Allogeneic PBSCT can be used in place of allogeneic bone marrow. However, the use of growth factors in healthy children or adults will remain controversial until the long term implications of their use are more fully understood. This is likely to remain an area of much research and interest in the near future.

Children with SCID, osteopetrosis and haemophagocytic lymphohistiocytosis (HLH) who have no sibling or matched unrelated donor may receive haploidentical transplants using both marrow and PBSC.

What are stem cells?

All blood cells are produced in the bone marrow and released into the peripheral bloodstream as required at various stages of maturity. Mature cells all originate from one cell type, known as the pluripotent stem cell. These are unlike other blood cells as they have the ability to replicate in unlimited numbers and can also differentiate into whichever mature cells are required (Walker et al., 1994) (Figure 14.1).

As shown in Figure 14.1, there are several lines of haematopoietic precursor cells arising from the pluripotent stem cell. The cells which are commonly counted at the time of harvest are the colony-forming units, granulocyte–macrophage (CFU-GM) which are committed to the neutrophil line. Burst-forming units–erythrocyte (BFU-E) are another indicator of the presence of haematopoietic stem cells. There are, however, only 0.1% of CFU-GM cells circulating at any one time, although 98% are found in the bone marrow (Fliedner & Steinbach, 1988). It is therefore necessary, by means of non-stem cell toxic chemotherapy ± colony-stimulating factors to mobilise these cells into the peripheral circulation.

The physical and psychological assessment of the child undergoing PBSCT is similar to that previously mentioned for BMT. An important aspect is the indication of normal renal function; this will be required prior to the high-dose chemotherapy, as reduced renal function may cause complications due the delayed excretion of the cytotoxic drugs used, especially melphalan.

There are significant differences between the use of peripheral stem cells and bone marrow cells for transplant purposes, as shown in Table 14.2.

Mobilising peripheral stem cells

Stem cells must first be mobilised from the bone marrow into the peripheral circulation in order to obtain a good yield. This is usually

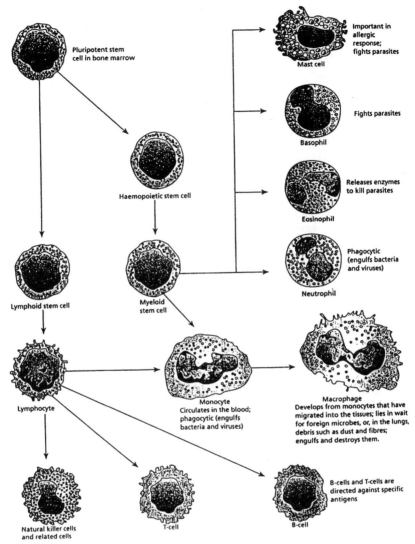

Source: Roberts, 1994.

Figure 14.1: How different white cells develop

achieved by the administration of a non-stem cell toxic drug, such as cyclophosphamide, approximately 10 days before the harvest is anticipated. This induces a degree of myelosuppression which, in turn, encourages new growth of the stem cell population. Given alone, this can increase the GFU-GM population by 10–18 times its previous level (Korbling, 1993) and BFU-E levels can increase eight-fold. With the addition of a haematopoietic growth factor, such as G-CSF, GM-CSF or IL-3, this can increase to as much as 370 times (Fliedner & Steinbach, 1988).

Table 14.2: Comparison of stem cell and bone marrow harvesting	
Peripheral stem cells	Bone marrow
Harvesting is painless	Harvest site may cause discomfort
General anaesthetic is required to insert rigid central venous access line	General anaesthetic is required
Can be collected with the child as an outpatient (in older children who can cope with collection using peripheral venous cannulation)	A short inpatient admission is necessary
Stem cell collection may need to be carried out more than once; sessions last 2–4 hours	Bone marrow is harvested in one session; session may last up to 2 hours
May result in a shorter inpatient stay due to quicker regeneration of neutrophils (14 days)	Neutrophils may take longer to regenerate (21 days)
Each stem cell collection requires individual freezing, increasing laboratory time and cost; adequate storage space is essential	Bone marrow can frequently be re-infused within 24 hours
The neutropenic phase is reduced and there is less need for supportive therapy such as antibiotics and blood products (Rosenfeld et al., 1996; Russel et al., 1996)	Due to the potential longer regeneration period, the use of blood products, especially platelets, may be increased
A suitable cell separator machine and trained nurse or technician are required, allowing for the treatment of very small children needing specialist paediatric care	A fully equipped and staffed operating theatre is required for a potential of 2 hours

A daily injection of growth factor, usually G-CSF, is given subcutaneously for approximately 10 days commencing the day after the cyclophosphamide. Studies looking at the most effective dose and combination of this with other growth factors, such as GM-CSF or IL-3, are under way (Vose et al., 1993; Testa, 1996). There exists some discrepancy between units at present as to which is the most effective protocol to use.

Although the dose of cyclophosphamide is relatively low (in some units the dose given is much higher) many units routinely give a dose of mesna and a minimum of four hours' hydration to prevent the risk of haemorrhagic cystitis. (If the higher dose is given, a 24-hour infusion of mesna will be required.) An effective antiemetic, such as ondansetron ± dexamethasone, is also recommended to prevent nausea and vomiting. The child will need to be in hospital as a day case, although some units prefer an overnight stay.

The injection of growth factor can be a daunting prospect for the child and the family as up to this point, it has been possible to give most medicines either by mouth or painlessly through an existing central line. It must be explained fully that the most effective way of giving this particular drug is by subcutaneous injection; there is the advantage that the child can remain an outpatient or, even better, have the treatment at home.

There may be a family member willing to learn the technique of giving the injection but if this is not an option, it can usually be arranged for a paediatric community nurse or GP practice nurse to administer the G-CSF, thus keeping hospital visits to a minimum. Some children may prefer such procedures to be undertaken by nursing staff; and there are some who trust only themselves. One such patient refused to let anyone give any of his injections. Instead, he preferred to practise on his favourite toys and an orange, and completed the full course with the help of some ethyl chloride spray.

Each unit will have its own policy and regulations for the administration of injections at home and these will vary throughout units. Often the first injection, if not the first two or three, will need to be given under supervision either in hospital, or at home.

For those parents who wish to give the injections, education given by nursing staff to support them in this role can be enhanced by various booklets and videos available from the drug companies which produce growth factors. Hospital play specialists are skilled in helping both parents and children with these procedures by the use of dolls or puppets in the play setting. Most families will opt to have the injections given at home and will indeed succeed in this, with support and education. The use of an ethyl chloride spray can be of considerable help, and EMLA cream is also thought to be of use in some cases, although there is some doubt about its anaesthetic effect below the skin. For some children, the use of EMLA cream has been seen to be of psychological benefit.

Venous access

Approximately 8–10 days following the cyclophosphamide administration, a full blood count should show a significant increase in the neutrophil population, indicating an appropriate time to commence the cell harvest (though approximately 10% of the general population will never mobilise enough stem cells, especially if they have received several intensive courses of chemotherapy prior to the stem cell harvest).

In order to achieve the cell harvest, a rigid leukopheresis line will be inserted temporarily (Vaux, 1996). The existing central venous line is unlikely to be sufficiently rigid or to have a wide enough bore to withdraw the required amount of blood volume without collapsing. If an extra line is required it will often be a temporary double lumen Vascath or apheresis line which may require a short general anaesthetic for insertion. It may be inserted into any of the following veins: subclavian, internal jugular or femoral. If a new line is necessary, the child must have a full explanation of why it is needed and be well prepared both for the line itself and a general anaesthetic.

Stem cell collection

Once venous access is achieved, the stem cells can be collected using an apheresis process through a cell separator machine. This is often a COBE Spectra which is the most suitable for use in small children. The machine removes blood from the child via the leukopheresis line, spinning it in a centrifuge. The machine will have been programmed to separate the blood into the different layers of red cells, white cells and platelets in the buffy coat, and plasma according to density. The buffy coat, containing the mononuclear cells, is then transferred into a collection bag while the remaining blood is returned to the patient. This process takes 2–4 hours to complete and it may be necessary to repeat it for 2–3 days, although one day is usually sufficient.

It is necessary to prime the lines in the cell separator machine before commencing the collection process. A saline solution is usually used for this but for children weighing less than 30 kg, it is necessary to prime the machine with blood to prevent shock developing from the sudden loss of blood volume. The packed red cells used should be fully cross-matched, CMV-negative and leukodepleted (Vaux, 1996).

To prevent the blood in the collection tubing from clotting, an anticoagulant, acid citrate dextrose (ACD) or heparin, is added, a small amount of which will be received by the patient in the return line. The citrate inhibits normal coagulation by binding to ionised serum calcium and can therefore reduce blood calcium levels resulting in hypocalcaemia, also called citrate toxicity (Hooper & Santas, 1993; Purandare, 1994). The first signs of hypocalcaemia are often numbness or tingling of the peripheries, particularly the nose, ears, fingertips or toes (Walker et al., 1994). It is rapidly reversed at onset with the administration of i.v. calcium gluconate or calcium chloride. If it is not treated with the onset of symptoms, the child may complain of painful muscle spasms, particularly in the hands or feet which may lead to muscle twitching and convulsions (tetany).

Cardiac arrhythmias may also be present. In some units, the child is encouraged to drink plenty of milk before and during the harvesting procedure to help to boost the calcium levels in the blood, although this will only have a gradual and ongoing effect and will not help when levels are already low. When any of the above symptoms are noticed, the cell separator machine should be slowed down to a level tolerated by the patient.

Another side effect which may be seen during this procedure is hypovolaemia, particularly when the child is first connected to the machine. As previously mentioned, it is necessary to prime the lines with blood for low weight children and baseline observations of pulse and blood pressure should be recorded. The platelet count can drop significantly after apheresis as the platelets may stick to the apheresis machine and not be returned to the patient (Hooper & Santas, 1993). A baseline blood count should be taken prior to apheresis and a platelet transfusion may be required if the level is less than $50 \times 10^9/l$.

On completion of each collection, a blood sample is taken to ascertain the stem cell concentration. This is usually counted initially by the number of mononuclear cells or CD-34 antigen-positive cells which gives an adequate indication of number of stem cells in the collection. (CD-34 antigen is found on the surface of early progenitor cells.) Although CD-34 antigen-positive cells do not measure the pluripotent stem cell, a count greater than $5 \times 10^6/kg$ is said to be adequate for successful engraftment (Vaux, 1996). The number of mononuclear cells required for engraftment are thought to be in the range of $3-10 \times 10^8/kg$ bodyweight (Vose et al., 1993).

Due to the length of time the procedure takes, it will be necessary for distraction therapy to be arranged to relieve the boredom for the child. This should be planned with the child in advance of the procedure. Some children may be quite content to watch a video or play computer games, but some will prefer interactive board games which can be played with parents, the play specialist or a nurse as available (Hooper & Santas, 1993; Vaux, 1996).

If the child is to continue with conditioning and re-infusion of cells within a few days, the harvested stem cells need only be refrigerated until the child is prepared for re-infusion. If the cells are to re-infused later, the cells require the addition of the cryopreservative, DMSO, and to be stored frozen in liquid nitrogen at approximately −200°C (Vose et al., 1993).

Following completion of the stem cell harvest the child may be discharged home for a short period or may continue immediately with the conditioning regime and the re-infusion. Conditioning will vary according to the underlying disease and may be over one day, i.e. melphalan, or as long as six days, i.e. BEAM (BCNU, etoposide, melphalan and cytarabine). This will be one factor which predetermines the need for cryopreservation of the stem cells prior to re-infusion.

Nursing care post-PBSCT

Each treatment unit will have its own guidelines for infection control and isolation procedures. The local policy must be explained fully to the family. Some units nurse children undergoing PBSCT in a side room, some on the open ward and some in strict isolation. There are at present no documented research studies which indicate which of these is the best, but the feeling is that many of these children are no more at risk of acquiring infections than those receiving high doses of immunosuppressive chemotherapy as part of their treatment regime. The main differences in treatment that will be faced by a child receiving PBSCT are those met in the initial period before and during the initial stem cell harvest. Although much of this can be achieved on an outpatient basis, it can be a very frightening procedure if not fully understood. The cell separator machine is very large and frightening, especially to a young child. At a convenient time prior to the first collection, the child and the family should visit the department, see the machine and meet the nurse or technician who will be involved in the harvesting process. It is sometimes helpful to see another patient connected to the machine as reinforcement of the explanation and reassurance that it really is a painless procedure. Ideally, a nurse and/or play specialist who the child knows well should stay with them for at least the first part of the collection until the child feels settled. In some hospitals, the machine may be transported to the child's bedside which may help to reassure them, but in many units, the machine is in a separate department, which may be more unsettling.

Chapter 15
Further developments in bone marrow transplant

Louise Soanes

Gene Therapy

This treatment option is presently undergoing clinical trials, although its future in clinical practice has yet to have any great impact. However, its role in the future treatment of adenosine deaminase deficiency ADA (a form of SCID) is most promising. It is hoped that the therapy will be applied to other forms of genetic diseases currently treated with bone marrow transplant (Abramovitz & Senner, 1995).

Gene therapy involves the insertion of genetic material into a patient's cells. In the case of ADA, the initial trial used genetically corrected T-lymphocytes from the patient. These lymphocytes were isolated and grown with the help of cytokines and monoclonal antibodies. The isolated normal gene was then inserted using a retrovirus as a carrier (vector). These transduced cells were then grown and re-infused to the patient. As these genetically modified T-lymphocytes have only a limited lifespan, at present, it offers only therapy for ADA rather than a cure. Research into the use of genetically modified bone marrow cells continues and has been used in very few patients (Morgan, 1993; Robinson et al., 1996).

Umbilical Cord Blood Transplants

Umbilical cord blood (UCB) has been shown to contain immature haematopoietic cells, though in fewer numbers than bone marrow.

These cells have been found to have high proliferative and expansion properties. This factor, combined with the increased number of NK cells (with their immunosuppresive function), may explain the reduced incidence of GVHD following umbilical cord blood transplants (UCBT) (Gluckman, 1995). Since the first UCBT in 1989 there have been over 100 transplants reported for a variety of malignant and non-malignant conditions (Apperley, 1994).

The collection of umbilical cord blood is made during or after the third stage of labour. Opinions vary as to which of these two times allows for the greatest yield of stem cells. The cord is clamped, cleaned and the umbilical vein is then cannulated and the sample collected into a blood transfusion bag containing an anticoagulant. The sample may then be stored in a refrigerator for a few days or frozen in dimethyl sulphoxide (DMSO) (Apperley, 1994). Red cell depletion of the UCB is used in some units, but as the sample is often small (approximately 100 ml) this is not thought neccessary by all units.

Many of the UCBT carried out at present use blood from siblings of the child receiving the transplant. However, many countries are now banking allogeneic cord blood. This collection is undertaken with the full informed consent of the mothers involved. Both mothers and cord blood samples are screened for viruses and genetic disorders before collection and, in the UK, follow-up of the child and mother for these investigations takes place when the baby is three months old. Though involving little risk for the mother and baby the ethical use of donated cord blood and its ownership is currently under debate.

Transplants using UCB as a source of stem cells may have a limited use in adults. However, application of the technique to paediatric BMT looks promising though evaluation of its merits in comparison to bone marrow have yet to be fully established. Some of the factors involved are shown in Table 15.1.

T-cell Infusion in Children who Relapse Following BMT

Relapse following BMT or failure of the marrow to engraft is a devastating event for the child and the family. Multiple transplants are not uncommon in the USA (Magarth, 1994), but are rare in the UK. Factors influencing the decision to proceed to a second transplant are assessed on an individual basis but may include:

- The availability and potential risks (both psychological and physical) to the donor
- The risk of toxicity to the patient in proceeding with the second transplant
- The probability of the second transplant being successful (Prentice et al., 1996).

Table 15.1: Advantages and disadvantages of the use of cord blood	
Advantages	Disadvantages
Greater availability of stem cells from ethnic minority groups	The donor initially will be unable to donate further cells
Cord blood less likely to contain viruses	Second transplants are impossible
Shorter preparation time of patient	Screening for all genetic disorders is impossible at birth
Banked cord blood reduces the search time for a donor; practical and financial implications are involved	Little evidence of GvL is shown in UCBT, therefore its use in children with leukaemia is uncertain

Donor registries do allow adult donors to donate marrow twice and to donate T-cells to the patient in light of a relapse (Gordon-Box, 1996), however, the use of G-CSF in unrelated adult donors is an area of current debate.

The use of sibling donors in these circumstances is a more difficult decision, on both moral and practical grounds. The use of central lines for small children unable to cope with leukopheresis from a peripheral cannula may expose these children to another general anaesthetic. The psychological stress involved for this tiny group of sibling donors is an area as yet unexplored. For those children who have a relapse of their leukaemia following a transplant the outlook is very poor (Pinkerton, 1993). If a second transplant proceeds, the increase in the GvL effect is attempted with the control of GVHD prophylaxis and possibly the use of a T-cell-replete marrow. The use of donor T-cells may also be used to bring about this response, however, this is an area of controversy within paediatric BMT.

The use of donor T-cells in the successful treatment of adult CML has been well established (Kolb et al., 1995). However, T-cell infusions for those in blast crisis have not been so successful; it may be this disease-specific response that limits the use of T-cell infusions in the treatment of leukaemia relapse following BMT. Those children thought to most likely benefit from T-cell infusions are those who have re-entered complete remission following further chemotherapy.

Chapter 16
Staff support in bone marrow transplant

Louise Soanes

Stress Management

Caring for children and their families facing BMT, as with other areas of high-dependency nursing, is stressful. Some sources of stress are common to nursing as a profession and others are unique to the speciality.

The principal stressors in nursing have long been identified and are also evident in the field of BMT. These stressors include workload, dealing with death and dying, poor interpersonal communications between groups of health care professionals, low morale, the erratic nature of nursing. The wider issues of the financial and corporate restraints of working life in health care (Tyler & Ellison, 1994) are also factors. These stressors can be compounded by those specific to BMT nursing and include working with children who face death as a result of their condition or due to the treatment given in an attempt to save their lives as well as those those identified by Patenaude et al. (1979):

- Uncertainty regarding the benefits and outcomes of the treatment
- Intensity of the emotional involvement with families and patients
- Ethical dilemmas surrounding BMT
- Interpersonal relationships and communication between staff and, in some cases, families.

The inherent nature of BMT being a treatment modality offered to children with life-threatening diseases and the potential risk of mortality due to iatrogenic complications is still a threat despite the advances in therapy and supportive care.

Children undergoing BMT often spend long periods of time on the unit. This results in families being separated for months at a time. This separation and dissipation of the family involves the temporary loss of usual support networks. In their place, relationships are often formed with members of nursing staff. While this may be therapeutic for both sides involved, it can be particularly stressful to the nurse as families form relationships in which the professional boundaries become blurred and this may contribute to the risk of burnout in staff (Emery, 1993).

The involvement of nursing staff in partnership with families of children undergoing BMT is a positive relationship (as previously discussed). The nature of BMT, however, has become, and is likely to become more complex. The intensity of treatment and therefore the length of the hospital stay is likely to increase, possibly leading to even more intense nurse/parent relationships.

Formation of such intense relationships may lead to the loss of professional boundaries, in which each party is unsure of their role (Peterson, 1992; Ruston et al., 1996). Over-involvement by the nurse may lead to advocacy giving way to paternalism. The nurse may lose sight of the need to involve the parents in the decision-making process, and in an attempt to protect the family, make decisions or offer opinions on their behalf. In some situations, this may occur without the family's consent or knowledge. Such situations are dangerous for all involved. The parents become disempowered in the care of their own child and the nurse takes on a role that cannot be maintained.

Over-involvement occurs slowly and is often a two-way process between the parents and nurse. Indications for such involvement include the refusal of parents to allow nurses other than the 'favoured' nurse to undertake care of the child, exceptions to ground rules being demanded from or granted to parents, nurses coming in when off duty to care for the child and the formation of an exaggerated sense of responsibility towards the child's care (Ruston et al., 1996).

Strategies to avoid such situations include a unit culture that is open and honest with both the family and the staff involved. This includes advocating the belief encompassed in the partnership model (Casey & Mobbs, 1988) that parents are autonomous and the child's prime advocate.

In situations of stress, such as BMT, the parents need to be supported by nurses who recognise their responsibilities and can fulfil their role within a partnership, demonstrated in the nurse's readiness to negotiate care and their ability to involve the parents in the decision-making process. The ability of nurses to reflect upon their actions and to identify situations where their professional role may be under threat by over-involvement is also an essential aspect of therapeutic boundary setting in BMT.

Patient care issues related to such complexities as the decision to withdraw from active treatment, are one of the most stressful areas of BMT nursing. Added to this is the uncertainty of the benefits and outcome of treatment versus quality of life for the child, so raising many concerns for nurses on the unit. Being involved with families from the time of preparation to discharge can be stressful even when things go well. Families may come to rely on the nurse; often confiding in them as an intense relationship forms. The failure of treatment or iatrogenic complications may cause previously healthy relationships between the nurse and family to break down, bringing emotional as well as professional stress to the nurse.

The nurse may have growing feelings of empathy with the family which lead to conflict with other health care professionals, most often the medical profession.

Medical treatment decisions can lead to difficult ethical problems in which the nurse may have little or no involvement but upon which they are required to act; for example the use of experimental drugs or the prolonged use of aggressive interventions. Situations such as these may give rise to feelings of guilt. The reasons cited for this stress is that it is often nurses who give the drugs who feel culpable for the numerous physical side effects of BMT.

The nurse's lack of involvement in the decisions made on issues such as resuscitation and palliative treatment concerning 'his' or 'her' patient is often seen as a source of stress. This may be compounded if differences of opinion between medical and nursing staff are not openly discussed. Interpersonal staff conflicts on BMT units have been identified as one of the main sources of occupational stress (Molassiotis & van der Akker, 1995). As with the partnership between parent and nurse similar partnerships are needed between members of the multidisciplinary team with each group of health care professionals recognising that they are an expert not the expert and respecting their boundaries of professional responsibility. Historically, nurses have the greatest contact time with patients and families. The advent of primary nursing has enhanced this contact time to include the nurse as coordinator of much of the child's care.

The knowledge required to practise and coordinate care in BMT is changing rapidly. It ranges from the small everyday issues of routines and practices within individual units to the larger issues of advances in the science and technology. The stressors for newly appointed staff to the BMT unit are likely to fall into the former, with the fear of contaminating sterile areas and causing infection to patients being a prominent source of stress. This may apply to previously experienced nurses in the allied fields of BMT moving to a new work place of pure BMT or due to sudden changes in practice or medical strategies arising in a short space of time. The nurse may find they change from proficient practitioner or even expert to novice overnight. The period of novice may be short-lived as previously learnt coping mechanisms come in to play, but even the temporary loss of role can give rise to stress (Benner, 1984).

The response to stress differs in new and experienced nurses (Hinds et al., 1994). Nurses with greater experience may have developed a variety of coping mechanisms than their newer colleagues. There are a number of factors which enable some nurses to cope and experience stress in a more effective manner. This includes personal characteristics, previously acquired coping mechanisms and features of the work environment, for example corporate strategies for recognising and dealing with stress. The nurse's own personality and social support system is instrumental in their ability to cope with stress but something which professionally they have very little control over. The use of stress management courses and workshops is gaining increasing popularity in some areas of the NHS in order to prevent expensive (both in human and financial terms) loss due to stress.

The features of the work environment are a matter of concern to nurses working in BMT. Creating an arena where views can be aired gives the carers a chance to be involved in the organisation of the unit. The establishment of multidisciplinary team meetings can help give staff an opportunity to discuss ethical and interdisciplinary issues with other team members in a professional setting. It also offers the managers of the unit insight into the needs of staff and their current stressors, enabling them to plan and implement changes within the unit (Coody, 1985).

If stress can be seen as 'held in emotion' then it would seem logical to share this emotion in a group as a method of stress reduction. Support groups can be seen as an element of self-care in stressful areas of nursing, reducing the risk of burnout and loss of staff due to dissatisfaction and isolation. A support group is the most convenient and easiest formal method of staff support, and staff can gain from the support of their colleagues recognising that they are not alone in facing the problems of paediatric BMT. Support groups can help to reduce the sense of emotional isolation, but if they are to function for the purpose for which they are intended, there should be some shared aims. Consideration should be given to the group's ground rules and to the choice of leader otherwise the weekly meeting of staff may be neither a group nor source of support.

The emotional cost of nursing on a BMT unit is very real. The creation of a supportive, caring environment involves simple as well as complex approaches where the aim of support moves from crisis intervention to crisis prevention. The appropriate handling of stressful life events occurring in the personal life of members of staff, positive feedback on performance at work, monitoring sick leave with concern for the staff members' health, can help to create a caring environment in which staff feel valued and of worth to their area of work.

The quality of care given to the family during BMT relies heavily on the extent to which the carers are cared for. The prevention and intervention strategies for dealing with stress are a valid area for development in the recruitment and retention of staff in the highly stressful areas of nursing such as paediatric BMT (Kennedy & Grey, 1997).

Educational Needs of Nurses in BMT

Lack of knowledge may initiate feelings of insecurity and incompetence, and is compounded by the few textbooks available on the subject of paediatric BMT. Nurses caring for the child and family are required to be effective in their care and for this, specialist education is required. Though education alone cannot create expert BMT practitioners, Benner (1983) notes that skilled nursing requires a sound educational base. The outcome of offering such a foundation means quicker skill acquisition and safer practice.

New members of staff will benefit from a period of preceptorship (UKCC, 1994) for a negotiated period of time in order to adapt to a new clinical area. This may then be extended to formal clinical supervision benefiting staff in both their professional and personal development (Butterworth & Faugier, 1992).

Carper (1978) claims that the rationale for nursing practice is derived from four components of knowledge: empirical, aesthetic, personal and moral. These offer a widely acclaimed and useful pathway to help nurses make sense of their practice and to perceive the dimensions of their personal knowledge.

Such knowledge is recognised as being untapped but difficult for the nurse to express in a quantifiable, scientific manner and therefore making it difficult to conceptualise (Clarke, 1986). If this knowledge is to be valued as a learning experience in order to enhance practice, it must be brought to life and utilised by the practitioners who own it, making what they do at the bedside valued and credible to paediatric BMT.

Specialist paediatric BMT courses are offered by some nurse education institutions throughout the country, at both diploma and degree level. The application of nursing theories involved in these courses can enhance the nursing knowledge of both inexperienced and experienced practitioners. The work of Benner (1984) and Schön (1991) identifies the use of structured reflection as a vehicle for nurses to rediscover and explore their practice and enable them to identify what makes the nurse effective (Benner & Wrubel, 1989).

BMT units need nurses capable of offering the multifaceted and holistic care required by children and their families. Nurses working in the area of BMT require research-based knowledge, in order to provide care that is relevant to the needs of the child and family.

SECTION THREE
GENERAL SURGERY

Chapter 17
General surgery

Rachel Hollis, Sharon Denton and Gillian Dixon

Introduction

Up until the early years of the twentieth century, and before the advent first of radiotherapy and then of chemotherapy, surgery was the only treatment available to children with solid tumours. Complete, radical surgical excision of a malignant tumour held the only chance of cure. This was only possible in the early stages of localised disease, where a tumour could easily be detected and readily accessed by the surgeon. Mortality rates at surgery were high and cure rates very low, only around 5% in Wilms' tumour for example, today one of paediatric oncology's greatest success stories.

The history of the treatment of Wilms' tumour (or nephroblastoma) illustrates the changing and developing role of surgery in the treatment of the solid tumours of childhood. Tumours of the kidney were first described in medical literature as early as 1814 (Biemann Othersen, 1986). There was a steadily growing recognition that a variety of differently described renal tumours were actually a single entity, nephroblastoma, and this was brought together in a definitive review by Max Wilms in 1899, of a tumour which continues to bear his name.

The first nephrectomy carried out on a child with a renal tumour was performed by Mr Jessop at the General Infirmary at Leeds in 1877. Excision, with a high surgical mortality, remained the only treatment available until 1915, when for the first time radiotherapy was given after surgical excision.

Radiotherapy developed alongside improved surgical techniques and in the 1940s survival reached around 20%. Chemotherapy was first used in the 1950s, with single-agent dactinomycin (actinomycin-D), followed by the addition of vincristine. By the 1960s a combination of surgery, post-operative radiotherapy and adjuvant chemotherapy had pushed survival rates to around 80%. The treatment of Wilms' tumour came to be a model for the development of multimodality therapy in childhood malignancy. Surgery began to be seen more clearly as one arm of treatment, used in association with radiotherapy and chemotherapy.

As national and international clinical trials began to look at the treatment of childhood cancer in a more coordinated way, it became apparent that paediatric tumours generally demonstrated a better response to radiotherapy and chemotherapy than adult malignancies. The role of surgery therefore changed in response to these developments. When used in isolation, the primary aim of surgery had always been complete resection of a solid tumour. Advances in paediatric surgery and the increasing expertise of the specialist surgeon have played their part in improving cure rates and decreasing morbidity in many forms of childhood malignancy. Part of the cost of those cure rates has been, in some cases, major and mutilating surgery, resulting in either loss of function, or major cosmetic insult, or both. As radiotherapy techniques have changed and as multi-agent chemotherapy protocols have proved effective across a range of diseases, the role of surgery has developed and become more defined. In some types of malignancy, such as bone tumours or soft tissue sarcomas, this has meant a more prominent role for sophisticated surgical techniques and a decreased reliance on radiotherapy for local control. In the field of general surgery there have been moves to minimise the late sequelae of surgical interventions without jeopardising the hope of further improving cure rates. The question in surgery has changed from 'Can it be removed?' to 'When should it be removed?' and even 'Should it be removed at all?' Surgery in paediatric oncology has an important role to play in the refining and tailoring of treatment for the individual child.

One of the most important developments in the treatment of childhood cancer has been the increased referral of children to specialist cancer centres (Stiller, 1988). The paediatric surgeons working in these centres have, therefore, been able to develop an expertise in their surgical management which has contributed to decreased surgical morbidity. It has also meant the greater integration of the surgeon into the wider multidisciplinary team caring for these children and their families. One of the greatest lessons of the recent past is the importance of the multidisciplinary approach from the earliest days of diagnosis. Paediatric surgery is a vital component of the oncology service and has developed several distinctive roles which will be explored below.

Surgery as an Aid to Diagnosis

In most paediatric solid tumours tissue analysis is of critical importance, not just in confirming the actual diagnosis but also in gaining further biological information as to the exact nature of the disease. This information is being used increasingly to modify or intensify treatment according to a particular child's prognosis. The role of the surgeon is vital in providing the pathologist with the best possible material in order to arrive at the most accurate diagnosis, so that the child may receive the optimum treatment.

Surgery as a Treatment Option

For many of the solid tumours of childhood, surgery remains the definitive and, in some cases, the only treatment in curing the disease. The timing and the nature of much surgery has been increasingly refined with developments in chemotherapy and radiotherapy. For most tumours surgery is a part of a controlled clinical trial or study protocol which aims for the best chance of cure, whilst trying to minimise long term effects of treatment, by preserving function and improving cosmetic effect. In surgery, the move generally has been away from mutilating surgery towards more conservative options. There are some tumours where more radical surgical options are used more and more, for example in tumours of the pelvis, and some head and neck surgery where plastic surgeons are able to carry out increasingly complex interventions.

Surgery as an Aid to Treatment

The supportive aspects of surgery in paediatric oncology are important across all treatment modalities. Without central venous access many of the aggressive multi-agent chemotherapy protocols now used in childhood malignancy would be impossible to administer. The supportive care that children require is equally dependent on robust venous access and developments in the use of central lines have been integral to the management of many forms of therapy.

As surgeons have become more integrated members of the oncology team they have taken an important role in helping to manage some of the short term effects of such treatment regimes, for example in the management of gut toxicity following chemotherapy, and the treatment of abscesses and colitis caused by infection.

The surgeon may be involved in the administration of radiotherapy by techniques such as brachytherapy. In this treatment modality there is a role for surgery in helping to minimise some of the associated toxicity, with the development of surgical techniques to move vital organ tissue out of the field of external beam radiotherapy. Surgical intervention may also be required in the management of late effects, such as strictures caused by radiotherapy.

As will be seen, the place of surgery in paediatric oncology has moved from an isolated, often heroic, intervention to being an increasingly integrated part of the overall management of children with cancer. This can sometimes lead to difficulties for nurses and families when the paediatric oncology patient requires a specific surgical intervention. The increasing specialisation of childrens' nurses is leading them to develop skills, knowledge and clinical expertise in particular areas. Paediatric oncology and paediatric surgery are two specialities in their own right and it is rare to have nurses who bridge the two. Children will often move, therefore, from a paediatric oncology ward to a surgical ward and back again, with perhaps a diversion to an intensive care unit at some point between the two. There are particular challenges here for the nursing teams operating in these two distinct, frequently geographically distant, settings. Communication between teams and individuals caring for these children is of vital importance in maintaining continuity of care and, for the family, confidence in both caring teams.

The move from one clinical setting to the other may be in either direction, from surgery to oncology or the reverse. Some children will initially be referred to the paediatric surgeon, either because there is no suspicion of cancer, or because the child presents with a number of differential diagnoses, resulting from a distended abdomen, for example. As the likelihood grows that the child has some form of malignancy some families may find it difficult to be on a ward where many children will be undergoing relatively straightforward surgical procedures. They will begin to look for further information and support from the oncology team. It is at this stage that good liaison is critical to ensure that the child and the family receive appropriate and consistent information as the process of diagnosis and staging continues. At some stage it will probably be appropriate for the child to be transferred to the oncology ward and this move should be negotiated with the family, who may react in a variety of ways. For some, it will give the opportunity to be in an environment with other families in the same position, where they perceive the expertise to be in treating their child. For others, however, it may be difficult to leave an area where they have made relationships with staff and found support. It may also mean confronting the reality of their child's diagnosis. Denial is a natural element of many people's reaction, and being on an 'ordinary' ward can reinforce that particular coping mechanism. Moving on to the oncology ward can be hard for some families and it may sometimes be appropriate to delay that move until they are ready for it. Sometimes a first course of chemotherapy may be given on the surgical ward, particularly if most treatment is likely to be as an out-patient.

The move from an oncology unit to a surgical ward is likely to take place at a later stage in the child's illness, at the time of primary tumour surgery. The issues involved in this transfer of care will be outlined below. However and whenever the change in clinical setting occurs, the most important factor for the child and the family will be good, consistent communication between themselves and the wider multidisciplinary team at this critical point.

Surgery as an Aid to Diagnosis

Tissue diagnosis is a critical component of the preliminary 'work-up' of a child with a solid tumour, and should be integrated with other investigations. The child and the family will be subjected to a range of procedures the aim of which is to determine the nature of the disease (diagnosis) and evaluate its spread (staging). Careful planning of the investigations and appropriate preparation of the child and family requires the cooperation and expertise of all members of the multidisciplinary team (Sepion, 1990; Pinkerton et al., 1994). The importance of the early referral of the child to a specialist centre cannot be over-emphasised and at this stage can help to prevent unnecessary or repeated investigations.

On first presentation of a child with a suspected solid tumour, a considerable amount of information can be gained without invasive procedures, through accurate history-taking and careful clinical examination. Determining whether a mass is palpable, if it is painful, whether it is mobile, if it has grown quickly or been there for some time and whether there are enlarged lymph nodes, can give early indications of differential diagnoses. Blood pressure may be raised in a child with an abdominal mass indicating either a Wilms' tumour or neuroblastoma. Phaeochromocytoma can also produce an elevated blood pressure, but this is rare in children. Pallor and bruising may indicate disease in the bone marrow and this would point towards a diagnosis of neuroblastoma, particularly where the characteristic periorbital bruising is evident.

Moving on from clinical examination, biological tumour markers may help to further the process of diagnosis. These markers are tumour-associated compounds found in either the serum or the urine of children with particular malignancies. Examples are the excretion of urinary catecholamines and their metabolites in neuroblastoma, alpha-fetoprotein (AFP) in the blood of children with hepatoblastoma, and AFP or beta-HCG (human chorio-gonadotrophin) in germ cell tumours. Such markers are of clinical significance at the time of diagnosis and can also be used in the evaluation of response to therapy. They may assist in the detection of minimal residual disease following apparent complete resection and in follow-up, the presence of a raised tumour marker may indicate tumour recurrence before this can be detected clinically.

The information obtained from a child's history and clinical examination will be used to determine the need for further radio-logical investigation and the most appropriate imaging techniques. The growth and development of medical imaging over the last 25 years has provided a range of methodologies on which to call. There is now a technique for most clinical problems and the challenge for the clinician, in consultation with the radiologist, is to identify the type of imaging suited to a particular tumour, both at diagnosis and for subsequent follow-up. Plain X-ray films retain their importance, especially in the detection of tumours of the chest, and bone, but have been superseded in many respects by more sophisticated developments. Ultrasound is of particular importance in the assessment of abdominal tumours. Computerised tomography (CT scanning) has played an increasing role in the documentation of the extent of the primary tumour and the accurate assessment of tumour response (Pinkerton et al., 1994). More recently, magnetic resonance imaging (MRI) has been used to great effect in certain situations, in particular where there is soft tissue involvement. CT and MRI scans are used predominantly in the evaluation of primary tumours, although they are also used to detect metastases, most notably chest metastases by CT scanning. In tumours that metastasise to bone, technetium bone scans are widely used to detect bony lesions. The use of radio isotopes in general has increased the quality of the information available to the clinician looking at the extent of disease. Within paediatric oncology, the use of isotope scanning has been particularly important in neuroblastoma. Metaiodobenzylguanidine (mIBG) is a compound taken up by tumours of the central nervous system, and so is a useful imaging agent in neuroblastoma (and phaeochromocytoma) where, labelled with radioactive isotopes, it has been shown to be effective in assessing the extent of disease and sometimes in locating the primary tumour. Scans and imaging provide a great deal of information about the nature and spread of a tumour and the interpretation of such information is an art and a science in its own right. The radiologist is an important member of the multidisciplinary team in the planning and interpretation of these investigations.

Some of the imaging procedures outlined above, in particular CT and MRI scanning, involve complex, frightening, sometimes noisy machinery, and require children to keep still for considerable lengths of time. For small children, this often means sedation and general anaesthetic. If scans are carried out under general anaesthetic other staging investigations, such as bone marrow aspiration and trephines, or lumbar puncture, should be carried out at the same time. If appropriate facilities and personnel are available tumour biopsy can sometimes be performed under that one anaesthetic.

In most types of solid tumour the definitive diagnosis is usually made on tissue biopsy from the primary tumour site. Even where diagnosis is almost certain on the basis of positive tumour markers and primary tumour imaging (as may sometimes be the case, for example, in neuroblastoma) biopsy will still be required. The accuracy of diagnosis in childhood cancer is of critical importance and can be difficult to make in some paediatric tumours, which may be poorly differentiated and require sophisticated analysis to arrive at a positive identification. It is recognised (Triche, 1992) that the more information there is available on the identification of a disease and the nature of a paediatric tumour, the more specific and effective treatment can be. It is not just the broad diagnosis, for example Wilms' tumour, which is required, but more specific information regarding the molecular and genetic make-up of the cells involved which can help the pathologist and the scientists to identify more clearly the nature of that particular tumour, in that particular child. Within Wilms' tumour, for example, it is necessary to distinguish between favourable histology and unfavourable histology. In rhabdomyosarcoma, the embryonal variant has a far better prognosis than the alveolar type. In neuroblastoma, the amplification of the oncogene N-myc has been shown to be a particularly poor prognostic feature (Look et al., 1991), and other significant biological features are increasingly recognised.

In order to obtain all the information required about a tumour, a range of tests will be required. Histology and immunochemistry can generally be carried out on fixed samples, but there is an increasing need for fresh tissue for cytogenetic and biological studies.

Where fresh biopsy samples are required by the pathologist and scientist, it is self-evident that there must be close collaboration with the surgeon carrying out the biopsy to ensure they are collected. It is important to make sure that the quality of the biopsy and the material gained is adequate for all the tests required in any particular tumour type. It is equally important that the technique used to carry out the biopsy is as safe as possible and appropriate to the child's clinical condition. There has been some disagreement amongst surgeons and oncologists on the most appropriate type of biopsy in certain paediatric solid tumours and the Surgical Group of the United Kingdom Childhood Cancer Study Group has attempted to define a UKCCSG consensus on the principles of tumour biopsy (UKCCSG, 1996). This paper makes the point that the primary role at biopsy is to make a diagnosis as a basis for individual patient treatment, but that biological research studies and the storage of tissue for future studies are also important in furthering the understanding of children's tumours, and so contributing to developments in treatment. The protocols of the UKCCSG for the treatment of particular tumours prescribe certain types of biopsy, which should be carried out in the context of national guidelines and, where appropriate, national and international clinical studies. The different options for biopsy are as follows:

- No biopsy
  This may be appropriate for some germ cell tumours where diagnosis can be made on tumour markers alone. In neuroblastoma, biopsy is preferred because of the importance of biological information, but occasionally the diagnosis will be clear from tumour markers, primary tumour imaging and bone marrow aspiration. If a child's clinical condition is such that a biopsy would be detrimental to them, it is hard to justify this further intervention. In the case of some lymphomas, examination of ascitic fluid or pleural effusion may produce sufficient cells for morphological analysis and immunophenotyping and so avoid the need for further tissue sampling (Pinkerton et al., 1994).
- Fine needle aspiration cytology (FNAC)
  In the UK this is rarely used, as such biopsies are held to provide inadequate samples, and lead to difficulties in interpretation. In

Europe, however, this technique is increasingly used as a less invasive intervention.

- Wide needle core biopsy (e.g. Trucut)
  This is usually a multiple biopsy, ideally under radiological guidance using ultrasound or CT. It may be used in liver tumours, Wilms' tumours and others.

- Laporascopic/thorascopic biopsy (needle or incisional)
  This specialised technique may be used where an open, incisional surgical biopsy is thought to be too invasive. It requires considerable clinical expertise, but is increasing in its application.

- Open incisional surgical biopsy ± needle cores
  This is the biopsy of choice for most types of solid tumours as it is the least likely to lead to diagnostic problems. Certain considerations should, however, be borne in mind when planning such a biopsy. Skin incisions should be planned to allow the scar to be excised at the definitive resection. A deep narrow wedge is generally preferable to a wide, superficial biopsy and if the biopsy can include the interface of the tumour with adjacent normal tissue this is often helpful to the pathologist.

- Complete resection
  This may be the only satisfactory biopsy in some germ cell tumours, certain cystic renal tumours, and ganglio-neuroblastoma.

All these biopsy techniques carry with them the potential risk of complications: bleeding from the tumour, damage to adjacent organs, or the subsequent development of adhesions. Any form of biopsy is also a form of rupture of the tumour and so brings the theoretical risk of local spread. The biopsy site should generally be placed where it will be excised at subsequent surgical resection. When identifying the type of biopsy to be carried out, the risks of the procedure should be taken into consideration and every attempt made to minimise distress to the child. It should also be remembered, however, that inadequate samples may lead to a delay in treatment and the need for repeat biopsies. The more accurate the information that can be gained on the nature of the tumour, the more closely treatment can be tailored to the need of the individual child. When preparing a child for biopsy, there are particular anaesthetic and surgical risks which should be identified and managed in order to minimise the risk of the complications of this procedure (Table 17.1).

Table 17.1: Risk factors prior to diagnostic surgery		
Physiological parameters	Potential problem	Possible treatment
Blood count	Anaemia. Thrombocytopenia Neutropenia	Transfuse if Hb< 8 g/dl. Platelet transfusion if <50 × 10⁹/l. Alert to risk of infection
Haemodynamics	Hypertension in, e.g. Wilms' tumour, neuroblastoma. Hypovolaemia from a ruptured tumour	Oral nifedipine or labetalol infusion depending on severity. Fluid resuscitation — colloid transfusion
Renal function	Acute obstruction due to tumour or early stage renal failure. Hypovolaemia may lead to acute renal failure; Tumour lysis. Spinal tumour may present with neurogenic bladder	Correction by fluid management or haemodialysis. Hydration and allopurinol. Indwelling catheter
Respiratory state	May be severely compromised if large chest tumour, or anaemia is severe	Humidified oxygen therapy. Chest X-ray and blood gas monitoring
Pain control	May experience pain exacerbated by fear and anxiety	Consider all suitable methods; liase with anaesthetist. Check contraindications in view of altered blood count
Gastrointestinal disturbance	Possible acute bowel obstruction caused by tumour causing vomiting and pain	Nil by mouth. Insertion of nasogastric tube and antiemetic therapy

Surgery as a Treatment Option

The primary objective in treating most solid tumours remains complete surgical resection. The removal of the primary tumour is held to be an important prognostic factor for many types of malignancy. The way in which this is attempted will vary widely, depending on the size, the location and the nature of the tumour. For some localised tumours, primary surgical excision remains the best and most satisfactory option. The greatest changes to surgical strategy have occurred in those tumours found to be sensitive to chemo-therapy and, to a lesser extent, radiotherapy.

When these other treatment modalities were first introduced, surgery remained the first line of treatment. Tumours were removed where possible and first radiotherapy and then chemotherapy were used to try to prevent any recurrence of disease (adjuvant treatment). If a tumour could not be completely removed, as much as possible was resected (debulking). Radiotherapy and chemotherapy were then used to treat residual disease, with varying degrees of success.

Current approaches to surgical management are generally more likely to involve pre-operative (neo-adjuvant) treatment with chemotherapy in order to shrink the tumour prior to resection. Developments in chemotherapy have introduced the possibility of reducing the size of many paediatric tumours, so facilitating complete tumour resection. Thus surgery is now more likely to achieve its primary aim, through an approach which brings other advantages in its wake.

Decreased local invasion by the tumour may allow greater preser-vation of adjacent healthy tissue and less risk of damage to neigh-bouring organs. There will be less risk of rupture of the tumour and because the blood flow to it is reduced there is also less risk of haemorrhage. With complete resection of the tumour, a child is less likely to require post-operative radiotherapy, with its attendant complications.

With the use of pre-operative chemotherapy, tumours that were unresectable at diagnosis will frequently become so. In some cases, there will be such a good response to chemotherapy that the residual tumour becomes unable to be detected clinically or radiologically. In such cases surgery may still be necessary, as there may be residual macroscopic or microscopic disease apparent at surgical exploration. It is important to define the extent of any remaining disease in order to plan subsequent treatment.

The timing of surgical intervention in the overall treatment of children with cancer remains the subject of much study, comparative work and disagreement among oncologists and surgeons. The studies and clinical trials coordinated by the UKCCSG and on an international level by the Societe Internationale d'Oncologie Paediatrique (SIOP) and other groups, include surgery as part of the overall management of children with particular diseases. In some of these studies, the correct place of primary surgery is one of the ques-tions to be asked. In such trials, the family faced with the devastating news of a diagnosis of cancer may be asked if consent will be given to their child being 'randomised' in a clinical trial of treatment. If the family agrees, the child will be randomly allocated to one of a choice of different courses of treatment, and this may take place at a very early stage in their child's illness. This decision can be very difficult for the family and raises important ethical questions about issues of informed consent in certain of the current treatment strategies.

The following is an outline of the role of surgery in the current management of the more common solid tumours of childhood and its relation to other treatment modalities. This will include a brief review of some ongoing studies and trials.

Wilms' tumour

Wilms' tumour, as outlined previously, has been one of the great success stories of paediatric oncology. It has been treated by the three major modalities of surgery, radiotherapy and chemotherapy, but the challenge remains; how to use them most effectively, how to continue to increase survival if possible, and how to reduce the effects of therapy on children with a good prognosis.

Historically, the surgical treatment of Wilms' tumour has always been immediate nephrectomy unless the tumour was either metastatic at presentation, spreading into the inferior vena cava and thus inoperable, or bilateral. European groups (through SIOP) have suggested benefits from pre-operative chemotherapy in reducing both tumour rupture and local spread, so that it becomes more resectable. This may 'down stage' a child with Wilms' tumour from Stage III disease to Stage I or II, thus reducing the need for subsequent chemotherapy and, in particular, doxorubicin which is cardiotoxic.

The disadvantages of this approach are that during the pre-operative chemotherapy there is obviously less information about the tumour itself. The diagnosis may prove to be inaccurate, the histological features which predict tumour response may be unclear, and the local extent of spread unknown. Because of this the American National Wilms' Tumour Study remains philosophically committed to the standard practice of immediate nephrectomy as providing the most accurate diagnosis and staging and the best surgical treatment.

In the UK, at present, a trial is in progress to compare these two approaches: to compare pre-operative chemotherapy with immediate nephrectomy in children with an operable tumour.

This particular trial brings up some difficult issues for all members of the team caring for the child and the family. Entry into the trial and randomisation into one of these two treatment groups must occur at a very early stage in the child's diagnosis. At this time the family is still reeling from the shock of the diagnosis of cancer, and are trying to come to terms with the enormous impact of their child's illness and treatment. They are then told that the specialists in whom they are hoping to put their trust 'do not know' which is the best way to treat their child. They are asked to try and understand the concept of the randomised clinical trial in the context of their child's treatment and prognosis. This is a discussion which both family and clinician will inevitably find hard and which calls for great sensitivity from all members of the team supporting the family. It raises some of the complex ethical dilemmas so often faced concerning the issue of informed consent. How 'informed' can that consent really be at this stage of a child's illness and treatment? Do we have the right to ask families and children, to make that sort of decision? Do we have the right to make it for them? These are questions which must be asked constantly and which show clearly that consent to treatment can never be a once-for-all decision. Rather, it should be a dynamic process at the heart of the relationship between the child, the family and the team caring for them.

In all situations, with or without primary chemotherapy, a child with a Wilms' tumour will eventually come to surgical resection. This may be complicated by intracaval tumour, where cardiac bypass procedures may be required, or by extensive bilateral tumour. There is a risk of renal failure following surgery for bilateral disease, and on rare occasions, a child may actually need a kidney transplant.

Soft tissue sarcomas

The most common form of soft tissue sarcoma in childhood and adolescence is the rhabdomyosarcoma. Treatment strategies have been derived from multi-institutional clinical trials, on a national or international basis. These trials have resulted in more sophisticated use of radiotherapy, more effective chemotherapy, and have looked at ways of combining these modalities with surgery to maximise survival and reduce treatment-related side effects.

The role of surgery has developed through this process, and the broad treatment strategy is now for biopsy or conservative initial surgery in the first instance. If, at presentation, the tumour can be removed completely, safely and without mutilation then primary excision is recommended. However, this is rarely possible; the main exception being in paratesticular tumours, which may be completely excised. Radical surgery, such as amputation of a limb or pelvic exenteration, are no longer used as primary treatment (Spicer, 1995) but may remain an option after chemotherapy. Chemotherapy is used both as treatment for possible systemic disease and to optimise local therapy, particularly with regard to organ conservation where possible, for example in tumours of the bladder. Secondary surgery is carried out following the shrinkage of the tumour by chemotherapy. Where tumours have failed to respond initially to chemotherapy the child may have radiotherapy before surgery, to further shrink the tumour before resection.

Where secondary resection is incomplete, or is not possible due to the site of the tumour, the child may go on to have further adjuvant treatment. Occasionally, the response to chemotherapy and radio-therapy may be inadequate to the extent that they will still require a mutilating procedure, such as amputation or pelvic exenteration, but such an outcome is increasingly unusual. Soft tissue sarcomas in different sites require variable methods of local control (Table 17.2).

Table 17.2: Local control in soft tissue sarcomas	
Site	Usual local disease control
Orbit	primary chemotherapy; radiotherapy if not complete response; surgery rare
Parameningeal — head and neck	primary chemotherapy; radiotherapy commonly used; surgical techniques complex but increasing in practice (plastics)
Non-parameningeal — head and neck	primary chemotherapy; surgery considered if resectable — may be specialised plastic approach; radiotherapy as second-line treatment
Bladder and prostate	primary chemotherapy; surgery if feasible — may be mutilating; radiotherapy if unresectable or residual disease
Paratesticular	immediate surgery; adjuvant chemotherapy
Limb	primary chemotherapy; on occasion immediate surgery; surgery for local control; radiotherapy for unresectable or residual disease

Advances in the pathological diagnosis of soft tissue sarcomas have identified other types, such as primitive neuroectodermal tumour, which respond in a similar way to rhabdomyosarcoma and are treated using the same strategies. Other types of rare soft tissue sarcoma are paediatric variants of adult tumours, for example liposarcoma and fibrosarcoma. They are less sensitive to chemotherapy and surgical management plays a more important role, with radiotherapy where resection is incomplete.

Neuroblastoma

Neuroblastoma is a malignant tumour derived from the sympathetic nervous system. It is the most common intra-abdominal tumour in children with a median age at presentation of two years. Surgery is extremely important in the management of neuroblastoma, but the timing and strategy for resection is dependent on the stage of the disease at presentation (Brodeur et al., 1988):

- Stage 1 and 2A
  Localised disease — essentially curable by surgery alone.
- Stage 2B
  Localised disease with evidence of nodal involvement — a short course of chemotherapy may be required before and following surgery, although this is a point of some dispute. Current studies are looking at the place of radiotherapy after surgery.
- Stage 3
  Localised tumour which crosses the mid-line or is unresectable at presentation — pre-operative chemotherapy will shrink the tumour enough for most children then to have surgery. If resection of the primary tumour is incomplete, children will go on to have radiotherapy. Aggressive surgery is indicated in this group and surgeons will go to great lengths to remove the tumour. This may result in damage to neighbouring tissues and possible organ loss, for example nephrectomy, splenectomy. Developments in chemotherapy, and improved surgical techniques, have led to better survival rates in this group (Pinkerton et al., 1994).
- Stage 4
  Dissemination of tumour to distant lymph nodes, bone, bone marrow, liver and/or other organs — the outlook for this group of children remains extremely poor. Because of this there have been questions over the role of prolonged and difficult surgical procedures in this group. With the use of more intensive chemotherapy protocols in these children it has become possible to obtain

clearance of identifiable metastatic disease and then surgical resection is recommended. This can be a complex procedure, with children needing intensive nursing support. Where resection is incomplete there are questions over the use of local irradiation, either external beam, or mIBG targeted therapy (Lashford et al., 1992). The use of high-dose therapy, such as melphalan, with autologous marrow or stem cell rescue is now accepted in Stage 4 neuroblastoma. Other treatment options are being explored for this particularly harrowing disease (Plowman & Pinkerton, 1992).

- Stage 4S

Localised primary tumour, with dissemination limited to liver, skin and / or bone marrow, but not bone — this usually occurs in infants under one year, and will frequently resolve spontaneously. The role for surgery is unproven, although resection is recommended by some authorities where resolution is incomplete.

There is a remarkable difference in the way this tumour behaves in most children who present under one year old regardless of the extent of the disease. Infant neuroblastoma carries a much better prognosis and so surgery is nearly always less aggressive than in the older child.

Liver tumours

Most primary liver tumours in children are malignant, the most common being hepatoblastoma, followed by hepatocellular carcinoma. The aim of surgical treatment of these tumours is complete resection. The increased use of aggressive pre-operative chemotherapy regimes, usually containing cisplatin and doxorubicin, has greatly improved the number of tumours that can be resected. At the same time as developments in chemotherapy there have been technical advances in liver surgery which have made resection an attainable goal in more of these tumours (Vos, 1995). This is directly related to segmented or lobal involvement of the liver where resection is not a possibility, but transplant may now be considered as a real option.

The combination of effective chemotherapy regimes and advanced surgical treatment has led to a dramatic improvement in survival in these relatively rare tumours. In hepatoblastoma survival is now around 70–80%, although it is less good in hepatocellular carcinoma at around 40% or less (Vos, 1995).

Germ cell tumours

The nomenclature of germ cell tumours can be confusing. They originate in embryonic cell division and arise from the pluripotent germ cell population which in foetal life migrated from the yolk sac endoderm to the genital ridge (Pinkerton et al., 1994). The tumour may, therefore, occur in the ovary or the testis, but may also be found in distant sites due to the aberrant migration of cells at an early stage in foetal life. In children, 70% of germ cell tumours occur outside gonadal sites, most commonly in the sacrococcygeal area but also the mediastinum and pineal region. Malignant germ cell tumours in children have histological features which reflect two cell populations, yolk sac cells that produce alpha-fetoprotein and trophoblastic, producing beta-HCG. These tumour markers are useful in monitoring the disease. Surgery has a clear role in the management of most of these tumours:

- Testicular teratoma — when there is no evidence of metastatic disease surgical excision is likely to be curative. This must use an inguinal approach. Children should be followed up closely after surgery. Most of these tumours in childhood are of predominantly yolk sac elements and so produce AFP which can be monitored as part of follow-up.
- Ovarian tumours — again yolk sac tumours are more common and AFP is a useful marker. With localised disease, unilateral salpingo-oophorectomy may be curative without the need for radiotherapy or chemotherapy. However, this is a chemosensitive tumour and where there is extensive disease, chemotherapy can be used to avoid the need for extensive, mutilating surgery.
- Sacrococcygeal teratomas — usually present in the neonatal period and are generally benign, with well-differentiated pathology. Complete resection is curative in most cases. Where presentation has more malignant elements they will generally respond well to chemotherapy.
- Mediastinal germ cell tumours — can be very bulky at presentation and difficult to treat by surgical means. Effective chemotherapy can shrink many of these tumours to a size where surgical resection is possible.

Hodgkin's disease

Historically, staging laparotomies have been carried out to identify abdominal disease, but this has had no demonstrable benefit. The role of surgery in Hodgkin's disease is therefore limited to tissue biopsy at diagnosis, although in the USA routine staging laparomtomies are still undertaken.

Non-Hodgkin's lymphoma

The primary role for surgery in non-Hodgkin's lymphoma (NHL) is also restricted to biopsy for tissue diagnosis, although this may be provided by bone marrow, ascitic fluid or pleural effusion cytology. NHL responds well to chemotherapy and there is therefore no role for initial debulking of abdominal disease, or attempted resection of the tumour; such intervention can cause unnecessary morbidity with no therapeutic effect. Occasionally, T-cell NHL can present with rapidly progressing upper airway obstruction, which may require an emergency tracheostomy. In general, however, this disease will respond so quickly to the initiation of treatment that such an invasive procedure will be unnecessary.

Intestinal NHL may present with bowel obstruction either because of the mass itself, or because the mass has become the basis for an intussusception. Limited resection to relieve the obstruction may be appropriate, but radical surgery is not indicated, and biopsy alone followed by chemotherapy may suffice.

Retinoblastoma

Retinoblastoma is a tumour of neuro-ectodermal origin which arises in retinal tissue. Its treatment depends on the extent of the tumour and is as conservative as possible, using sophisticated radiotherapy techniques and adjuvant chemotherapy in certain settings.

Enucleation of the eye is now relatively uncommon, but is recommended if:

- The tumour involves more than half the retina
- There is evidence of glaucoma
- No useful vision is likely to be retained with conservative treatment.

It is mandatory if:

- Conservative treatment has failed
- There is involvement of the optic nerve.

Enucleation is clearly a specialist intervention, as is the overall management of this tumour. Most children with retinoblastoma are seen in two specialist centres in the UK, where such surgery is carried out. By this centralisation children receive the specialist care they require, and families receive appropriate support in dealing with surgery and its effects.

Surgical Treatment of Metastases

The most common site of metastases in paediatric solid tumours, both at presentation and at relapse, is the lung. If control of the primary tumour can be achieved then surgical treatment of metastases may be attempted, and has produced good results (Plaschkes, 1986). This will generally involve thoracotomy, and where bilateral treatment is required this will usually be carried out on two separate occasions. Localised metastatic lesions in the liver may also be treated with surgical resection.

Preparing the Child and the Family for Surgery

The child undergoing planned surgery for excision of a tumour requires extensive physical and psychological preparation. The following areas of care need consideration:

- Psychological care of the child and the family
- Change of clinical setting
- Pain assessment and control
- Physical preparation of the child for a general anaesthetic.

Psychological care of the child and the family

In the early stages after the child's diagnosis the parents may experience a sense of numbness and shock precipitated by the sight of their child appearing acutely ill. Information and advice given at this time may need to be repeated and emphasised regularly (Evans, 1993a). Where possible, the surgeon and oncologist should both be present to give details of the treatment required. A nurse should also be present to ensure continuity of information. Other members of the team may be introduced at a later stage.

Throughout the child's stay, it is important to remember that they are part of a family unit and therefore care should include close family members. Parents should be encouraged to continue their role in care. Siblings should not be forgotten as their lives, too, will change dramatically. Everyday routines will be disrupted whilst their brother or sister may endure lengthy hospital stays, intensive treat-ment and frequent clinic appointments. Siblings may feel insecure, and confusion is common (Dominic, 1993). In order to avoid long-lasting emotional and behavioural problems siblings should receive special care and attention as soon as the diagnosis has been made.

Help from the play specialist should be sought early for the child, brothers and sisters. They may be seen by the child as a non-threatening member of staff and the playroom thought of as a 'safe area' where only pleasant things happen. Age-appropriate play can be invaluable in preparation for surgery. Teaching the child and family the correct use of central lines can be made easier by using dolls, teddies or puzzles which are available with functioning central lines in place. Role play can help to prepare the child for surgery and the dressing-up box can include uniforms, oxygen masks, theatre hats, stethoscopes and much of the paraphernalia of surgery. Coping mechanisms can be introduced in the form of play, for example, using play dough to squeeze, or visual imagery during painful proce-dures. Relaxation techniques can be valuable for both the child and the family and there are numerous tapes and videos available for this purpose, for example, water music and whale sounds.

Very few hospitals have a teenage unit at the present time, there-fore alternative accommodation must be sought (NAWCH, 1990; House of Commons Select Committee, 1997). If possible, teenagers wanting privacy should be nursed in a single room, ideally with their own bathroom facilities. If they wish to stay on the main ward, then having a group of similarly aged teenagers together may be consid-ered. Relaxation of ward rules will inevitably occur if their particular needs are to be met, for example, watching TV later in the evening, having groups of friends to visit and free access to recreational activi-ties when the playroom is closed to younger children.

Change of clinical setting

It is important that the transfer from the oncology ward to the surgi-cal unit is as smooth as possible. This will avoid unnecessary stress and worry for the family who have built a rapport with the team on the oncology unit. An unfamiliar environment with many new faces may produce 'a crisis of confidence', leading to increased fear and anxiety about the impending surgery. Nursing staff should endeav-our to promote continuity of care and extend support from the new members of the multidisciplinary team. Because of the close links between the two wards there is a need for comprehensive documentation which will aid transfer, with the obvious benefits of having standardised clinical charts and assessment tools. Before transfer, the designated named nurse (Department of Health, 1991) from the surgical ward should have a pre-operative discussion with the family at which relevant information can be exchanged and a plan of care made. There should be liaison between named nurses from both areas, and note should be made of any specific considerations for the child, in particular the need for pre-medication prior to blood product transfusion, whether in-line filters are used, previous allergies and dystonic reactions, and previous pain history (McGrath, 1989).

Pain assessment and control

The admission procedure may be an appropriate time to discuss the assessment and management of pain (Taylor, 1996). Pain assessment and relief has improved greatly and many units are now able to offer a comprehensive 'pain service'. To gain understanding of the child's previous pain experience it may be useful to document words that the child and the family use (Llewellyn, 1993a, b). This will help when using the chosen pain assessment tool (Llewellyn, 1996). The tool should be appropriate to the child's cognitive developmental stage and easy to use. Ideally it should be introduced prior to surgery and before the child experiences pain. As it is widely accepted that fear of the unknown can increase a child's perception of pain (Rodin, 1985) it is important that the child is given relevant explanations of what to expect following surgery. The amount and depth of information given should be tailored to each child according to age and comprehension. This may be successfully introduced in the form of story-telling by the play specialist (Hahn, 1987).

The anaesthetist should explain the various methods of pain relief that are suitable, for example, epidural infusion, patient-controlled analgesia (PCA) and continuous opioid infusion. The pain history may indicate low pain thresholds and drug tolerance; therefore the usual dosage prescription may require review. Advances in pain relief mean that it is unnecessary for a child to receive intramuscular injections as a route for analgesia. A child may choose to suffer increased pain quietly for a long period of time rather than consenting to a painful injection. Also, absorption of intramuscular analgesia is irregular compared with the intravenous route and the likelihood of the child experiencing peaks and troughs in pain relief is increased (Llewellyn, 1993a, b). The ideal should be to provide continuous pain relief with the ability to deal with breakthrough pain

with supplementary oral medication or bolus doses of the appropriate infusion.

Epidural analgesia is the introduction of local anaesthetic, with or
without an opioid, into the epidural space via a fine catheter
accessed by the anaesthetist prior to the surgical procedure. The
solution is delivered to specific nerve roots to provide a band of analgesia (epidural block) corresponding to the site of entry to the
epidural space (McShane, 1992). If the epidural is ineffective, alternative analgesia should be established and the epidural disconin-
ued. Successful epidural analgesia should be discontinued once it
has been agreed that oral/rectal analgesia will offer effective pain
relief. Epidural analgesia is not without side effects and knowledge of
these, by experienced nurses with the appropriate training, allows for
early identification of problems. When caring for a child with an
epidural infusion hospital protocol should be strictly followed.
Observations should include: pulse oximetry monitoring, hourly
blood pressure and pulse recording, epidural site and block checks,
limb sensation and movement checks and strict pressure area cares.
Awareness of side effects should minimise potential complications,
such as brachycardia, hypotension, respiratory depression, nausea
and vomiting, pruritus, paraesthesia, limb weakness and urinary
retention.

In addition to the more conventional types of pain relief available in the hospital setting, nurses should be aware of the contribution complementary therapies have to offer (Mantle, 1992);
parents may express a wish to be involved in providing massage,
relaxation or aromatherapy for their child. This may be implemented into the child's plan of care following local policy,
provided there are no medical contraindications. The use of
complementary therapy requires a skilled practitioner who has
received appropriate training.

Physical preparation of the child for a general anaesthetic

On admission the child will require similar preparation to that for
any child requiring routine general surgery. This should include the
allocation of a named nurse, introduction to the plan of care and a
tour of the ward and playroom. Baseline observations of vital signs
and pulse oximetry should be taken and an accurate height and
weight recorded.

In the pre-operative period, details will need to be given regarding fasting. Traditionally, patients used to fast from diet and fluids for

a minimum of six hours. Research indicates that clear fluids may be taken up to two hours pre-operatively (Bates, 1994). During the fasting period the continuation of mouth care should be encouraged. This maintains the child's comfort by keeping the mucosa moist and also serves to reduce the feeling of thirst.

The theatre team may provide an opportunity for the child and the family to visit the anaesthetic room and parts of the theatre suite. If it is likely that the child will require a period of time in the intensive care unit then arrangements should be made for the family to visit this area, to meet the nursing staff and to familiarise themselves with the 'high-tech' environment.

The parents should be allowed to accompany their child to theatre and, if they wish, provision should be made for at least one of them to stay with the child in the anaesthetic room until they are asleep (Turner, 1989). Repeated general anaesthetics can lead to psychological problems due to fear and anxiety for the child. Pre-operative preparation, as discussed previously, is of paramount importance, as is a calm, efficient but welcoming environment in the anaesthetic room.

The aim of pre-operative care is that the child is in optimum health to undergo the anaesthetic and the surgical procedure. The blood picture should be as near normal limits as is possible. This may entail pre-operative transfusions of blood and platelets or supplementary therapy of electrolytes such as potassium.

The type of tumour may indicate the anaesthetic care. For example, in the case of neuroblastoma the tumour may secrete catecholamines. Careful monitoring of blood pressure and the administration of antihypertensive agents may be necessary. In the case of phaeochromocytoma, sudden gross hypertension may cause cardiovascular collapse, at the time of surgery. Tumours of the central nervous system, or the presence of cerebral metastases, carry a risk of raised intracranial pressure; signs to look for are headache, drowsiness, vomiting, papilloedema or bulging fontanelle. If there is raised intracranial pressure, mechanical, rather than spontaneous, ventilation, may be indicated during general anaesthesia. Tumours involving the airway, for example nasopharyngeal rhabdomyosarcoma, have the potential for pre-, peri- and post-operative compromise of the airway.

Bone marrow suppression, caused either by the disease, for example leukaemia, or chemotherapeutic agents can cause potential problems for the anaesthetist (Table 17.3).

Table 17.1: Bone marrow suppression	
Symptom	Problem
Low haemoglobin level	Reduction in oxygen carrying capability of the blood Possible need for pre-/peri-operative blood transfusion
Low platelet count	Bleeding/clotting problems Difficulty in maintaining haemostasis during operation Possible need for pre-, peri- and post-operative transfusion of platelets
Low white cell count	Susceptibility to infection especially chest infections Need for pre-operative X-ray May require oxygen therapy and physiotherapy post-operatively May lead to oxygen dependency post-operatively If severe chest infection may require ventilation ICU post-operatively

The medication required by the child with cancer can alter anaesthetic management. Steroid therapy can lead to adrenosuppression and intravenous hydrocortisone may be necessary in the perioperative and immediate post-operative period. Bleomycin, in the presence of oxygen therapy, can cause pulmonary fibrosis and may lead to respiratory failure. Thus minimum oxygen concentration must be administered to maintain oxygenation. Doxorubicin can cause cardiomyopathy and thus compromise cardiac function. Assessments must therefore be made prior to anaesthesia; these include chest X-ray and echocardiography. Other chemotherapeutic agents may cause renal toxicity. Urine and blood assays are taken to establish the child's renal function; if necessary the appropriate changes in the child's fluid balance and electrolyte management are made. If the tumour is enlarging it may begin to occupy vital organ space and this may lead to a mediastinal shift, with chest tumours or splinting of the diaphragm with abdominal tumours. This may cause respiratory or cardiac compromise and thus the surgeon and anaesthetist may not have the luxury of time for the child to be in optimum health due to a developing emergency situation.

During the operation the anaesthetist and surgeon will be aware of complications that may arise and should be prepared to adapt their procedures accordingly. This may include rupture of major blood vessels requiring grafting or rupture of the tumour which may indicate further adaptation to the treatment regime.

Parents should be kept informed of progress as far as possible. Once the surgery is complete, it is important that the surgeon visits and provides a comprehensive description of the findings and the procedure. A prolonged anaesthetic may result in a longer stay in the recovery area, thus increasing the time the child is away from the ward. When the condition of the child allows, the parents should be allowed to stay in the recovery room until transfer is appropriate (Brown, 1995).

There are specific nursing considerations which are dependent on the site of the tumour requiring surgery.

Tumours of the Chest

These include primitive neuroectodermal tumour (PNET) and chest metastases. The main post-operative consideration with all chest surgery is to maximise respiration and oxygenation. In the immediate post-operative period, this may entail ventilatory support in the intensive care setting. Observations of respiration should include rate, depth, effort and pattern of chest expansion. It would be pertinent to monitor oxygen saturation continuously. Oxygen therapy, if required, should be given with caution and titrated to maintain oxygen saturation levels, as agreed by the anaesthetic team. The oxygen given should be humidified; thus promoting comfort by keeping the mucosa moist and aiding expectoration of secretions. If there are chest drains, they should be managed according to guidelines developed locally by the surgical and nursing teams. Continuous low pressure suction on chest drains is sometimes indicated, requiring clear definition of the negative pressure and careful monitoring. Chest drains should be observed for bubbling and/or swinging with respiration and for signs of bleeding. Any excessive blood loss via chest drainage may be replaced intravenously with colloid. Thoracotomies are painful incisions therefore effective pain management is a priority. Thoracic epidural infusions are the method of choice and should be maintained until the chest drain(s) are removed. Alternative analgesia methods may be employed, for example PCA or continuous opiate infusion combined with regular analgesia. Physiotherapy is very important after chest surgery to prevent the development of a chest infection by helping the lungs to reinflate. It should therefore be planned to coincide with optimum pain relief.

Tumours of the Abdomen

These include Wilms' tumour, neuroblastoma, hepatoblastoma and germ cell tumour. Resection of tumours in the abdomen can lead to a prolonged paralytic ileus. This may be exacerbated by chemotherapeutic agents, for example vincristine, and opiates such as morphine. Prolonged ileus may be an indication for total parenteral nutrition (TPN). The site of the tumour may indicate the need for stoma formation (either permanent or temporary) depending on the amount of gut involved. This leads to specialised nursing care, education of the child and the family, close liaison with the stoma nurse and consideration of the effect of altered body image. In the case of Wilms' tumour and neuroblastoma, hypertension may be a problem pre- and post-operatively. This should be controlled with a calcium channel blocker, such as nifedipine, or a betablocker, such as labetalol. Depending on the extent of the tumour involved with the vascular system there may be an indication at surgery to graft major blood vessels. Post-operative observations should in this case include circulatory observations of the limbs especially the lower extremities. In the case of surgery to the liver, liver function tests and clotting assessments should be performed. Alteration to dosages of drugs, whose main route of elimination is the liver, should be considered.

Tumours of the Pelvis

These include rhabdomyosarcoma, PNET and teratoma. They may involve the urinary tract and/or the reproductive system.

Urological nursing often involves caring for indwelling catheters (urethral or supra-pubic) and ureteric stents. Bleeding is very common and clots may lead to blockage of the drainage system. Stents and catheters may need irrigation or flushing to maintain patency. Securing the drainage tubes helps to prevent dislodgement, stents and catheters may be sutured in place at surgery. Bladder spasm is very distressing for the child and may be treated by oxybutynin and diazepam as prescribed. Extensive urinary surgery may lead to the formation of a urinary stoma.

Surgery to the reproductive system may bring to light issues related to fertility and this will be discussed later in this section.

Post-operative Nursing Care

Recent advances in surgery have resulted in children requiring high dependency care from nurses with advanced skills. Specialised nursing care allows for a safe and full recovery from the anaesthetic and surgical procedure. During this post-operative period the care of the child progresses from a high level of nurse dependency to a greater emphasis on family-centred care which requires nursing support rather than management. Care should be tailored to meet the individual needs of the child and the family. There are general considerations which must be acknowledged to promote this recovery (Table 17.4).

Discharge Planning

Discharge from hospital is planned in advance to enable a smooth transition from the surgical ward to the community or home. It may warrant a further change in the clinical setting by, for example, transfer back to the medical oncology ward. Close liaison between all parties should be encouraged to ensure that timing for discharge is appropriate and occurs when the child is deemed fit for discharge by parents, nursing staff, surgeons, oncologists, and the child concerned.

The child and parents are given verbal advice on wound care, medication and return to activities such as contact sports and school. A contact number for advice and queries should also be given. An outpatient appointment will be made at a combined surgical/medical oncology clinic, for follow-up assessment of the child.

Paediatric oncology outreach nurse specialists have a vital role in ensuring a smooth transition from ward to home and a strong link between the two. They liaise with the surgical team before the child's discharge and coordinate community services. They may visit the family at home shortly after discharge, or offer telephone support. This service is valued by families, because they feel vulnerable and unsure as to how to care for their convalescing child.

Late Effects of Surgery

Stoma formation

Occasionally the surgical treatment for bladder tumours is total cystectomy, this will mean that a urostomy or an ileal conduit will need to be formed. The psychological preparation of the child requiring stoma formation should begin as soon as the surgeon is aware that a cystectomy is the treatment of choice. Preparation includes clear and concise explanations about the care of the urostomy; it is helpful if the stoma specialist nurse is introduced at the earliest possible time. For a very young child or baby, explanation and teaching should be directed at the family members who will be performing the care. The older child, who has more awareness of body image, will require more direct involvement and counselling and may benefit from meeting another child with a stoma (Johnson,

Table 17.4: Post-operative care considerations

Problem	Aim of care	Nursing care	Family involvement
Potential respiratory difficulty following general anaesthetic	Safe recovery	Maintain airway and consider possible ventilatory support	Reassure re: child's conscious level May be aware of change in child's colour Can help with moving and changing child's position
Potential bleeding and hypovolaemic shock	Early detection of any deterioration of child's condition	Record blood pressure, pulse and colour Observe and record signs of irritability Record drainage from wound drains Safe transfusion of blood and platelets as required Check peripheries and capillary refill Give colloids as necessary	Give explanations about wound, drains and what is expected in regard to amount of drainage
Pain due to surgery	Control and relieve to allow for rest and movement	Care of chosen system, e.g. epidural, PCA, morphine infusion Assist in achieving a comfortable position and promoting an environment conducive to rest Provide distraction and relaxation Liaise with play specialist Consider complementary therapies, e.g. massage	Help with assessment tools Give comfort and support Help with diversion and play therapy Provide comfort from home, e.g. blankets, toys, pictures, etc.

(contd)

Table 17.4: (contd)

Problem	Aim of care	Nursing care	Family involvement
Reduced oral intake due to gastrointestinal disturbance	Maintain hydration	Nil orally until condition dictates Care of i.v. infusion as per protocol Monitor fluid balance Invasive monitoring care: CVA line Care of nasogastric tube: record aspirate type and amount Administer antiemetic therapy Check for hypovolaemia and oedema Monitor blood sugars Consult dietician re: nasogastric feeding, TPN	Perform mouth care Encourage drinks and order favourite food from dietician
Potential deterioration in renal function	Monitor urine output: aim for 0.5 ml/kg/hour	Care of catheters Weigh nappies Monitor for retention of urine (epidural complication) Monitor urea and electrolytes	Encourage child to sit on a potty or toilet Help in changing nappies Give teenager privacy

(contd)

Table 17.4: (contd)

Problem	Aim of care	Nursing care	Family involvement
Potential wound infection	Prevent infection and promote healing	Monitor body temperature Complete wound assessment chart Remove wound dressing after 24 hours if wound not visible Observe for inflammation and discharge Obtain swab for culture and sensitivity	Provide support and comfort during dressing changes Teach care of line, catheters and stoma bags as appropriate
Reduced mobility	Maintain skin integrity and meet hygiene needs	Provide regular pressure area care Use of pressure-relieving aids Ensure good pain management Liaise with physiotherapist Provide for hygiene needs	Assist with washing, cleaning teeth, brushing hair Provide cool, comfy nightwear Take the child for walks around ward in pushchair/wheelchair
Boredom and anxiety	Provide reassurance and stimulation as appropriate to physical condition and developmental stage	Provide toys, books, games, music, etc. Privacy for teenagers Explain all procedures Enlist the help of play specialist, school teacher and psychologist	Presence at bedside and involvement as much as desired Encourage the child to take periods of respite away from the ward Arrange for close friends to visit

1992). After surgery, the programme of education about the care of the urostomy continues, and dolls or teddies are often useful in demonstrating procedures. The stoma specialist nurse can offer support to the child and the family in grieving, and in coming to terms with the child's altered body image (Dickinson, 1995). Children should be encouraged to help with their stoma care as soon as is possible, as familiarity may help lead to a sense of normality. Extensive bowel resection may also result in stoma formation and issues of general management will be the same.

Bladder neuropathy

Due to the effects of the tumour, surgery or treatment with chemotherapy or radiotherapy, the child may have a resultant bladder neuropathy. In the past, the treatment of choice was continuous urethral catheterisation. However, this has associated complications of urethral erosion, urinary infections and fears of leakage or disconnection and the embarrassment of wearing a catheter bag. Nowadays, intermittent self-catheterisation (ISC) is favoured.

ISC is performed throughout the day at regular intervals. The child (or carer) empties the bladder by the insertion of a catheter which is then immediately removed. The aim is to enable the child to control their bladder rather than have the bladder controlling them (Winder, 1994). The child and the carer are taught by nurses who have specialised training. Videos and leaflets are available to reinforce the advice given by the nurse. The child is taught the anatomy of the urinary system and the nurse explains the procedure of ISC, including the care and supply of catheters and observes the child/carer perform ISC.

Nursing note:

A mirror is often helpful when identifying the urethral opening in girls.

This programme of education continues until the child/carer is able and confident to perform ISC on their own. ISC leads to a more normal pattern of bladder emptying and, as a result, can improve the child's body image and lifestyle. In addition, it offers some control over the body (Seymour, 1996).

Infertility

Surgery to the reproductive system, necessitating organ removal, will bring to light issues of fertility. Infertility may also be caused by some

chemotherapeutic agents and radiotherapy which may compound
the surgical problem. In the very young child this may be a difficult
concept for the parents to cope with and may be seen as a low priority. In future life, however, it may be of paramount importance to the
survivor of childhood malignancy who can barely remember the
original illness. Sensitivity in broaching this subject is important and
referral to a specialist team, which may include a counsellor, psychologist and gynaecologist, may be appropriate. Nursing staff should be
aware that for teenagers, infertility may be viewed as a high priority
but embarrassment may prevent them from discussing it.
Opportunities should be provided for the subject to be discussed and
then at the appropriate time the various options available can be
considered.

Malabsorption

Resection of large amounts of intestine may lead to malabsorption,
resulting in nutritional deficiency. The child may require long term
nutritional support at home, for example TPN through a central line
or enteral feeding using modular products. Care should be aimed at
providing the required feed at home, with the aid of the dietician,
general practitioner and the paediatric outreach nurse specialist
(Sidey, 1995).

Adhesions

Formation of bowel adhesions due to scar tissue is a common
complication of all abdominal surgery. The child may present with
acute abdominal pain and severe dehydration due to persistent
vomiting, indicating intestinal obstruction. Intravenous fluid
replacement therapy should be commenced immediately to prevent
hypovolaemic shock and to correct any fluid and electrolyte imbalance. The pain experienced may vary in nature from being
described as mild and cramp-like, to severe, continuous and
localised. This will depend on the type of obstruction and if the
obstruction does not resolve with conservative management, i.e. 'nil
by mouth' and a nasogastric tube, surgery will be indicated to divide
the adhesions.

Body image

When the surgeon is considering the type of surgical procedure to be
used, attention should be given to the placement of the incision to

minimise the effect on body image. Scarring cannot be avoided, but careful planning can reduce the cosmetic insult, perhaps with a scar placed where it can be covered by clothing, for example a 'bikini-line' incision, or an incision in a natural skin crease. Occasionally future plastic surgery may be needed to reduce surgical scarring.

Surgery as an Aid to the Management of Treatment

As surgeons have become more closely integrated members of the multidisciplinary team caring for the child with cancer, so the contribution they can make to the overall management of children has been more widely recognised within the team. Surgery has a distinctive part to play in certain aspects of a child's clinical management.

Central venous access

The introduction and continuing development of indwelling central venous access devices (CVADs) has been essential to the advances in treatment seen in paediatric oncology over the last two decades. The administration of aggressive multidrug chemotherapy protocols and the complex supportive care they necessitate, would be impossible without the availability of robust, permanent venous access (Hollis, 1992). The types of central venous access devices now common in clinical practice have brought great benefits to children, but are not without risk. They bring with them a number of potential complications and, in particular, carry significant morbidity related to infection and sepsis (Corbally, 1993).

There are two types of central line in common use. The external catheter (Hickman or Broviac type) is composed of cuffed silastic tubing, tunnelled under the skin from the anterior chest wall into the cephalic subclavian or internal jugular vein, with the tip lying near the right atrium. The line is held in position by a dacron cuff, which encourages the formation of fibrous tissue ingrowth into the cuff, and has an external segment. It may have one or more lumens. The alternative is a wholly implantable subcutaneous port, attached internally to a silastic catheter, accessed by insertion of a needle. In recent years there have been developments in both types of line arising from the increased sophistication of both medical technology and surgical techniques of line placement. These developments have given rise to a number of clinical features which should be considered when choosing the most appropriate line for a particular child (Table 17.5).

Table 17.5: Comparison of the clinical features of central venous access devices

External catheters	Implantable ports
'Hickman' or 'Broviac' type	'Portacath' type
Designed for continuous use	Designed for intermittent use
Dual and triple lumen readily available	Dual lumen port available but have been limited in practical application
Regular dressing required	Dressing required only when port is in use
Some restriction on activity (e.g. swimming) and lifestyle	Less restriction on activity and more 'normal' lifestyle
Some restriction on dress	Minimal restriction on dress
Dislodgement possible	Dislodgement rare
No needle required for access	Needle required for access; needle dislodgement possible, possible extravasation
Significant impact on body image	Less impact on body image
?Higher infection rate	?Lower infection rate

The choice of line will be influenced by a number of factors, taking into account these clinical features. A child undergoing a particularly complex or aggressive treatment regime, who is likely to require continuous access over weeks or even months, would be better with a multilumen, external catheter. A child with a solid tumour, or acute lymphoblastic leukaemia, receiving 'standard' intermittent chemotherapy may find an internal port less restrictive. Older children and teenagers, for whom body image is of particular importance, may find an internal port less intrusive.

For some children, particularly those with a developed needle-phobia, the accessing of the internal port via a needle would be a major disadvantage. The use of local anaesthetic applications on ports is, however, very effective and children should be assured of this. In addition, it is the training of the operator (i.e. person accessing the port) that will make a difference to the overall discomfort that is felt as most discomfort results from compression of the soft tissues between the base of the port and the ribs; too much prodding and pressure will culminate in increasing discomfort. For some younger children the process of changing dressings on an external catheter can be a distressing experience, whereas when the internal port is not in use, no intervention is needed. There is some clinical evidence that the risks of infection are greater in external catheters than internal ports. This is probably related to the fact that the exit site is a portal of entry for skin flora, and that the port of access is inevitably exposed (Shapiro, 1995).

All these factors need to be taken into account when considering the insertion of a central venous access device. Historically, external catheters have been more widely used in paediatric oncology patients, and this remains the case in most centres within the UK, as has been shown by recent data from an audit looking at central line use (PONF/UKCCSG, 1996). Implanted ports, however, have recently been evaluated in a number of studies (Shapiro, 1995) which show they can be used successfully in children with leukaemia as well as solid tumours and may offer certain advantages. The lower infection rates reported in implanted ports appears significant. Quality of life may also be improved, with fewer restrictions on activity and less maintenance of the catheter. Certainly for teenagers they appear a more attractive option with a more 'normal' lifestyle and minimal alteration to body image. When clinical condition and treatment plan permits, the child and the family should be given a choice of what sort of line they will have.

The information needed to make that choice is an important first step in the process of preparing the child and the family for the insertion of a central line. They need first to understand what a central line is and why it is necessary. For children, play can be very important in this process (Leese, 1989). Dolls or teddies with central lines in place can demonstrate the difference between the types of line (also helpful to parents!) and help children to become familiar with them. So, too, can seeing other children with lines in place and the family will often find it useful to discuss this with another family and hear 'first hand' about their effect and use. Information given must clearly be tailored to the age of the child or young person and the understanding of the family. For teenagers, offering a choice of line can be helpful in restoring a measure of control in their treatment and it is therefore of critical importance that youngsters receive the information they need to help them make the right choice. Pictures, diagrams, models and the 'real thing' may all be helpful in this process.

Before surgery consideration should be given to the siting of the catheter, as the impact on physical appearance and body image can be minimised by careful surgical placement (Daniels, 1995). This also affects ease of access, particularly with internal ports. Central lines should be inserted by an experienced surgeon who carries out this procedure on a regular basis, in order to minimise potential complications. Where it is possible, line insertion should be carried out when the child is neither neutropenic nor thrombocytopenic, in order to reduce the risks associated with bleeding, bruising and infection. This is clearly not always possible, as the child's clinical condition and the need for treatment will often dictate the need for a line. When the child has a low platelet count, the administration of pre- and post-operative platelet transfusions will be required to try to avoid these problems. The issue of pain control should be discussed before surgery, in order that it may be effective post-operatively.

Surgical techniques for the insertion and fixation of central lines have developed alongside the growing expertise of those carrying out these procedures. Increased collaboration between surgeons working in the regional centres treating children has led to moves towards standardising these techniques, and formulating national guidelines. Part of the impetus for this has come from a national study in the UK, looking at the management of central lines in paediatric oncology. This study was first set up in 1993 as a collaborative venture between nurses and doctors working in the speciality under the umbrella of the Paediatric Oncology Nurses Forum (RCN) and the UKCCSG, to audit practice and establish guidelines in this important aspect of supportive care (Leese et al., 1997).

There are at present wide local variations in the type of line used, the way it is inserted, the way it is secured, and the different aspects of subsequent management. Whilst it is hoped that national guidelines will be established in the future to address these issues, there are certain basic principles essential to good practice in the handling of central venous access devices (Crow, 1996). Aseptic technique is of paramount importance from the time of insertion onwards. The frequency with which lines are cleaned and dressed subsequent to insertion is a local variable, as is the type of dressing used. Recent data regarding the frequency of early dislodgement of external lines (Tweddle et al., 1997) indicates the importance of a robust method of securing lines in the early days after insertion, allowing time for the exit site to heal and the cuff to become established *in situ*. There is at present no good clinical evidence as to whether gauze and tape or occlusive film dressings, or any variation on these themes, is superior when it comes to the securing of lines, or the prevention of infection. There is a pressing need for research to be carried out in this important area of care to provide evidence to compare against time-honoured custom and practice. There is some evidence that chlorhexidine is the most effective antiseptic when cleaning exit sites (Maki et al., 1991).

Central lines are capped by a variety of different obdurators and connectors, many of which aim to provide a closed system for both blood sampling and the administration of drugs and fluids. There has been no convincing study to show the benefit of these devices in preventing infection, but they are widely used in clinical practice. It should be remembered that many of these devices are guaranteed for only a limited number of punctures, records need to be kept of this and obdurators changed on a regular basis. All those handling such devices need to be aware of the need for a sound non-touch technique in all areas of clinical management.

There remains discrepancy over the flushing of central lines when not in use. There is clinical evidence that a Hickman-type line only needs to be flushed once a week with a heparinised saline solution and indeed there are centres which do not routinely flush these catheters at all (Hollis, 1992). An implanted port should be flushed with a heparinised solution once a month.

There are many ways of guarding against accidental damage to central lines.

Nursing note:

In some small children, who may tug an external catheter and even pull it out, it may be better to insert the line into the back, rather than the chest wall, so that it is well out of reach. Lines must always be well secured and many families and the staff caring for them, have devised a range of 'pockets' and pouches in which to keep the line out of the way. Others simply tuck it into a vest or a 'crop-top' for added security. Some children who have an external catheter in place may wish to go swimming. Again, an ingenious range of methods of protecting lines has been devised using occlusive dressings and even urine collection bags into which a line can be coiled, and then secured to the chest wall.

Swimming appears to carry a significant risk of infection, although unproven, and this must be balanced against the benefit of the child doing one of the 'normal' activities they enjoy. A child who enjoys swimming may be better with an internal port where this is possible.

Once the central line has been established, the family and the child need to be taught how to care for it, in accordance with local policy. This teaching needs to be carried out in a standard way, at the pace of the individual child or family, well-supported by the nurse caring for them (Pike, 1989). By encouraging them to become involved with treatment in this way and take on this aspect of care, the family or the child themselves can regain some sense of control over the process. This may be one of the first steps in transferring some of the child's care from the hospital setting back to home. Learning to care for the line themselves, helps the older child or teenager to accept it in a more positive way.

Complications of central venous access

The major complications of central venous catheters are early dislodgement, infection, sampling problems and blockage.

Infection

There are several distinct types of infection related to central venous catheters. Superficial infections at both the tunnel and the exit site are often an early complication, although they can occur at any time during the life of a line. Infection can also occur at the pocket of an internal port. Catheter-related infections are frequently signalled by fever and rigors associated with use of the line and may be identified by positive blood cultures which can indicate colonisation. As stated previously, a number of studies have shown overall lower rates of infection with internal ports in comparison to external catheters (Shapiro, 1995). As this author points out, however, this may be partly related to the population of patients in each group. As external catheters tend to be used in patients with leukaemia and those undergoing intensive chemotherapy regimes, they tend to be more at risk of infection associated with prolonged and profound neutropenia.

There has been, and continues to be, much debate about the treatment of catheter-related infections and the indications for the removal of an infected catheter (Shapiro, 1995). It is frequently possible to treat catheter-related bacteraemias with antibiotics, although the reappearance of a particular organism on more than one occasion would be reason to remove the line. Certain organisms, notably *Staphylococcus aureus* and species of *Candida* are almost impossible to eradicate with antibiotics alone and removal of the catheter will then normally be required. When lines are removed because of infection, an interval should be left before a new line is inserted, as otherwise it too is likely to become infected. Any serious infection of the tunnel of an external line, or the pocket of an internal port, is likely to lead to its removal.

Sampling problems

Sampling or blood withdrawal problems can occur in both types of central venous access device, and may be caused by the formation of a fibrin sheath which acts as a sort of one-way valve at the catheter tip, or because the tip is up against the wall of the blood vessel. Repeated flushing and aspiration of the catheter, change of position of the child, or the instillation of 5000 units of urokinase into the catheter may solve this problem.

Blockage

The instillation of urokinase may also help to clear a line that has become completely blocked. Lines are particularly likely to block with prolonged parenteral nutrition, and lipid clots can be cleared with the use of alcohol instilled in the line. Where precipitation is thought to have occurred in the line, hydrochloric acid or sodium bicarbonate may also be used to free a blocked line. Such interventions should always take place according to a properly formulated protocol. There is an increasing recognition of the risk of venous thrombosis formation on the end and around the catheter in the superior vena cava, with the consequent potential of pulmonary emboli. Imaging and an echocardiogram should be considered to establish the cause of the occlusion in an occluded catheter, particularly in the presence of infection.

The risk of potential complications associated with central venous lines can be minimised with the development of a sound policy for handling and training whether it is aimed at health care professionals (Dougherty, 1996), parents, or children themselves. Research is needed to develop evidence-based practice in all aspects of the management of central lines.

Central venous access is essential for the administration of chemotherapy regimes, and for the management of the side effects of such treatment and subsequent support of the child. As well as providing the route by which much of that supportive care is given, surgery may be needed at other times to treat the complications associated with treatment.

Management of Infection

Mucositis is a common side effect of many cytotoxic drugs, particularly in the combinations used in some of the multidrug regimes in paediatric practice. When children become neutropenic they are very much at risk of infection affecting the mucosa of the intestine. Enterocolitis may present in a particularly severe form as a typhlitis, with paralytic ileus and large loops of inflamed distended bowel. This will produce many of the signs of an acute abdomen in the child and on occasion can lead to perforation of the gut. In the face of profound neutropenia and thrombocytopenia, management of this condition will, where possible, be by the conservative measure of resting the bowel, to allow healing to take place. On occasion urgent surgical intervention will be required. An experienced surgeon should, therefore, be involved in the child's management from the onset of such symptoms and decisions about treatment taken in close cooperation and consultation with the oncologist. The surgeon should be clearly identified as an important member of the multi-disciplinary treatment team. There are other occasions when surgery may be required, for example in the surgical treatment of abscesses or other localised manifestations of infection.

Nutrition

Central venous access is required for the administration of parenteral feeding, but surgeons may be involved in methods of enteral feeding as well. Where children are going to require long term enteral nutritional support, nasogastric feeding is usually the first option. For some children, because of problems related to the tumour or disease process, or to side effects of treatment, this is not an option and then a gastrostomy may be considered (Corbally, 1993). As gastrostomies are only rarely encountered in oncology patients, the expertise of surgical nurses and nutritional support teams will need to be brought in to support these families.

Surgery to Avoid the Complications of Radiotherapy

In the planning of external beam radiotherapy, consideration is always given to normal tissue structures and the radiation dose they will receive. In certain situations there is a role for surgery in actually moving certain critical organs to ensure that they do not receive high doses of radiation with attendant damage, and repositioning them for the duration of treatment.

Several mechanisms have been devised, using tissue expanders, for moving normal bowel out of a radiation field. This has a particular application in pelvic Ewings' sarcoma, where it is necessary to target the tumour with a high dose of radiation. Another technique, of ovarian plication, has been developed to 'hitch' the ovaries out of the area of pelvic irradiation (Tait, 1992).

In some children brachytherapy will be used, where a radio-isotope is placed within the tumour, or in close proximity to it, in order to give a continuous, concentrated dose of radiotherapy. Here the surgeon may be required to carry out physical placement under the guidance of the radiologist.

Future Trends in Surgery

The continual development of treatment for children with cancer has focused on two major aims, to improve cure rates for the 35% of children who do not survive; and to reduce long term effects of treatment and improve the quality of life for those who do. Future trends in surgery, alongside the other treatment modalities, will address these issues in the different areas identified in this section.

As scientific progress is made in the process of tissue analysis, and the understanding of tumour biology, so the requirements of tissue biopsy will become more clear, with the possibility of less invasive techniques and thus reduced risk of complications for children. The development of guidelines in biopsy techniques will help to improve consistency on a national level, and contribute to developing expertise in surgeons involved in this process.

The increased role of surgeons in the setting up and conduct of clinical trials in the treatment of paediatric solid tumours has led to a more defined understanding of the place of surgery in the overall clinical management of children. As the understanding of such tumours continues to grow, increasingly, treatment will be tailored to the needs of the particular tumour in the particular child. In some cases this may mean a greater role for surgery in the complete resection of tumours. In other cases it may mean identifying groups of children who should not be operated on, as in non-Hodgkin's lymphoma in recent years.

As surgeons develop further expertise in particular fields there will be continued improvements in surgical techniques, with the hope of increased collaboration and communication leading to more standardised procedures based on best clinical practice.

There have been moves away from mutilating surgical treatment to more conservative options, for good reason and with positive effects. As the late effects of radiotherapy and chemotherapy and their associated toxicities become more apparent, it may be that the role of surgery will be re-evaluated, but with surgeons working much more closely as part of the multidisciplinary treatment team. In some areas, such as tumours of the pelvis, and of the head and neck, more radical surgical options are already being explored.

Surgery can be in many cases one of the most emotionally critical points of treatment for the child and family. It is a very definite and concrete intervention with a clear aim, and often immediate results. It thus presents an enormous challenge to nurses working in both the oncology and the surgical setting to ensure that the child and family are prepared for, and supported through this stressful event.

Chapter 18
Neurosurgery

Lindy May and Jane Watson

Introduction

Rickman Godley performed the first successful craniotomy for removal of a brain tumour in 1884; however, the patient died of meningitis 10 days later (Ainsworth, 1989). The procedure of craniotomy is believed to be 20 000 years old, when primitive man used this method in an attempt to rid sick tribal members of demons. Today, craniotomy/craniectomy is used for the removal of brain tumours and surgery still constitutes the primary therapy for tumour irradication. Nowadays, however, it is often just the starting point of treatment, which consists of radiotherapy and chemotherapy in addition to surgical resection.

Review of Literature in Relation to Current Treatment of Brain Tumours

Paediatric brain tumours are the most common solid tumour found in children and the second most common neoplasm (Shiminski-Maher & Shields, 1995). Paediatric brain tumours account for 20% of all paediatric cancers (Tobias & Hayward, 1989). Historically, these tumours have been treated with surgery and/or radiotherapy, but more recently chemotherapy has been utilised, either on its own or more usually in conjunction with the above treatment. Chemotherapy, long thought to be ineffective in the treatment of these tumours, has changed from its previous usage as a palliative treatment, to a more actively utilised and recognised treatment (Ryan & Shiminski-Maher, 1995). Chemotherapeutic agents used in the treatment of brain tumours may, however, have a neurotoxic effect on the developing brain (Moore, 1995). Influencing factors in the treatment regime today include the child's age, the degree of surgical resection and the histological characteristics of the tumour. The length of survival following the diagnosis of a paediatric brain tumour, and the quality of that survival, have been influenced by the recent advances in neurosurgery, anaesthesia, chemotherapy and radiotherapy (Packer et al., 1989). Neuroradiology and, in particular, MRI scanning have been essential aids in these advances.

Along with the increased survival time for the child with a brain tumour comes the recognition of significant long term consequences of the treatment, and these include intellectual and endocrine functions (Johnson et al., 1994).

Aetiology of Brain Tumours

Tumours of the brain comprise about one-fifth of all cancers during childhood and there has been an increase in their incidence, in the last 15 years, of 15%. This response may be due to better diagnostic services rather than any real biological changes. The only known factors that predispose to the development of brain tumours are certain genetic factors, such as neurofibromatosis types 1 and 2, tuberous sclerosis and Li-Fraumeni syndrome (Byrne, 1996). Radiation, including exposure *in utero*, is known to increase the risk of tumours. Environmental factors may be important and electromagnetic fields have been the subject of numerous recent studies, following the increased incidence of central nervous system tumours in areas close to high-power lines in America (Byrne, 1996). The results of these studies are as yet inconclusive.

Tumour Types

Fifty to sixty per cent of childhood brain tumours originate in the posterior fossa and these include astrocytomas, medulloblastomas and ependymomas; the remaining 40–50% are supratentorial and include optic pathway tumours, hypothalamic tumours, cranio-pharyngiomas and astrocytomas (Wisoff & Epstein, 1994). Primitive neuroectodermal tumours (PNETs) can occur at any site.

Astrocytoma

This tumour comprises about 33% of all paediatric brain tumours and most originate supratentorially. Signs and symptoms depend on the anatomical position of the tumour and its histological grade: tumours originating in the occiput will result in visual field defects; those in the motor cortex may result in a hemiparesis and seizures; the deep-seated astrocytomas, such as hypotholamic tumours, produce endocrine disturbance. Approximately 20% are malignant; these tumours are treated with surgical resection where possible, followed by chemotherapy and/or radiotherapy, but the outlook remains bleak for the majority of children with them. Low-grade astrocytomas which are totally resected surgically should result in long term survival and probable cure for the child; low-grade astrocytomas which are not totally resectable may require further treatment with low-dose chemotherapy and/or radiotherapy in the expectation that tumour growth will be halted or reduced.

Prognosis: a cure should be achieved if a benign astrocytoma is completely removed surgically, and the prognosis is good, although these tumours have occasionally regrown. With an incomplete removal of a benign astrocytoma there is a higher risk of tumour regrowth. With a malignant astrocytoma a long term cure remains unlikely.

Medulloblastoma

This is the most common malignant brain tumour in children and accounts for 20% of childhood brain tumours. These are posterior fossa lesions, originating in the cerebellum and often involving the fourth ventricle (with resulting hydrocephalus) and the brain stem; dissemination of tumour cells down the spinal column occurs in 25–45% of all children (Geyer et al., 1980). Symptoms include early morning vomiting, ataxia, headaches and sometimes visual disturbance.

After surgical resection, craniospinal irradiation has been the treatment of choice, resulting in a 20–60% survival rate over the past two decades (Shiminski-Maher & Shields, 1995). The value of chemotherapy is continually being assessed and several trials are currently in progress, yet to be evaluated.

Prognosis: medulloblastomas respond well to treatment and treatment regimes are continuing to improve the prognosis for this tumour group. These tumours are known to recur, however, and the presence of spinal metastases at diagnosis increases this risk and lowers the overall chance of survival.

Ependymoma

This tumour originates from the ependymal cells of the ventricular lining and usually involves the fourth ventricle; hydrocephalus is therefore common and spinal metastases often occur (less than 10% at diagnosis). Treatment is by surgical resection of the cerebral lesion. The grade of an ependymoma has not been proven to be of prognostic significance and a 'watch and wait' policy would occasionally be implemented in a non-metastatic, totally resected tumour. After surgical resection, all other children would receive radiotherapy (if over three years old) and chemotherapy (if under three).

Prognosis: depends on the degree of surgical resection and the presence or absence of metastases.

Brain stem tumours

Symptoms include multiple cranial nerve involvement and, occasionally, hydrocephalus. The development of MRI scanning has allowed for better visualisation of the brain stem, and although the majority of brain stem tumours are malignant with a poor outlook, there are a small number which are cystic, focal and operable. Radiation is the main treatment for all brain stem tumours regardless of whether tissue diagnosis is obtained; chemotherapy may also be used.

Prognosis: remains poor for children with these tumours, and although not proven, those with tumours of a lower histological grade may have a longer survival.

Mid-line tumours

The anatomical site of these tumours, plus their histological diagnosis, make the signs and symptoms they exhibit very variable; the treatment given is based on their histology. Included are deep-seated tumours, such as craniopharyngiomas, germ cell tumours, optic pathway, hypothalamic and pineal tumours. Their symptoms include endocrine abnormalities, visual disturbance, cognitive impairment, personality and memory changes. Although most of these tumours are benign, their position makes surgical resection difficult or impossible and radiotherapy and/or chemotherapy may be the only treatment possible. Craniopharyngiomas are the most common of these tumours, accounting for 6–8% of all childhood brain tumours. They are difficult to resect and there is usually significant long term endocrine disturbance. Radiotherapy is sometimes used, as are intracystic radioactive implants.

Prognosis: a complete surgical resection of these complex tumours offers the highest chance of cure, but often results in significant physical and cognitive changes. These tumours are persistent and an incomplete resection reduces the chances of long term survival.

Presentation of Brain Tumours

The variations in presentation exhibited by the child with a brain tumour are dependent on the following factors:

- Compression or infiltration of specific cerebral tissue
- Related cerebral oedema
- Development of raised intracranial pressure.

Depending on the type and location of the tumour, one or all of the above symptoms may occur. The diagnosis of a brain tumour is often difficult to establish in a child, since many of the signs and symptoms may mimic those of the more common childhood illnesses. This delay in diagnosis will frequently lead to anger and/or guilt on behalf of the parents, and much reassurance is required to allay the fears that an earlier diagnosis may have led to a better outlook, which in reality is rarely the case.

Signs and symptoms may further vary depending on the age and development of the child, in addition to the size and location of the tumour, although most children will suffer headaches. Supratentorial cortical tumours are commonly associated with hemiparesis, visual disturbance, seizures and intellectual difficulties. Supratentorial/mid-line tumours are commonly associated with pituitary disturbance, visual changes and raised intracranial pressure due to hydrocephalus. Posterior fossa tumours are also frequently associated with hydrocephalus and, in addition, with ataxia, vomiting and nystagmus. Brain stem tumours may involve any of the above plus cranial nerve involvement (Figure 18.1).

Midsagittal Section

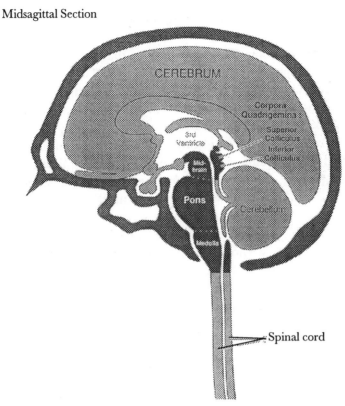

Figure 18.1: Brain stem: midbrain, pons and medulla

Increased intracranial pressure and hydrocephalus

If any of the three components in the skull (blood, brain and cere-brospinal fluid) vary in volume due to oedema, haemorrhage or hydrocephalus, the intracranial pressure varies. This results in an increase in head circumference in the baby whose skull sutures are not yet fused. In the child with fused sutures this results in symptoms such as headaches, vomiting, papilloedema and an altered level of consciousness. Tumour growth can cause a direct volume increase, resulting in raised intracranial pressure, or can cause a block to the normal flow of cerebrospinal fluid, with resulting hydrocephalus. The surgical treatment of increased intracranial pressure involves removal of the tumour, where possible, which may resolve the hydrocephalus by releasing the local blockage. An external ventric-ular drain may sometimes be used as a temporary measure and a ventricular peritoneal shunt inserted in those children where hydro-cephalus does not resolve. Occasionally, a third ventriculoscopy may be performed, thus eliminating the need for a shunt (Drake, 1993).

Hydrocephalus refers to the progressive dilatation of the ventricles due to production of the cerebrospinal fluid (CSF) exceeding its rate of absorption. Thirty to forty per cent of children with brain tumours will require a permanent shunt for secondary hydrocephalus (Bonner & Siegal, 1988) and consequently the neuro-oncology nurse must have an understanding of the mechanics of shunts and their possible complications. These complications may include infection, blockage or disconnection; very occasionally, tumour dissemination may occur via the shunt (Berger et al., 1991).

Shunt malfunction may mimic the signs of the brain tumour (such as vomiting, headache and drowsiness) and diagnosis may well be impossible without a scan. This may necessitate either sedation or general anaesthesia in the uncooperative child, followed by surgical replacement of the shunt if required. Children presenting with pyrexia and neutropenia who have a shunt must have the possibility of a shunt infection assessed. CSF is only taken for culture if such infection is strongly indicated, as the risk of introducing infection by sampling is a possibility. In a study of patients with intraventricular reservoirs placed for chemotherapy delivery 8.2% had positive CSF cultures, although they were clinically asymptomatic (Brown et al., 1987). This raises the discussion of treatment for infection.

The child with a brain tumour presents additional concerns when receiving chemotherapy requiring hyperhydration; the risk of increased intracranial pressure from hyperhydration must be balanced against the risk of chemotherapy side effects due to inadequate hydration. The presence of a ventricular-peritoneal shunt for the treatment of hydrocephalus might be an asset in the presence of hyperhydration, assisting in reducing raised intracranial pressure. The administration of an antiemetic with a sedative side effect must be balanced against the possibility of the drowsiness caused by shunt malfunction. Both parents and nurses must be encouraged to report subtle changes in the child's behaviour promptly, so that appropriate investigations can be instigated if necessary. Repeated absence from school, the effects of hospitalisation and the underlying disease in the child with hydrocephalus and a brain tumour, may result in cognitive and psychosocial impairment. The neuro-oncology and liaison nurses alongside the community children's nursing services can assist in communicating with the schools about the special needs of the child with a shunt.

Nursing note:

Once a shunt has been fitted for the treatment of hydrocephalus, it is there for life; working shunts are rarely removed. With a shunt *in situ* the child can still fly in an aeroplane without any ill-effects. Routine childhood immunisations can be given to the child with a shunt after discussion with the consultant. Sports are not contraindicated, but activities such as boxing and rugby are not recommended.

Investigations into Brain Tumours

Radiology

CT scan

Computed tomography (CT) has been the cornerstone of neurological diagnostic procedures and continues to be of huge importance. The head is scanned in successive layers by narrow X-ray beams that pass through the skull and are transmitted or absorbed depending on the tissue density. The X-rays are converted into light photons by an array of scintillation crystals (the 'scanner'). The photons are, in turn, converted to electrical signals that are stored on a computer. The information is digitised and manipulated by the computer and the resulting display image photographed on polaroid or standard film. A CT scan will illustrate changes in the location of structures, abnormalities and displacement of these structures and changes in tissue density.

MRI scan

Magnetic resonance imaging (MRI) is perhaps a less invasive technique than the CT scan since no radiation is used, and it is becoming more widely available. MRI provides more accurate pictures than the CT scan, particularly of the posterior fossa and spine. The patient is placed in a strong magnetic field and is then subjected to precise bursts of computer-programmed radio frequency waves. The magnet causes atoms with an odd number of nuclei protons to line up in a uniform manner and when further energy in the form of radio frequency waves is applied, the nuclei can be predictably tipped out of alignment. Once the radio frequency waves are turned off, the resonating nuclei will relax back again to their original position; momentary radio frequency signals are emitted as the nuclei relax, which the computer uses to construct images of the tissue. MRI scans are images of the hydrogen distribution in the body, since this is the most abundant atom in human tissue, and has a single proton (i.e. an odd number) in its nucleus. MRI is effective in detecting tumours, necrosis and central nervous system degeneration. The images received are extremely accurate in their detail of anatomical information and the physiology and biochemistry of living tissue.

The child requiring either a CT scan or MRI may require sedation if they are unable to lie still for the required time. This may pose problems for the child who has raised intracranial pressure and a general anaesthetic may be safer in these situations. An appropriate explanation, using photographs of the scanners, relaxation techniques and diversion therapy can often result in a successful CT scan without sedation; but the noise of the equipment and the length of time required to keep still for MRI means that most toddlers and young children will require sedation or anaesthesia.

Nursing note:

MRI can be performed when metal clips are still *in situ*. However, it is advisable to discuss this with the neuroradiologist first.

Neurological assessment

The purpose of the nurse's neurological assessment is different from that conducted by doctors and it is performed to determine the following:

- Identify the presence of any central nervous system dysfunction and hence anticipate further dysfunction that may be aggravated by surgery.
- Compare existing data to determine any changes (this may be particularly appropriate in a child with a brain stem tumour, where deterioration may be sudden and consequent treatment should be prompt).
- Detect any life-threatening situations (children with secondary hydrocephalus may quite suddenly reach a level of raised intracranial pressure which is no longer acceptable and respiratory arrest will occur without intervention).
- Provide a profile on which further nursing assessment will be based.

This neurological assessment should comprise a recognised coma scale, such as the Glasgow coma scale, or associated coma scales, such as the Great Ormond Street Hospital for Children NHS Trust Coma Chart (Figure 18.2). The latter was research-based and utilises one concise chart for all patients. It is based on cognitive rather than chronological age.

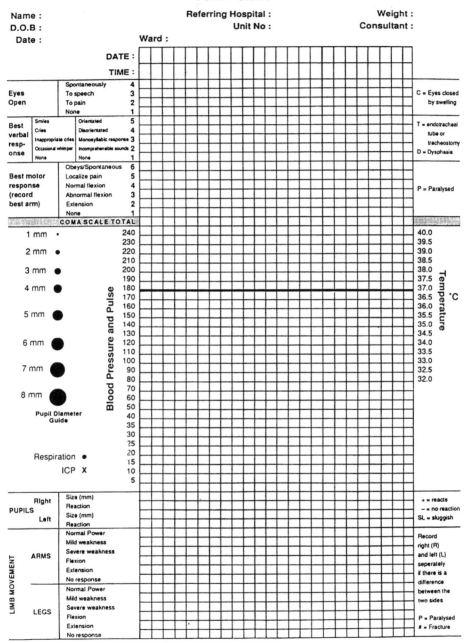

Figure 18.2: (a) Coma chart, (b) coma scale and (c) comments chart
(From the Great Ormond Street Hospital for Children NHS Trust.)

(contd)

GREAT ORMOND STREET HOSPITAL FOR CHILDREN NHS TRUST
COMA SCALE

The coma scale is scored on a total of 15 points. A total of less than 12 should give rise for concern. This is a universally accepted tool for measuring coma. A decrease in coma scale will be associated with a decreased level of consciousness. This needs to be considered along with the patient's vital signs.

A Eyes Open
If eyes closed by swelling, please write 'C' in relevant column, in red biro, thus indicating reason for lower score.

B. Best verbal response
In the left hand margin are two separate scales: the far left is the scale for babies and infants, and on the right is the scale for older children.

The following section gives an explanation of the best verbal response of infants.

a) **Smiles**

This can be used to describe an alert contented infant, as not all will smile at a stranger. The interaction between parents and infant should therefore be taken into account.

b) **Appropriate Cries**

The infant may be unable to settle.

c) **Inappropriate Cries**

The infant may have periods of being drowsy, but at times is heard to cry out. This is not always associated with being disturbed. The cry maybe high pitched.

d) **Occasional Whimper**

Less frequent than above and may be associated when deep painful stimuli is required to gain motor response.

e) **None**

No verbal response.

C. Best Motor Response to Stimuli
The age and cognitive abilities of the child must be taken into account.

D. Pupils
When recording pupils size it is important to remember the effects of drugs; eg morphine will cause pinpoint pupils, and atropine drops will dilate pupils for up to 6 hours.

E. Limb Movememts

a) If a child has a permanent hemiparesis, please indicate such in the relevant column - eg weakness, even though it is normal for this child.

b) A child with a severe developmental delay, may score lower on the coma scale, as his motor response may be poor.

Figure 18.2: (contd)

GREAT ORMOND STREET FOR CHILDREN NHS TRUST

COMMENTS CHART

NAME   UNIT NUMBER

DATE	TIME	SIGNIFICANT OBSERVATIONS (Eg. headache, ataxia, vomiting)	SIGNIFICANT EVENTS (Eg. seizure, sedation)	SPECIAL INSTRUCTIONS (Eg. EVD height, positioning)

SB 1996 NEUROSCIENCE'S   To be used with Coma chart

Figure 18.2: (contd)

Coma scales standardise observations for the assessment of level of consciousness; pupillary signs and motor function of the upper and lower extremities are based on assessment of eye opening, best verbal response and motor response. Observations of vital signs must also be recorded in conjunction with the neurological observations and these may alert the nurse to problems caused by or in association with a change in intracranial pressure. Although there is a recognised association of raised intracranial pressure with a lowered pulse and raised blood pressure this is often a late sign in children, and a drowsy or irritable child with slow pupil reaction should alert the nurse to a rise in intracranial pressure. Infants and small babies with tachycardia and a low blood pressure may be displaying signs of systemic hypovolaemia following surgery, or their symptoms may be due to a sudden loss of cerebrospinal fluid resulting in a reduction in intracranial pressure; neurological observations in conjunction with recordings of vital signs will help ascertain the cause and the necessary treatment to be given.

Respiratory patterns will change with both raised and lowered intracranial pressure and in the extreme situation intubation and ventilation may be required to assist the child until the situation is corrected. Hyperpyrexia is not uncommon, due to damage to the hypothalamus (following surgery or trauma); the presence of blood in the CSF is also known to result in pyrexia, although the reason for this is unknown. Whatever the cause, pyrexia must be treated promptly, as the resulting rise in metabolic rate increases the oxygen and metabolic requirements of an already compromised brain.

Play Therapy

A play specialist is often the best person to discuss anxieties with a child and play is an excellent medium through which the child can display their fears (Belson, 1987). The provision of play therapy is one of the top priorities in providing for a sick child's recovery and well-being (Brimblecome, 1980). Preparation for surgery is essential and should be performed whenever possible as it reduces some of the child's fears, and prepares the child for the post-operative period; children cope better with the anticipated, however brief the explanation may have been. They have huge fears of the unknown and many of these fears are based on fantasy which can be alleviated once discovered. Play also provides an emotional outlet for the child and enhances his coping mechanisms (Harvey, 1980). Play is seen by the multidisciplinary team as a vital contribution to the child's recovery since it promotes normal development in both sickness and health and provides a comforting sense of normality which helps the child to adjust to a strange environment. Although the value of play therapy has not yet been demonstrated by research studies, the reduction of stress in patients, parents, doctors and nurses is being recognised when a play therapy programme has been established (Harvey, 1980).

The Multidisciplinary Team

Clearly, the multidisciplinary team is required from the time of the child's admission. Once the diagnosis of a brain tumour has been established by scanning, various medical and nursing teams will need to assess the child. Initially, the child will have been referred to a neurosurgeon; an endocrine assessment may be relevant, the opinion of a neurologist sought, and a neuropyschologist involved. The oncologist and radiotherapist will be aware of the child, but will not become involved at this stage unless surgery is inappropriate as the initial treatment.

The clinical nurse specialist will not be involved until a definite histological diagnosis has been reached, however, the ward nurse is involved at this stage. The anxiety and uncertainty at this early stage of the disease will cause enormous distress and exhaustion to the family and the nurse can assist by listening to their worries, answering their questions where possible and supporting them at this traumatic time. Anxious parents will result in an anxious child; appropriate information needs to be given, including details of procedures and surgery. Hospitalised sick children will often behave in a manner younger than their years, and the location and effect of the tumour may add to this; information, therefore, needs to be appropriate for the child's developmental and emotional state.

Pre-operative Care

The child with a newly diagnosed brain tumour, and their family, will have been overwhelmed with information and explanations. They will also have met many new people at an exhausting, confusing and very frightening time. It is therefore understandable that explanations need to be repeated and be consistent as the full implication of diagnosis and prognosis is impossible to take in at once (Stedeford, 1984). The family needs to be encouraged to take one step at a time.

Reassurance must be given where possible and allowances made for perhaps irrational or unpredictable behaviour. Much time is given to the child, but the family (parents, siblings, grandparents, etc.) also have needs which must be met if the welfare of the child is to be maintained. The shock of diagnosis and the uncertainty of the outcome, coupled with the grief and loss of a healthy child, can be shared with the nurse, who can then guide the family through the next few hours and then days, providing support through surgery, the post-operative period and the anxiously awaited histology results. A unique relationship can often form at this time between the family and the nurse, and is of invaluable assistance to the family.

Once the operation has been explained and consent obtained, the play specialist will prepare the child psychologically and the nurse can prepare the parents. Preparation of the child starts by discovering what they themselves perceive as their illness and what they think is going to happen. From there, the play specialist can explain to the child, in a way which they understand, what the operation involves: for the toddler, this may include use of a doll to demonstrate what a head bandage or an intravenous infusion looks like, and for the older child, preparation may include looking at appropriate books or photographs. All preparation must be assessed on the individual's needs, and questions should be encouraged and answered as fully and honestly as is appropriate.

Preparation of the child's parents will include explanation of the monitoring equipment which will be used, the time of surgery and a description of how the child will look on return from theatre. Whatever details are given to the parents, nothing will prepare them adequately for seeing their own child post-operatively, although some of their fears may be lessened by familiarisation with the equipment.

Once the parents have accompanied the child to the anaesthetic room, their long and anxious wait begins, and encouraging them to go off the ward for a while is usually beneficial. This time away from the ward can be seen purely as a distraction technique for the family, but it also alleviates the anxiety about every incoming phone call to the ward, which is often incorrectly interpreted by anxious parents as a message from theatre concerning their child. During this time, the bed space will be prepared for the child and the monitoring equipment checked. Comfortable chairs for the parents to sit near the child can be organised later, once the child is stable and without impeding access to the child and emergency equipment.

During Surgery

During anaesthesia, controlled ventilation provides optimum operating conditions for performing craniotomy/craniectomy, by reducing intracranial pressure. There is no ideal anaesthetic agent for neurosurgery since all the drugs presently available have side effects, or may cause unpredictable problems (Hickey, 1992). Considerations include the effect drugs have on cerebral metabolism, cerebral blood flow, intracranial pressure and vasomotor tone. Other intraoperative concerns include the introduction of controlled hypothermia (thus decreasing cellular metabolism and the need for oxygen), hyperventilation (thus reducing brain bulk intracranial pressure) and venous air embolus (a potential problem associated with the sitting position frequently used for posterior fossa surgery). Surgery may take several hours and it is the responsibility of the theatre nurse, in addition to the anaesthetist, to ensure correct positioning of the child both to allow access for surgery and to ensure the patient's protection; this includes positioning of the limbs, protection of the eyes by closing and covering them, and the usual attention to theatre protocol, such as the use of diathermy. The theatre nurse needs to be familiar with the constantly new and updated neurosurgical equipment such as microscopes, stereotactic frames, neuroendoscopes, the Cavitron and the Wand. Correct assembly, cleaning and maintenance of this equipment is essential and involves appropriate training.

The anaesthetist and the neurosurgeon work closely during surgery. Any sudden haemorrhaging must by supported by the anaesthetist by prompt and appropriate replacement of blood/blood derivatives. An increase in intracranial pressure must be treated by hyperventilation or the administration of appropriate drugs such as mannitol. Any interference with the vital areas of the brain stem will produce an immediate irregularity or abnormality to the child's pulse and blood pressure, and the anaesthetist will report this reaction immediately to the surgeon, who can then stop or proceed with caution. Should the child's condition deteriorate, the anaesthetist will advise the neurosurgeon whilst attempting to stabilise the child's condition. The theatre nurse can alert the ward nurse as to any difficulties which might have arisen during surgery, although a detailed description should also be given by the anaesthetist. Analgesia can be given prior to the child's return to the ward and, if appropriate, the theatre/recovery nurse can clean any excessive blood/betadine off the child, in an attempt to lessen the shock to the parents when they first see their child.

Post-operative Management

After surgery, the child will be taken to the recovery room, the intensive care unit or the high dependency paediatric neurosurgical ward, depending on their condition, the individual hospital's organised layout, and medical and nursing expertise available.

The objectives of immediate post-operative nursing management are:

- Regular neurological assessment and early recognition of raised intracranial pressure
- Recognition and control of factors which could result in a rise of intracranial pressure
- Recognition of potential complications and administration of the required intervention
- Safety of the child
- Administration of regular analgesia
- Comfort and support to both the child and family.

Numerous problems can occur following surgery for a brain tumour and these are identified in Table 18.1.

Long Term Concerns

These include:

- Personality changes (often permanent and caused by surgery to the frontal lobes or the pituitary gland)
- Change of body image
- Change of family dynamics
- Quality of life
- Long term prognosis.

With so many potential complications, the child must have very close observation for the first 24–48 hours after surgery; emergencies may be sudden and the nurse's observation and clinical skills have a vital role in the child's well-being (Ainsworth, 1989). It is also essential that observations are recorded consistently, thus ensuring communication and continuity of care throughout.

The implications of these complications can be profound and the multidisciplinary team, both in hospital and in the community, will be closely involved with the family, working alongside the liaison nurse.

Table 18.1: Post-operative nursing management

Problem	Aim of care	Nursing care	Family involvement
Respiratory complications — due to airway obstruction, pneumonia	Ensure adequate oxygenation	Maintain a clear airway Appropriate positioning Suction as necessary Observe colour Observe and record respiratory rate Monitor oxygen saturation	Encourage child to cough and expectorate, if appropriate
Altered level of consciousness	To monitor and control intracranial pressure Ensure safety	Elevate the head 30° Frequent re-assessment of vital signs and neurological observations Assess deficits and administer basic care needs Ensure safety by supervision and use of cot sides	Encourage participation in providing care needs, alongside the nurse Supervision of the child in ensuring safety
Cardiac arrhythmias — due to brain stem irritation or blood in CSF	Early intervention if required	Observe for arrhythmias on the cardiac monitor	—
Haemorrhage (subdural, epidural, intracerebral or intraventricular)	Maintain haemodynamic stability	Observe for signs of haemorrhage Record vital signs Record Redivac drainage and replace with appropriate i.v. fluids	Family to provide reassurance

(contd)

Table 18.1: (contd)

Problem	Aim of care	Nursing care	Family involvement
Hypovolaemia	Rehydrate with appropriate fluid	Administer packed cells/albumin	—
Seizures	Maintain airway Prevent physical injury	Record episodes Position for maintenance of airway Administer oxygen Administer prescribed anticonvulsants	Once family are familiar with seizure activity they can record and report episodes
CSF leak	To prevent further leakage and reduce the risk of infection	Apply sterile dressing and inform medical staff	Inform nurse if they notice the dressing to be wet
Electrolyte imbalance due to surgery or diabetes insipidus	To maintain electrolytes within normal limits	Record fluid balance and replace fluids as prescribed Monitor urine specific gravity and report changes	Involve the family in recording of fluid balance following the acute post-operative period
Headache	To reduce/eliminate pain To detect any change to type, intensity and duration	Assess for signs and symptoms of pain (restlessness and tachycardia) Give analgesia as prescribed	Facilitate promotion of a quiet environment Encourage the child to relax Use relaxation methods such as stroking, talking, listening to quiet music

(contd)

Table 18.1: (contd)

Problem	Aim of care	Nursing care	Family involvement
Gastric irritation	To reduce symptoms	Administer appropriate therapy as prescribed	—
Neurological deficits (may be early and late sign): motor, sensory, communication	Ensure safety Encourage early rehabilitation	Provide care and stimulation until the child is self-caring Involve the multidisciplinary team, particularly physiotherapist and occupational therapist Work with speech therapist, introduce picture boards and writing boards	Family encouraged to assist in the child's care
Hyperthermia	To reduce temperature	Apply fan and give antipyretics	Can undertake tepid sponging under nursing instruction
Diminished gag reflex	To ensure safety	Suction as necessary Keep nil-by-mouth Gag reflex checked by medical staff before introducing oral feeding	Reassuring and comforting the child
Periocular oedema	Relieve periocular oedema	Nurse upright if appropriate (some centres use moist eye patches)	Provide ongoing reassurance

(contd)

Table 18.1: (contd)

Problem	Aim of care	Nursing care	Family involvement
Visual disturbances (late sign)	Minimise distress and utilise alternative senses	Maintain a safe environment Provide constant reassurance Following instructions from the ophthalmologist, apply an eye patch Involve the multidisciplinary team	To reassure the child and assist in providing suitable books and toys as a distraction
Inadequate nutrition	Establish cause Maintain adequate nutrition	Establish nutrition plan as soon as possible Involve the dietician Administer prescribed drug therapy	Assist at meal times and offer ongoing encouragement
Altered bowel function	To maintain normal bowel function	Monitor stool frequency Give aperients as necessary	Encourage fluids and dietary roughage
Hydrocephalus	Early recognition and reduction of symptoms	Provide appropriate analgesia and regular neurological assessment	Provide a quiet environment

Taking into consideration the potential problems following surgery as previously outlined and relating them to the area of the brain involved, it is possible to anticipate specific events. Many of the events outlined can, of course, occur after any neurosurgical operation but described below are some of the complications related to specific sites of surgery.

Infratentorial complications

The child is operated on in the sitting position and is nursed at a head-up tilt of at least 45° after surgery. Good alignment of the head and neck allows good venous drainage from the brain, but is difficult to achieve in the agitated toddler. Potential cranial nerve dysfunction may involve the glossopharyngeal and vagus nerves and oedema to these nerves will affect the child's gag reflex and swallowing. Consequently, following posterior fossa surgery all children are electively kept 'nil by mouth' for a period of a minimum of 12 hours post-surgery (may vary between centres). After this time the gag reflex will be tested and oral fluids commenced if appropriate; any excessive dribbling of saliva should be reported and physiotherapy given at an early stage if required. Other potential cranial nerve involvement includes the occulomotor, trochlear and abducens nerves, resulting in deficits in extraocular movements. The facial nerves may be involved and also the acoustic nerve. Cerebellar dysfunction is not uncommon following posterior fossa surgery and although in many cases this is temporary, some residual ataxia or loss of fine movement may be permanent.

'Posterior fossa syndrome' occurs in a small number of children and includes mutism among its symptoms; this syndrome will be described in more detail in the case history that follows.

Nausea and vomiting is particularly prevalent following posterior fossa surgery and this is thought to be due to irritation to the fourth ventricle; antiemetics can be given and intravenous fluids will be necessary alongside careful monitoring of the child's electrolytes and urine output.

The child will need constant supervision in the post-operative period, not only because of the potential problems outlined above but also because of the need for ensuring his safety at a time when they are agitated, ataxic and visually disturbed, and when their parents are not functioning in their normal protective role.

Supratentorial complications

Following surgery the child is nursed at a 30° head-up tilt to allow for good venous return from the brain; correct positioning of the Redivac drains is necessary to allow for drainage without the syphoning effect caused by placing the drain too low beneath the patient's head.

Potential cranial nerve dysfunction may include the following: the optic nerve; the occular motor nerve; trochlear and abducens, resulting in deficits in extraoccular movement. Diabetes insipidus may occur if the hypothalamus has been involved. Seizures and hemiparesis are the other major areas of concern in addition to the main points listed.

The following case history outlines the assessment, treatment and short term outcome of a child diagnosed with a posterior fossa tumour.

Case history: Thomas, an inpatient perspective

Thomas was a seven-year-old boy, the second of three children of healthy unrelated parents. His sister was three years old at the time of Thomas's diagnosis, and his brother nine. All the family had previously been well and there was no family history of any malignant disease.

Thomas was born at 39 weeks' gestation by vaginal delivery, following a normal pregnancy. His developmental milestones were normal. He smiled at 6 weeks, crawled at 10 months and walked at 14 months; his first words were at about a year of age and he now attended a mainstream school where he was said to be a bright pupil, who liked sports. Thomas had received all routine vaccinations and apart from having chickenpox as a toddler, he had been a healthy child.

Three months prior to his hospital admission, Thomas started vomiting in the early morning. Initially these episodes lasted for two or three days at a time, following which he would be well; he then had an episode of diarrhoea and the general practitioner put it down to a viral illness. However, Thomas continued to vomit shortly after awaking most mornings, and when he began to complain of headaches, his mother returned to the doctor where she was reassured and sent home. Eight weeks following the onset of vomiting, Thomas's parents thought he was a little wobbly on his bike, but presumed it was because it was a fairly new bike and perhaps a bit big for him. However, when he fell in the playground, knocking his head in the process, he became unsteady on his feet and complained of double vision; his mother took him to an optician who noticed papilloedema and referred him back to the GP. She was told that Thomas had some swelling behind his eyes which required further investigations, but it was not until she was told to go straight to casualty, that she realised there might be something seriously wrong. Having phoned her husband and made arrangements for the other children, she awaited the paediatrician at the local casualty. Thomas was again examined and told that he required a special scan of his head later that day. Thomas was admitted to the paediatric ward, a little confused as to his admission there and keen to return to school. His mother, desperate for some indication as to Thomas's illness, asked both doctors and nurses as to the reason for scanning her son and was told it was possible Thomas had a 'growth of some sort in his head'. She describes the next few hours as 'a blur'; Thomas was scanned, a lesion found, and he was transferred to a paediatric neurosurgical unit.

On arrival, Thomas was accompanied by both parents; although he felt reasonably well, he was becoming increasingly worried by his parents' behaviour. A nurse sat down and talked to him, showed him the playroom, and the ever-popular computer games and videos. Slightly reassured, Thomas was again examined by a paediatrician and was found to have gross bilateral papilloedema, nystagmus on left gaze, but no apparent palsy; all other cranial nerves were normal; he had mild ataxia, but could heel/toe walk without stumbling and sit upright without leaning over; he complained of early morning vomiting and mild headaches, but no tiredness or drowsiness. His CT scan showed a posterior fossa enhancing mass, with obstruction to the CSF flow and resulting hydrocephalus. Thomas was occupied by the play specialist whilst his parents were spoken to by the neurosurgical senior registrar, accompanied by a nurse. They were told Thomas had a brain tumour and that surgery would be the starting point for treatment and that it was probable that further treatment in the form of radiotherapy and possibly chemotherapy, might be necessary.

There were many questions from his shocked parents, about how the tumour had occurred, how they felt guilty about not pushing harder for an earlier referral and the consequences of that delay, whether he would be brain damaged, whether he would die.

At this stage, both parents became deeply distressed and it was not appropriate to continue the discussion. The surgeon explained he would be available to talk to them at another time, later that day if they wished. They were left undisturbed for a while. The nurse who had been present during the discussion then returned to answer further questions.

The importance of this same nurse returning is that, since she had heard the previous discussion, she could reiterate what had already been said (parents often forget much of what has been explained during a time of deep distress); families will often look to the nurse for coordination of care and the integration of information (Shiminski-Maher & Shields, 1995) and this is the beginning of this process. In addition, the paediatric neurosurgical nurse is an expert in her own field and can offer suggestions and advice; finally, she can form a unique and supportive bond with the family, an invaluable part of this family's holistic care. This 'link nurse' became the parents' access for advice, reassurance or just the opportunity to talk, and with someone who did not require explanation or pretence.

Explanations to parents usually need to be repeated, perhaps several times, and terminology used that is understood.

After discussion with Thomas's parents (June and David), it was decided that Thomas himself needed some explanations; his parents wished to tell him themselves, but in the presence of their nurse in case of difficult questions; June and David asked Thomas why he thought he had headaches, to which he answered that since he had had a scan of his head, it must be a problem with his head, but he didn't know what. June told him he had a lump in his head which should not be there and that he needed an operation to remove it. Thomas continued playing with his game for a while as if he had not heard them and then asked his mother if she had been crying and where she had been. June explained she was sad that Thomas was unwell and needed an operation, and reassured him that she was not leaving him on his own in hospital; this resulted in a torrent of questions from Thomas about how they would get into his head and if it would hurt; when this would happen and when he could go home; whether he could still go on his school outing next month and if he could go out to McDonald's!

The play specialist joined the discussion with Thomas, to enable her to work with him in preparation for various procedures including surgery. He was started on oral dexamethasone to reduce the cerebral oedema around the tumour, and since he had never taken any medicines before, he was nervous of being able to swallow the tablet and it was crushed to reduce any additional anxieties for him. Once he had settled again, Thomas was allowed to go out to the nearby park with his parents.

An MRI scan was scheduled for the following day and the play specialist showed Thomas photographs of the scanner and prepared him for an unsedated scan. Thomas seemed agitated and frightened by the prospect despite this and was consequently sedated for the scan. The 'magic' anaesthetic cream (EMLA) was applied before inserting an intravenous cannula for the necessary contrast medium which would enhance the tumour; blood was taken at the same time for routine analysis and cross-matching. Thomas was duly sedated using both intramuscular and oral sedation after being given an explanation of the procedure and the use of relaxation techniques (and the 'reward' box, a much-valued item on the ward!).

Once recovered from sedation, it was necessary to prepare Thomas for surgery the following day. Much of this was done by the play specialist, who gave him a cognitively appropriate explanation of what was to happen; this covered what time he would have his last drink, how much of his hair would be cut, where the scar on his head would be, reassurance that he would not wake up during surgery, that his mum would be there when he woke up, and some explanation of the monitoring equipment and the 'drips' which he would have. This time is invaluable in allowing the child to express his fears (which he may not do in the presence of his parents who he may try to protect), and to ensure his understanding. A boy once told by the anaesthetist he would be 'put to sleep' for his surgery, became very withdrawn: discussions with him revealed that his dog had been 'put to sleep' at the vet's the week before; time and patience is necessary to reveal and allay such misconceptions.

The consultant neurosurgeon spoke to June and David and consent for surgery was obtained. The parents were made aware of the potential complications of the operation, including neurological deficits which might be short or long term, and the unlikely possibility of Thomas dying during surgery. The surgeon explained that he would discuss with them after surgery how successful he had been in removing part or all of the tumour, but that he would be unable to tell them its histology for several days.

The idea of waiting for histology is difficult for parents, and the nurse, having once again been present during the discussion between the neurosurgeon and June and David, tried to guide them into coping with one day at a time for the next few days, and in being strong for their son when he needed them most.

The nurse explained the equipment to be used and its purpose; she discussed how Thomas might appear, feel and behave on his return from theatre; how June and David could best help him; and the practical issues of where they might sleep if he was moved temporarily to a high dependency unit. She also elicited information about who was caring for their other children and when they might visit their brother.

The usual physical preparation for theatre having been performed and the psychological aspects of the procedure having been attended to, Thomas was given a premedication of atropine (a sedative premedication was inappropriate due to the drowsiness it would cause afterwards, therefore confusing his neurological status). He was accompanied to the anaesthetic room by his mother and the nurse. Following the induction of anaesthesia, June returned to the ward.

Surgery was uneventful. Following a minimal hair shave, a midline posterior fossa incision was performed. An incomplete removal of tumour was achieved, due to the adherence of the tumour to the floor of the fourth ventricle. The frozen section taken at the time of surgery was a medulloblastoma.

Once surgery was finished, the ward nurse received a handover from the anaesthetist, the surgeon and the theatre nurse; once satisfied with Thomas's condition, she returned with him to the ward. Having seen him briefly, his parents were asked to wait outside whilst Thomas was assessed. He had been returned directly back to the ward without a period in theatre recovery and, consequently, the nurse's attention was directed to Thomas rather than his parents.

Full monitoring equipment was attached to Thomas, including an oxygen saturation monitor (he did not require oxygen). His pulse, blood pressure and respiration rate were within normal limits. His neurological status was good with a coma scale of 12, and he was obeying commands, although not vocalising. He appeared to be in pain and was given intramuscular codeine phosphate with good effect (research is under way to ascertain an alternative method of administering analgesia, but to date, most adult and paediatric neurological centres use intramuscular codeine phosphate in the initial post-operative period). Intravenous fluids were commenced and arterial monitoring set up. Thomas immediately removed his own nasogastric tube and it was decided against passing a new one due to the distress it would cause him.

June and David then sat with Thomas, deeply shocked initially, but also greatly relieved to see him safely returned from theatre and conscious. They asked appropriate questions about the equipment and how and where they could touch Thomas; they sat holding his hand and anxiously awaited news from the surgeon.

Thomas was agitated and distressed during the afternoon, despite further analgesia (rectal paracetamol and diclofenac); he disliked being handled and was miserable when disturbed. Nursing him in the appropriate position with his head in alignment with his body and at a 45° upright tilt, became increasingly distressing for him and, despite attempts by his nurse, Thomas curled into a ball, further increasing the pain and stiffness to his neck muscles. His parents became correspondingly distressed and needed much reassurance that this behaviour did occasionally occur following surgery to this area. His vital signs and neurological status remained stable, although his temperature rose to 38.5° (this is a normal occurrence after craniotomy) and responded to the use of a fan.

Thomas had a nurse in continual attendance for the post-operative afternoon and night. Regular turns were performed despite his protestations and attempts were made to position him comfortably; regular analgesia was given. Observations were taken less frequently as his condition improved; he was to be kept nil by mouth until his gag reflex was checked the following morning and mouth care was given by his parents, who were encouraged to participate in his care. Intravenous fluids were continued and his urine output monitored.

The surgeon examined Thomas in the early evening and was happy with his progress; he reassured June and David that Thomas's agitation was distressing but not of medical concern. They were shattered on hearing that the surgical removal of the tumour had been incomplete, but grateful that no serious neuro-logical harm was apparent.

June and David slept little that night, since Thomas remained agitated and was slightly calmed by their presence; they were encour-aged to alternate their time with him, thus enabling each parent to get some sleep and respite from the exhaustion of their agitated son. Thomas himself slept intermittently, his neurological status remained stable; however, he was noted to be dribbling saliva constantly and it became evident that he had lost his gag reflex and was therefore unable to commence oral fluids — a further source of irritation to him.

On day 1 after surgery, Thomas's condition remained stable but he continued to be irritable and mute. His pyrexia subsided, but his nystagmus persisted and he appeared to have a weakness of both upper and lower extremities; physiotherapy was commenced to both his chest (the likelihood of a chest infection was increased due to his inability to swallow, and the pooling and dribbling of saliva) and to his limbs; gentle movements to his neck also lessened the stiffness of his neck muscles and his mother was taught these exer-cises. His electrolytes were checked and his intravenous fluid regime changed accordingly. Due to his agitated state Thomas's arterial line was removed for safety; the monitoring equipment was also withdrawn. Despite regular analgesia and reassurance, however, Thomas remained agitated so a CT scan was performed to rule out any post-operative complications. The scan demon-strated enlarged ventricles but no haemorrhage; a lumbar punc-ture was therefore performed to reduce the intracranial pressure and to help clear the blood in the CSF, thus hopefully reducing his distress. It was thought appropriate to sedate Thomas for the procedure and his parents were in agreement with this. Thomas slept for much of the afternoon following this, which gave his parents a much needed break.

There are several recognised symptoms which comprise 'posterior fossa syndrome' and it was assumed that Thomas was suffering from this syndrome; symptoms include difficulty verbalising, mutism, emotional lability, irritability and nystagmus (Kirke et al., 1995). The aetiology of this syndrome is unknown, although it is associated with hydrocephalus, cerebellar insult, resection of a mid-line cerebellar tumour and vascular disturbances. It can last for many weeks or even months and since it is thought that these children can process information but are unable to communicate orally, their frustration can be understood. Early recognition of the syndrome and appropriate intervention, such as speech therapy and communication tools, are essential, coupled with support and reassurance to both the family and the child that this condition is temporary.

The days after surgery continued to be traumatic. Nasogastric feeds were established as Thomas was still unable to swallow. He remained mute and appeared reluctant or unable to use communication methods or boards. He remained ataxic and disliked his physiotherapy sessions, preferring to lie in bed. Nothing appeared to please or appease him which was increasingly exhausting and frustrating to his family; even the appearance of his siblings did little to cheer him. His parents were encouraged to spend some time off the ward whilst the play specialist attempted to interest Thomas in something.

Histology confirmed the diagnosis of medulloblastoma. Unfortunately, the MRI scan performed prior to surgery had demonstrated spinal metastasis. Thomas would therefore require further treatment and his exhausted parents were told that with further treatment, the aim would be to cure him, but that his long term future could not be guaranteed.

Despite their suspicion that this might have been the diagnosis, June and David were distraught. They requested and were given relevant literature about medulloblastoma and all possible treatments. Although they still obtained much support from the nursing staff, both parents were clearly exhausted and were encouraged to spend a night at home. Granny stayed with Thomas during their absence.

Although Thomas continued to make some progress, a further CT scan showed hydrocephalus, and a ventricular-peritoneal shunt was inserted three weeks after the initial surgery. Although this represented yet another setback in June and David's view,

Thomas recovered from surgery so rapidly in contrast to his last operation that they felt reassured. In addition, Thomas seemed more settled and more alert following his shunt insertion and his parents could at last see some improvement in his condition. Thomas was nursed flat initially following his shunt insertion, but over the next few days as he was nursed in a more upright position, it became evident that he was less ataxic. Thomas vomited for two days following his shunt insertion and was maintained on intravenous fluids, but gradually the vomiting subsided and he tolerated nasogastric feeds. His parents were encouraged to take him out of the hospital as much as possible and to encourage his siblings and school friends to visit.

Meanwhile the next stage of Thomas's treatment was being planned via the multidisciplinary team, which had initially been made aware of Thomas's history some weeks before. The clinical nurse specialist, having already met the family following confirmation of the histology as a medulloblastoma, now became involved in their care.

Although much of the child's history was obtained from his notes, additional information concerning Thomas's own awareness and understanding of his illness, plus the emotional status of both Thomas and his parents, was obtained from the ward nurses and the play specialist. These facts were of benefit in understanding what this family had already undergone both physically and emotionally, and assisted in a smoother transition to the next stage of treatment.

Case study: a follow-up perspective

The role of the neuro-oncology clinical nurse specialist is complex and variable; promoting a flexible and responsive approach to the individual needs of children and their families. As stated by Bass (1993), the clinical nurse specialist is an experienced practitioner who exhibits clinical competence and advanced knowledge of physiological, psychosocial and therapeutic components. These are essential to the provision of good quality nursing care.

The care of children with brain tumours is complicated and extremely challenging. The speciality bridges many disciplines, including neurosurgery, oncology, radiotherapy, endocrinology, neuropsychology, physiotherapy, play therapy, speech therapy and dietetics. The pivotal role of the clinical nurse specialist facilitates the care of these children and their families throughout multiple treatments and long term follow-up by providing constancy and continuity (Ryan & Shiminski-Maher, 1995).

Thomas had been diagnosed with a medulloblastoma of the central nervous system, and his parents, June and David, were seen after the histology had been confirmed. This appeared to be a good time to establish their understanding of the situation so far, especially as Thomas had experienced a complicated and drawn-out post-operative period, and had been found to have residual tumour.

Buckman (1992) has suggested that there should be no attempt to introduce new information until it has been clearly established what parents already know or perceive. At this stage, it was important to clarify information which had already been given to June and David, bearing in mind that distressed relatives can only absorb a small amount when they are in a state of stress and shock (Buckman, 1992). It is also reassuring for parents to know that information can be repeated often, so that they feel confident to support each other and their immediate family.

June and David were helped to 'tell their story'. They needed an opportunity to express their grief about the loss of their healthy child. Parents often suffer a double loss in that they lose a healthy child at diagnosis followed by a possible loss to death (Ryan & Shiminski-Maher, 1995). This family had also lost their previous 'normality' and at a later stage, when there was a clearer picture of the family, these aspects could be explored in greater depth.

The diagnosis of a brain tumour is often difficult to establish, because the presenting symptoms may well mimic those associated with many common childhood illnesses (Shiminski-Maher & Shields, 1995). It was difficult for June and David to appreciate this however, and when Thomas's diagnosis was delayed, feelings of anger and mistrust at their local community services had to be explored with them. It was crucial at this point to help the parents to regain confidence and re-build relationships with the community services, as they would come into contact with them at a later date.

It was important to assess whether June and David had understood the ramifications of Thomas's diagnosis, by the way that they recounted their situation and by observing their body language. It would be necessary to repeat this process during subsequent sessions to facilitate further exploration and understanding. The professional is then able to clarify whether information is being absorbed effectively or not; this is an important element of communication skills as described by Buckman (1992). Another key factor which required consideration during the initial session, was information about Thomas's unique family unit. June and David were encouraged to give a detailed description of their nuclear and extended family, their employment status, the age and developmental stages of siblings and the family medical history. It was also important to find out if the family were dealing with any other problems at this particularly difficult time.

Noll et al. (1993) suggest that the identification of child and parental strengths and coping skills is critical; thus open-ended questions were used to establish the dynamics and interactions of all the family members. It is also helpful if the professionals are in a position to understand the family's social circumstances and note where additional input might be required to enable the family to use its own resources.

Insight into the family created a clearer picture as to how much individual members were aware of the seriousness of Thomas's condition; and that, of course, included Thomas himself. Thomas was suffering from 'posterior fossa syndrome' (Kirke et al., 1995) and, as a result, was irritable and mute. The family was naturally very upset by this and needed reassurance that other children had suffered in a similar way; and that this particular condition is temporary.

> **Nursing note:**
>
> **It is sometimes helpful to introduce the child to another child who is already receiving treatment. If the child's speech has been affected picture or word boards may aid communication.**

Benner (1984) has suggesed that almost no intervention will work if the nurse–patient relationship is not based on mutual respect and genuine caring. The initial session with June and David and their family was the beginning of a professional relationship in which a mixture of trust, support and flexibility could slowly develop and grow.

Another meeting was arranged for the following day, to allow June and David time to rest and recuperate, because the session had been very draining for them. They remained in a state of shock and acute anxiety and were very tired. There was a marked improvement in June and David's emotional state over the next few sessions. They had been seen by the medical staff and told that Thomas required further treatment in the form of chemotherapy and radiotherapy; and now they needed information and practical advice. Sanger and Copeland (1989) have explained how children and families who receive information about treatment show greater compliance and acceptance.

> **Nursing note:**
>
> **Be up to date on current media information to be able to answer parents' queries.**

At this stage, an added stress for the family could be related to coping with the issues and the dilemmas surrounding drug trials and protocols. Lowes (1993) has highlighted the importance of collective decision-making in such ethical dilemmas; and it is essential that professionals have come to a decision about their personal standpoint, so that they are in a better position to help the family.

The treatment prescribed for Thomas's metastatic disease was a combination of chemotherapy and radiotherapy. The parents were given a copy of the booklet, *Childhood Brain Tumours — A Guide for Parents* (Salkeld, 1992) and the literature regarding Thomas's case was also discussed.

The aim, as stated by Black (1995), was to provide time and space for the family to reflect on their experiences, understand what was happening, and adapt to the reality of the illness and treatment; at the same time, providing a safe place for the expression of fear, anger, anxiety and sadness.

Information and preparation for chemotherapy were now required for the family. June and David had the best idea of Thomas's needs at this stage in his preparation, but it was suggested to them that they should be open and honest with Thomas. They agreed to this and time was then spent with Thomas, discussing his past experiences and preparing him for the following stages of treatment. Information had to be set at a lower level than his chronological age, because of his general medical condition and his present inability to communicate. Over the following weeks, Thomas slowly began to communicate better and became less withdrawn and irritable.

At this stage, it was also possible to take the opportunity to spend time with Thomas's siblings, Mark and Clare. The children were often seen individually, because of their age difference and, with their agreement, it was possible to feed back difficulties or progress to their parents. Eventually, family sessions were facilitated, enabling all members to openly express their feelings and thoughts.

Treatment

Chemotherapy

The use of chemotherapy has increased the survival rates of children with malignant brain tumours as much as twofold (Albright, 1993). In addition, new developments in the management of children with tumours of the central nervous system, are multidimensional and are much more aggressive than those of the previous decade. Definitive surgical procedures, irradiation therapy and combination chemotherapy protocols, plus the introduction of long term supportive care, have now taken into account the unique needs of patients with intracranial lesions (McGuire Cullen, 1995).

An outline of how chemotherapy works and how its side effects can be treated was given to June and David, who were reassured that they would be taught and supported at all stages of treatment.

The protocol used for Thomas meant that he would receive a combination of agents. June and David were told that these drugs needed to be administered by intravenous injections or infusions, but that the use of a central venous access device makes this much easier.

The family was introduced to the staff on the neuro-oncology unit. This would include the i.v. team, nurses who would show them the central line and would use a teddy bear with lines in situ for play preparation and visual explanations. It is well known that play is an excellent medium through which the child can display fears (Belson, 1987). In time, the i.v. team, would teach June and David how to care for the line.

Initial side effects of chemotherapy

The side effects of chemotherapy have been discussed previously (see Chapter 3), but there are particular issues which should be mentioned concerning the care of a child with a brain tumour.

Nausea and vomiting

The use of antiemetics that act as serotonin antagonists, such as ondansetron, has greatly improved the quality of life for all children undergoing cancer treatment. Their greatest advantage has been in the treatment of chemotherapy-associated nausea and vomiting in children with brain tumours, as this allows accurate ongoing neurological assessment which is crucial in these children (McGuire Cullen, 1995). Nausea and vomiting may be associated with chemotherapy, or may be associated with increased intracranial pressure. Clearly, the correct diagnosis of the cause is of great importance, especially, as in Thomas's case, where a ventricular-peritoneal shunt was *in situ*.

Hydration

During the administration of chemotherapy, supportive care for children with a brain tumour is slightly different from those with other types of cancer because of the risk of increased intracranial pressure. As highlighted by Shiminski-Maher and Shields (1995), hydration for children with brain tumours is aimed at maintaining an isovolaemic state; thus avoiding fluid and electrolyte shifts that may result in cerebral oedema.

Alopecia

Hair loss can be particularly difficult for children with brain tumours because they are likely to have their hair shaved for surgery as well as losing it through the use of chemotherapy and radiotherapy. It may never grow back properly or there may be permanent thinning or bald patches.

Steroids

Weight gain — if there is an increase in cerebral oedema, Thomas could require the ongoing therapeutic use of steroids. This can create problems with body image due to weight gain, and is highly likely to cause him psychological difficulties. Time would be spent with Thomas to tackle this issue as soon as was medically possible. The common goal would be to reduce the steroid dose and discontinue the use of these agents at the earliest possible date (McGuire Cullen, 1995).

Weight loss — children often lose their appetite during aggressive chemotherapy and this is particularly true for children with brain tumours who may suffer severe nausea and vomiting. Thomas was also likely to be affected by the distress that would probably be felt and shown by his mother. June herself could have feelings of guilt and a sense of failure about nurturing her child. A psychological vicious circle could easily have occurred, if all members of the family had not been well supported. Thomas needed to be encouraged to snack frequently and to maintain an adequate fluid intake. June needed help to reduce her anxiety about this complex issue.

Nursing note:

In the event that the child continues to have problems with swallowing, the following suggestions may be helpful:
- **Place teaspoons in the fridge as it is easier to control mouth and swallowing actions when an implement is cooler than body temperature.**
- **Thicker fluids, e.g. yoghurt/ice-cream, are easier to control than clear fluids.**
- **Use a straw for clear fluids.**
- **Use foods with a high water content, e.g. melon/sorbet.**
- **Offer puréed foods with a high calorie content at frequent intervals.**

Family stress

Problems associated with the ongoing stress and the insecurity of an unpredictable outcome can be a heavy burden for families (Noll et al., 1993). It was important to take time to discuss the effect of long term treatment on family life. This included the effect on siblings and the relationship between June and David, as well as Thomas's isolation from his friends and peers, due to absence from school. Home tuition and school links should be instigated at a very early stage.

June and David were told about the philosophy of 'shared care' with their local hospital. This would reduce the number of visits to the centre and allow them closer access to home if inpatient treatment was required. They were informed that they would receive their own personal record book, which would contain details about the planned treatment, dates of required blood tests and other associated tests for safe administration of drugs such as regular GFR and audiology assessments. It would also state when MRI imaging would be carried out to assess the effect of treatment. Their record book would also contain relevant contact numbers for help, advice and support.

Noll et al. (1993) have strongly recommended that one person should be introduced as early as possible to each child and family, as a primary psychosocial professional. In this way, continuity of services can be maintained throughout treatment and a rapport and trust can be established and maintained. During Thomas's intensive chemotherapy, the role of the liaison nurse would be to maintain contact, offering emotional support and advice when required.

Radiotherapy

Radiation treatment is the oldest form of treatment for brain tumours (McGuire, 1993). Craniospinal irradiation has been the standard treatment for medulloblastoma with a five-year survival rate of 20–60% (Shiminski-Maher & Shields, 1995). Since radiation was part of the treatment required by Thomas, the family needed a clear explanation as to how radiotherapy works and about its side effects. At this stage, the family would be more likely to retain knowledge than at the outset of treatment. It has been shown that play provides an emotional outlet for the child and enables him to use his acquired and previously learnt coping mechanisms (Harvey, 1980).

The neurosurgical unit at Great Ormond Street Hospital for Children NHS Trust has produced a play pack which was used to prepare Thomas and his family for radiotherapy. It contains a parent's guide to play preparation, covering a five-day programme and a children's picture and story folder; portraying a child from preparation, through treatment to completion and recovery. The bag contains a flannel with eye holes to use at bathtime, to prepare Thomas for the wet and cold feeling associated with the application of the plaster of Paris used as a mould for the head mask. The completed mask would be worn daily, to facilitate precise and accurate radiotherapy treatment and to allow the greatest protection of delicate eye structures. There is also a large doll with a fitted mask, a pre-made child's mask and a packet of plaster of Paris, to be used in role play at home. June and David would be encouraged to get Thomas (with the doll lying prone beside him) to lie on his stomach for storytimes, so that he became accustomed to this position, which would be used daily for treatment.

> **Nursing note:**
>
> **Children can take a favourite toy into the radiotherapy room.**

The side effects of radiotherapy are covered in section four of this book and only those peculiar to children with brain tumours will be discussed here.

Steroid therapy at the commencement of cranial radiation may be appropriate if cerebral oedema occurred. If Thomas were to complain of headache then a short, sharp reducing course of dexamethasone might be required. If the course of radiotherapy is short, it is unlikely to cause undesired side effects (McGuire Cullen, 1995).

As in many institutions, Thomas's course of radiotherapy would be given in a different hospital to his previous treatment. It would, therefore, be important to meet the family once a week to maintain continuity of care and to be available to discuss any issues or problems that might have arisen. It would be during one of these sessions that the clinical nurse specialist would discuss in detail with June and David the long term side effects of treatment.

Long Term Side Effects of Treatment

Due to the increased survival rate of children such as Thomas, it is important that all children with brain tumours are provided with long term follow-up and assessment in order to determine the effectiveness of treatment and to monitor side effects. It must be remembered that survival alone is not indicative of quality of life. The adverse effects of surgical treatment are usually apparent soon after surgery; whereas the effects of chemotherapy and radiotherapy may take years to appear. As long term survival increases, it is already becoming clear that late effects will present new problems for these children in the future (Duffner et al., 1988).

Effect on intellect and education

A retrospective study into the long term educational performance of 25 children treated for medulloblastoma, who were a minimum of 5 years post-treatment showed that the majority of the children demonstrated a decline in their school performance over time (Phipps, 1996). It also demonstrated that a child's school performance in the first 2 years post-treatment is a poor long term predictor of their final school performance/attainment. The study found that 68% of the children reached a plateau in their school performance at 5 years post-treatment, rising to 76% at 7 years post-treatment.

The results confirmed previous findings that the younger the age of the child at presentation, the more severe were the intellectual problems following treatment (Duffner et al., 1988). Children who have received the same treatment as Thomas often have problems associated with poor short term memory and recall. If teachers and/or parents were to observe a decline in Thomas's ability to keep pace with his peers it would be necessary for him to have a statutory assessment for a 'Statement of Special Educational Needs'. An educational Statement is a legally binding obligation (Department of Education, 1993; Department of Education and the Welsh Office, 1994; Education (NI) Order, 1996; Scottish Office, 1996). Where possible, any special help required by a child (special educational provision) is provided within a mainstream state school alongside children of the same age.

Endocrine problems

Long term endocrine problems in children with brain tumours can be varied and complex (Lew et al., 1995). Many studies have found that cranial irradiation plays a central role in causing endocrine dysfunction, but it is impossible to avoid irradiating the hypothalamic –pituitary axis in the treatment of children with medulloblastoma. As discussed by Lew and LaValley (1995), the mechanism of radiation damage to the endocrine system is not well-known. It may be related to direct injury to the cells responsible for hormone secretion, injury to the stroma or injury to the vascular channels that transfer hypothalamic hormones to the pituitary.

The most common problems are:

- Short stature due to both growth hormone deficiency caused by the effect of cranial irradiation and the effect of spinal irradiation on vertebral growth
- Hypothyroidism due to the involvement of the thyroid gland during spinal irradiation.

With both the availability of synthetic growth hormone and its demonstrated ability to minimise growth retardation, and access to other relevant replacement therapies, it is essential that children like Thomas are seen at recognised growth centres from the time of diagnosis and at regular intervals thereafter. If replacement therapy is required, its administration can greatly enhance the child's general quality of life (Thomson et al., 1992).

Depending on the effect of radiotherapy on hormone production, some children may need medical support through puberty and as adults they may require fertility counselling and treatment; again, highlighting the need for long term follow-up facilities.

Hair re-growth

Hair thinning or hair loss is a very visible consequence of whole brain irradiation. (In 12 years of experience at Great Ormond Street Hospital for Children NHS Trust it has been noticed that most children have had a satisfactory re-growth with a thinning over the areas that received a boosted dose of irradiation. Sadly, there have been four cases where there has been an unsatisfactory re-growth of hair which has led to associated psychological problems.)

Second malignancy

Miké et al. (1982) estimated the risk of a second malignancy to be 10–20 times the lifetime risk of the general population. (In the same 12 years' experience at Great Ormond Street Hospital, two children have been seen to develop a second unrelated malignancy.)

Research

The complexity of the long term effects of radiotherapy on children such as Thomas makes it vital that research into both treatment and side effects is carried out.

Storr (1988) has suggested that the application, testing and reporting of research findings in practice could promote progression in research expertise and personal research skills. The clinical nurse specialist should be able to interpret research findings and act as a role model, making use of research to solve nursing problems.

Comprehensive knowledge of families and accurate record-keeping, makes it possible to collect and pass on relevant data to the neuro-oncology database, which has recorded 1100 children with tumours of the central nervous system, covering the period from January 1980–1997. Such data enables progress to be made not only with active treatment but also in reducing adverse side effects in paediatric patients.

Discharge Planning

Thomas and his family have remained under the care of this service throughout his long treatment and maintenance follow-up. He will have numerous transfers and discharges from hospital to community care during this time. These include:

- Internal transfer from the neurosurgical unit to the oncology unit
- Oncology unit to community, awaiting radiotherapy treatment
- Completion of radiotherapy treatment to community, awaiting chemotherapy treatment
- Discharge to community after each in-patient course of chemotherapy
- Discharge after any emergency admissions due to complications of treatment
- Completion of treatment to community for maintenance care.

As discussed by Holt (1993), communication across disciplines and agencies provides continuity; and communication must exist within and between each multidisciplinary team (Shiminski-Maher, 1993).

Throughout these changes, it is important that professionals are aware that the primary responsibility for the coordination of care may alter from one subspeciality to the next during the course of treatment. It is clearly essential that the child and the family know which team, or which individual, is responsible for coordinating care at each stage. At discharge, the relevant ward or unit will follow its individual discharge planning protocol and the role of the clinical nurse specialist will be to act as a link in a large multidisciplinary team involving both hospital and community. The role will also involve the provision of advice and support to individual members of the teams. From the time of diagnosis the clinical nurse specialist will make contact and remain in communication with the following people:

- General practitioner
- Health Visitor/Special Needs Health Visitor
- Community paediatric nursing teams/District nurses
- School/Education Authority
- Social worker
- Local hospital personnel
- Any other professional or support agencies who are involved with ongoing care.

Thomas and his family continue under the care of this service for continued surveillance, with the support of other agencies where appropriate.

Relapse

Between 25% and 40% of children with medulloblastoma will relapse (Byrne, 1996). If Thomas were to fall within this number the team would have the advantage of knowing the family, would have prior knowledge of its strengths, weaknesses and coping mechanisms, and would have knowledge of the family's views about further treatment or palliative care. Noll et al. (1993) suggest that establishing a rapport and trust with the family is essential to providing support at the time of a relapse.

The clinical nurse specialist would facilitate meetings for the family with members of the multidisciplinary team, to discuss the following:

- Diagnosis and confirmation of the spread of recurrent disease
- The possibility of further treatment, including the effect on the child's quality of life
- Second opinions
- Palliative and terminal care.

Following this, discussion and reflection would be needed to talk through the outcome of such a meeting. The family needs to feel well-supported by all members of the team in its decision.

Palliative Care

If the child should require palliative care, the aim would be to help the family to achieve goals in relation to care and the place of death. In addition to symptom control and pain management, the role of the clinical nurse specialist would be to prepare the whole family, including the child, for the child's likely deterioration and imminent death. Although some parents may want to 'protect' children from the knowledge that they are going to die, children who are terminally ill usually know. Silence can result in unnecessary suffering and many fears (Noll et al., 1993). With support, children of a very young age are able to work through their fears and anxieties, and obtain a sense of peace. Some children even have the ability to make their wishes after their death known to their family.

During bereavement, it is widely recognised that siblings benefit in the long term from being involved at an early stage. If they do not deal with their grief in childhood, it may result in complex problems later in life (Hill, 1994; Black & Judd, 1995).

After bereavement, the clinical nurse specialist would support the family with visits and telephone calls for a minimum of one year in order to cover all their personal anniversaries. This support is often required into the second year. A point of contact is always made available, but it is essential for the professionals to withdraw, and not hinder the family's endeavours to make progress.

As Noll et al. (1993) discussed, professionals who work with children with cancer are often in the midst of human tragedy that can result in personal emotional pain. It is essential that strategies for support exist for professionals to lessen the impact of distressing events, and before long term harmful reactions occur.

The case study has shown how difficult it can be to obtain a swift diagnosis of a brain tumour in a paediatric patient. It highlights the complex and protracted treatment that such children and their families have to endure and how the effects of treatment can extend into adult life.

With regard to the role of the clinical nurse specialist, it has demonstrated the advantages of a primary professional person maintaining continuity of care. As discussed by Houston and Luquire (1991), interventions by the clinical nurse specialist have been found to directly affect patient outcomes. The improved outcomes include decreased complications, decreased length of hospital stay, reduced re-admission rate, an increase in efficiency and quality of care, and improved patient satisfaction.

'The unique aspect of the clinical nurse specialist's role is in its versatility. For the clinical nurse specialist, whose primary intention is to retain the focus of patient care, the role provides all of the best worked into one; clinician, consultant, educator, researcher and clinical leader' (Sparacino, 1992).

Overall, in relation to palliative care, it is important to recognise that every child and family are unique, and will approach their child's illness and death in their own way. Families need to know that whatever setting they are in, home, hospital or hospice, they will have skilled, sympathetic help to manage their child's symptoms (Goldman, 1994).

Chapter 19
Primary bone cancer in young people

Chris Henry

Introduction

The knowledge and treatment of primary bone cancer in young people has advanced considerably over the last 20 years. Two main types occur, namely, osteosarcoma and Ewing's sarcoma. In 1970, only 15% of patients with osteosarcoma survived for five years. Ewing's sarcoma was considered to be so rapidly fatal that most patients were only treated with radiotherapy (Mankin et al., 1988). The use of adjuvant chemotherapy combined with conservative surgery and/or radiotherapy has markedly increased the young person's chance of survival. This improved combination of treatments has allowed about 60–70% of young people with both these conditions to survive for five years (Jurgens et al., 1992; Ornadel et al., 1994).

Little is known about the cause of primary bone cancer and therefore few risk factors have been identified. High doses of irradiation have been linked to bone cancer, however, there was no increase among the survivors of the atomic bomb in Japan (Piasecki, 1987). Radiation-induced bone sarcoma is more likely to occur in children as a complication of cancer treatment. Osteosarcoma of the jaw was reported to be more common in workers in the luminous watch dial trade, who frequently put their brushes, contaminated with radioactive material, into their mouths (Souhami & Tobias, 1986).

The incidence of bone cancer in young people is low, only approximately 150 new cases being seen in the UK each year (Souhami & Tobias, 1986). The incidence peaks during adolescence and is slightly more common in males than females. It has been suggested that there could be a link with the rapid rate of growth in limb bones at this time and research has shown that a significant number of young people with osteosarcoma are taller than their average peers (Jurgens et al., 1992). It would appear that the site of the tumour in the skeleton may have a bearing on the prognosis; patients with distal tumours seem to have a better outlook than those with more proximal tumours (Chalmers, 1988; Schwartz et al., 1993).

The highest incidence of osteosarcoma has been seen in Brazil. There is also a high rate in Italy, Finland and among Black Americans in the USA, whereas low incidences occur in Japan, India, Hungary and Cuba (Mertens & Bramwell, 1994). Ewing's sarcoma is rare in Africans, Black Americans and the Chinese population (Souhami & Tobias, 1986; Schwartz et al., 1993).

Current research into the molecular origins of cancer shows that young people with a history of hereditary retinoblastoma have an increased risk of developing osteosarcoma as a second primary tumour, as both tumours have the same genetic deletion in the same DNA sequence (Pasecki, 1992). It has also been shown that osteosarcoma is one of the tumours liable to occur in families with the Li-Fraumeni syndrome. The main features of these families are soft tissue sarcomas in young people, with the early onset of breast cancer in their mothers and close relatives, and are due to a p53 gene germline mutation (Porter et al., 1992).

A variety of chemotherapy drugs, including methotrexate, cisplatin, doxorubicin, ifosfamide and etoposide, have been shown to be effective against both osteosarcoma and Ewing's sarcoma. Previous studies from the European Osteosarcoma Intergroup (EOI) have indicated that dose-intensity, i.e. the amount of drug given in a period of time, may be an important factor in disease-free survival (Ornadel et al., 1994). It has been possible to increase the dose-intensity of certain drugs by the availability of haemopoietic growth factors, such as the granulocyte colony-stimulating factor (G-CSF), which reduces the duration of myelosuppression. Trials are also in progress to ascertain the value of post-operative chemotherapy and the optimal length of treatment.

Primary chemotherapy following diagnosis was established to allow time for an endoprosthesis to be made and it has enabled the study of the effect of chemotherapy on the tumour at the time of its resection. It is accepted that a 10% viable tumour at the time of surgery indicates a good response to pre-operative chemotherapy, and more than 10%, a poor response (Jurgens et al., 1992).

The increasing success of achieving tumour necrosis through the use of chemotherapy has resulted in a decrease in the need for amputation and the wider use of limb conservation surgery and its subsequent development. Studies show that limb conservation surgery, using allografts or endoprostheses, offers the same chance of survival as amputation, although there is a small risk of local recurrence. The use of allografts, however, was associated with more complications, especially in relation to infection and non-union (Roberts et al., 1991).

A review of young people with pathological fractures from osteosarcoma showed that although there was a correlation between local recurrence and the margins of resection in limb conservation surgery, this did not affect long term survival when compared to patients treated by amputation who had no local recurrence (Abudu et al., 1996). Endoprostheses have evolved, with extendible sections allowing for equality of growth, which require minimally invasive techniques to lengthen them. However, debate continues as to the minimum age at which they should be used (Jurgens et al., 1992; Pasecki, 1992).

Advances in surgical techniques have had an important effect on the treatment of young people with pelvic tumours. Wide local excision and bone grafting or the insertion of an endoprosthesis is now possible and this has had a positive effect on both the function and prognosis of these patients. Previous localised treatment by radiotherapy alone led to an increased risk of recurrence, especially if the tumour was Ewing's sarcoma.

The treatment of localised lung metastases in young people with osteosarcoma has improved with surgery involving a metastasectomy via single or bilateral thoracotomies, sometimes combined with further chemotherapy, using additional drugs to the trial. Jurgens et al. (1992) suggest that this is of little value in patients with Ewing's sarcoma, as the presence of metastases is a reflection of resistance to chemotherapy at other sites.

Types of Tumours and Their Presentation

Osteosarcoma

Osteosarcoma is the commonest primary bone tumour, arising in the medullary cavity, usually in the metaphysis, or end, of long bones. The commonest sites affected are the distal femur, proximal tibia and proximal humerus (Salisbury & Byers, 1994). The tumour consists mainly of malignant bone-producing cells, called osteoblasts, which are subject to wide variations. These cells invade and destroy the cortex of the bone and then find resistance to the outer covering of the bone, called the periosteum. As the tumour continues to grow within a restricted area, a sun-ray pattern of new bone is formed. The periosteum responds by laying down a wedge of bone at the angle where it is pushed away from the bone, this angle of elevation is called the Codman's triangle (Figure 19.1). Both these phenomena can be seen on plain X-ray films, the tumour bone sometimes giving the appearance of 'cotton wool'.

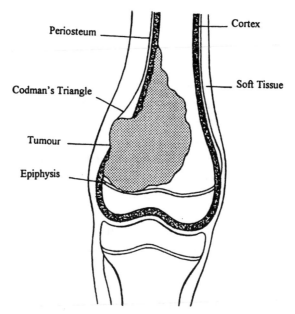

Figure 19.1: Osteosarcoma in the distal femur

Ewing's sarcoma

Ewing's sarcoma is the fourth most common primary bone tumour, but the second most common in young people. The tumour usually arises in the diaphysis, or shaft, of a long bone, but can also affect the scapula and pelvis. It consists of round cells of unknown aetiology and has a mottled and patchy appearance on X-ray, showing necrosis of existing bone (Salisbury & Byers, 1994). Sometimes the periosteum resists the tumour and is shown as having an 'onion skin' layered appearance, but it may also show a Codman's triangle. Ewing's sarcoma usually spreads into the soft tissues quicker than in osteosarcoma and may be extensive (Pringle, 1987). Unlike osteosarcoma, this tumour is sensitive to radiotherapy as well as chemotherapy which, although no longer used as first-line treatment, may be introduced later.

Bone marrow aspiration may be performed to screen for bone marrow infiltration. If present, these high risk patients may be considered for very high-dose chemotherapy with autologous bone marrow or peripheral blood stem cell support (Souhami & Tobias, 1986). Although high response rates have been recorded with the use of melphalan-containing regimes, the role of very high-dose chemotherapy with bone marrow rescue is still uncertain (Jurgens et al., 1992).

The clinical features which may indicate a poorer prognosis in Ewing's sarcoma are tumour size of more than 8 cm, a high white blood cell count, the presence of metastatic disease and a raised erythrocyte sedimentation rate (Schwartz et al., 1993; Salisbury & Byers, 1994).

Patient History

Commonly, young people see their doctor after a minor trauma which has drawn attention to a painful area. They first notice an ache in the affected part, which increases in severity to become painful enough to wake them at night. The pain is usually localised to the tumour but may radiate if it causes pressure on a nerve, especially in the sacral area of the spine. If the onset of pain is sudden then a pathological fracture may be present.

Because of the rarity of the tumours, a complaint of discomfort above or below the knee may not be immediately investigated and regarded as muscular strain from sporting activities. A study by Grimer and Sneath (1990) showed that, on average, a young person with osteosarcoma waited 6 weeks before consulting a doctor about the initial pain and it was then a further 7 weeks before a diagnosis was made. With Ewing's sarcoma, the youngsters waited 21 weeks before deciding to consult a doctor and 31 weeks for a diagnosis. The causes of delay in diagnosis were a low level of suspicion, inappropriate treatments and failure to detect the condition from X-rays. One of the possible consequences of delay may be related to the research statistic, that the greater the bulk of tumour present at diagnosis, the poorer the prognosis (Jurgens et al., 1992).

A swelling at the tumour site may be present, which will be warm and tender to touch. If the tumour is near a joint, there may be limitation and guarding of movement. Other symptoms may include night sweats and recent weight loss. At this stage, when plain X-ray films indicate a lesion, the young person should be transferred to a bone tumour specialist service to ensure speedy and appropriate treatment. Because of the rarity of these tumours it has been suggested that the pre-operative staging and biopsy are performed by the team involved in the surgical removal of the tumour (Souhami & Tobias, 1986; Grimer & Sneath, 1990).

Staging

Staging of tumours may be carried out in outpatient clinics or the young person may be admitted to the ward for a few days. If the latter option is chosen, nursing staff are able to prepare both the patient and the family for the various investigations, by ensuring that correct information is given, that it is age-appropriate and adapted to the young person's pace and level of understanding and by introducing them to the support of the bone tumour team. Inpatient admission also facilitates a thorough assessment of pain and optimum relief. This may require the use of opiates if the pain is severe and well-established, or the use of non-steroidal anti-inflammatory drugs (NSAIDs) which are very effective in relieving mild to moderate tumour pain.

Teenagers particularly value an individual approach as it helps them to keep some control over a new and very frightening situation. The nurse may play a key role in disseminating information while supporting, listening and understanding the wide range of emotions that the teenager and the family may express. Teenagers want to live and may show feelings of anger and resentment that this could be under threat. They may have difficulty expressing themselves and hide behind antisocial or risk-taking behaviour. If they do not have the opportunity to talk about secret fears and anxieties and offload some of their emotional burdens they may become isolated (Peck, 1992).

Sharing information with teenagers poses problems of confidentiality, autonomy and truthfulness and Brykczynska (1989) suggests that it is important to assess the level of parental involvement in the adolescent's life. Anger may be a strong feeling expressed by a teenager who has witnessed parents being taken to a separate room to be given information and they may not believe that they have been told the whole truth. It can be underestimated how well teenagers are able to absorb and cope with difficult concepts, and this ability is reflected in the deep and searching questions they often ask. Trust can only be earned by the sharing of accurate and honest information. One of the most devastating effects of cancer on a teenager is the loss of control over life and body; choices need to be made available for them to make decisions about treatments and future management (Peck, 1992).

A full assessment of family and peer relationships, support systems, coping strategies, education and leisure needs is required before implementing the staging programme. This assessment should be transcultural in nature, with special attention paid to existing beliefs and attitudes to cancer. Theories about the cause of cancer can be significantly affected by culture which, in turn, can influence the family's cooperation with the treatment plan (Sensky, 1996). Child-rearing practices, family dynamics and the role of women will vary between societies, all of which need consideration when giving information (Bird & Dearmun, 1995).

Families who have a young person with cancer are a high-risk group for family dysfunction, due to the severe stress involved. If family conflict existed prior to diagnosis, the illness increases the tension, making the risk of dysfunction more likely (Friedman, 1987). Honest and open communication can help to prevent isolation and distancing of relationships within families and helps individuals to adapt to the inevitable changes in roles and responsibilities.

Language is another important consideration. Young people and their families may not feel confident about communicating in English, and this may lead to additional stress and frustration (Bird & Dearmun, 1995). In this case, access to interpreters will need to be arranged. Sometimes another member of the family is suggested, but whoever is chosen will need careful consideration, as this person is given a heavy burden of complicated, difficult and emotional information to impart. Inevitably, they will find this distressing at times and will need support and guidance.

Investigations

Routine investigations include plain X-rays, MRI and CT scanning of lesion and chest, radionuclide bone scan of the skeleton, blood tests and needle biopsy.

MRI scanning will show the extent of the tumour in the medulla of the bone and soft tissues and must be taken before any treatment is commenced as it can be used to assess cessation of tumour growth following initial doses of chemotherapy. The MRI scan is also important to ascertain any tumour involvement around nerves and blood vessels. If limb conservation surgery is advised these scans are used by the biomedical engineering unit, with measurement films of both affected and unaffected limbs, in the manufacture of custom-made endoprostheses, allowing for the optimal resection of tumour, including 5 cm of non-tumour bone.

Nursing note:

Although the MRI scan is non-invasive, young people need to be prepared that they may feel claustrophobic in the tunnel, it can be noisy, but most important of all, because the scan can take up to 45 minutes to complete, they may become stiff and experience considerable tumour pain. Adequate analgesia cover is required.

The bone scan will detect or exclude additional lesions in the skeleton. The injection of a radioactive marker, intravenously, three hours before the scan, is the much-hated part of this procedure, despite the use of a local anaesthetic cream. However, this can be a useful scenario to return to when promoting the virtues of a central line in chemotherapy.

The need for CT scans of the chest introduces the necessary discussion about the possibility of metastases and their first-line involvement of the lungs. This may be difficult to deal with before a proven diagnosis is established, but teenagers will appreciate the explanation and it can lead into a discussion about the reasons for the use of chemotherapy. Approximately 10–20% of young people will have visible lung metastases on their first CT scan (Jurgens et al., 1992), another reason for the gentle preparation.

Unfortunately, the presence of lung metastases at the time of diagnosis indicates a poorer prognosis. This increases the need for support and information about the recent innovations in the successful management of lung metastases, in order to maintain a positive approach to treatment.

Routine blood tests are carried out, including serum alkaline phosphatase (SAP) and serum lactic dehydrogenase (LDH). SAP levels may be raised above the parameters set for young people and it has been shown that these levels were significantly higher in patients with metastatic disease than in those with localised disease (Mertens & Bramwell, 1994). Serum LDH may be used as a prognostic factor during treatment. A reduction in the level during chemotherapy may indicate tumour response to the drugs. A significantly higher level may be present at recurrence (Salisbury & Byers, 1994).

The final piece in the jigsaw of investigations is the biopsy. A number of problems have been reported in relation to inexpert biopsy. The biopsy may be incorrectly sited so that conservative surgery cannot encompass it, or correctly positioned for surgical incision, but in a site causing muscle contamination (Kemp, 1987). Grimer and Sneath (1990) found that problems relating to biopsy were ten times more common if they were carried out before referral to a tumour treatment centre. Cannon and Dyson (1987) found that local recurrence of tumour occurred in 38% of cases in which the biopsy site could not be excised. A review of 208 procedures by Stoker et al. (1991) showed that a needle biopsy, performed by experienced practitioners, was both safe and accurate, causing minimal disturbance to the tumour and reduction in morbidity, and an increased potential for limb conservation surgery.

Nursing note:

From the teenager's point of view, a needle biopsy may be a painful procedure if performed under local anaesthetic. When a painful swelling is already present, extreme discomfort from pressure on the tumour when taking the sample, rather than from the actual piercing of the skin, has been reported. For this reason a general anaesthetic or heavy sedative, such as diazemols or midazolam, may be considered, in spite of the associated risks. The young person also needs to be reassured that following biopsy there may be some residual bleeding into the tumour, causing further swelling, and that this is not the tumour visibly growing.

Treatment Options

When all the investigations are complete, a decision has to be made promptly about treatment. With the rare exception of a low grade tumour, all young people diagnosed with either osteosarcoma or Ewing's sarcoma will be referred immediately to a specialist centre for chemotherapy, for a period of about six to nine months. The aim will be to necrose the tumour, reduce its volume and have an immediate effect on any micrometastases which might be present (Grimer & Carter, 1995). Combined with this will be some form of surgical excision, generally after 2–4 cycles of chemotherapy, depending on the protocol, with radiotherapy being introduced, if appropriate, in the later phase of treatment.

This rapid referral for treatment underlines the importance of adequately preparing young people and their families before the diagnosis is established. Part of this preparation involves discussing the possible options for surgery. If the tumour is growing in close proximity to major blood vessels then the possibility of amputation needs to be mentioned, even if limb conservation surgery is planned. Failure to mention this very emotive subject will result in loss of confidence with treatment and practitioners if amputation becomes a reality, and does not allow adequate psychological preparation before surgery. The level of tumour response to chemotherapy will determine the options for surgery.

One of the most upsetting side effects of chemotherapy treatment that teenagers have to cope with is the inevitable loss of hair. The fact that this is temporary is of little consolation at this early stage and ideas about how other teenagers have adapted to this major change, such as cutting their hair into a shorter style and the use of caps, hats, scarves and wigs may help to lessen the impact.

Another difficult topic which needs to be raised at this stage is the possibility that the young person may become subfertile or infertile following chemotherapy. This is an issue which can be very upsetting for teenagers. Sperm banking facilities exist at most oncology centres but are not always offered to young teenagers on paediatric oncology wards which lack provision for them. Careful and sensitive assessment of sexual maturity, involving discussion with the parents (if appropriate) will need to be made to determine which individuals should be counselled for sperm banking. The facility for storing eggs is not available as yet, because the length of time required to harvest and store them would not be practicable (Spears, 1994).

These are very difficult concepts for a teenager to cope with. However, the rapport built on honesty, sensitivity, empathy, availability and, at times, humour, with the team and especially with their named nurse, will remain a valuable source of continuing support throughout the long and arduous treatment.

Limb conservation surgery

Limb conservation surgery involves the wide excision of tumour bone and adjacent soft tissues. This bone may be replaced by the insertion of an endoprosthesis, sometimes with an extendable section, which, in young people with osteosarcoma, often includes a hip or knee joint to give adequate clearance from the tumour (Figure 19.2).

Endoprostheses are most commonly used to replace tumours in the proximal and distal femur, proximal tibia and proximal humerus. In some instances it may be necessary to replace the whole femur or humerus. Part of the ileum, including the acetabulum and proximal

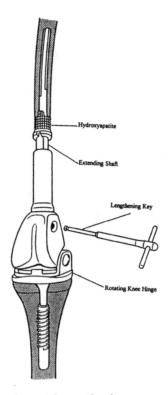

Hydroxyapatite

Extending Shaft

Lengthening Key

Rotating Knee Hinge

Figure 19.2: An extending femoral prosthesis

femur, may be replaced in pelvic tumours. Alternatively, if the tumour is above the acetabulum, excision of part of the ileum and grafting with the patient's own fibula, called a hemipelvectomy, may be performed. If the tumour is in the pubic ramus or fibula, a local wide excision is all that is required.

Tumours in the diaphysis of the bone, more commonly seen in Ewing's sarcoma, where margins of excision do not involve a joint, may be treated surgically without the use of endoprostheses. These tumours may be excised and bone transported from another area to be used as a bone graft. For example, the patient's own fibula may be used for grafting, following excision of a section of tibia. These autografts are much more successful than allografts, which have problems becoming incorporated into the host bone and re-achieving an adequate blood supply (Grimer & Carter, 1995).

Pre-operative issues

The timing of surgery between phases of chemotherapy requires close cooperation between oncologists and surgeons. Issues of infection and immunosuppression need to be resolved so that the young person is as medically fit as possible to cope with the procedure and anaesthetic.

Teenagers may want to discuss their fears relating to the anaesthetic and surgery. The most common questions relate to waking up during surgery; not waking up at the end; post-operative pain; length of time in bed; and restriction of activities. They are usually pleased to be having the tumour removed but are very keen to know what happens to it and look forward to a break from chemotherapy. This demonstrates one of the positive aspects of using separate areas for surgery and chemotherapy. For a while the young person becomes one of a number of teenagers undergoing surgery to correct a defect. They may establish friendships with peers who do not have cancer, but possibly an equally distressing condition and they can forget about the smells and routine they associate with chemotherapy.

Options and choice for pain management should be discussed pre-operatively, together with the advantages and disadvantages of each method. The possibility of urinary retention and how this may be resolved, needs to be included.

Nursing note:

The possibility of catheterisation is an issue teenagers feel very strongly about and, if given a choice, many would prefer to be catheterised in theatre rather than face the possibility in the immediate post-operative phase. In the case of pelvic surgery, catheterisation in theatre should be routine.

Concerns may be expressed about the position and size of the projected scar and a feeling of repulsion about having a large amount of metal inserted is not uncommon initially, especially if a knee joint is also being replaced. It may be helpful for teenagers to be able to handle a similar type of prosthesis and show it to friends and family. Photographs of previous patients, showing scars, appearance and involvement in normal activities such as riding bikes and swimming, are very helpful in allaying fears and misconceptions.

Nursing note:

A metal prosthesis will not set off the alarms at the airport.

Reduced serum calcium and magnesium levels are usually present if cisplatin is one of the protocol drugs and these may need to be supplemented. Cardiac arrythmias are a possible complication of doxorubicin administration and an ECG is taken pre-operatively.

Lack of appetite and weight loss are other issues that may cause concern and poor nutritional status is less favourable to healing. Emesis, taste and smell aberrations, mouth ulcers from chemotherapy and the psychological effects of cancer can all contribute to diminished food intake and consequent malnutrition. Ewing's sarcoma has a 67% probability of malnutrition, and osteosarcoma a 10–15% risk (Tebbi & Erpenbeck, 1996).

Another period of hospitalisation for surgery, the anaesthetic and post-operative pain may also decrease the desire to eat. It is therefore important to discuss and consider the use of dietary supplements and to try to provide a tempting menu suitable to the adolescent's needs. Poor intake of food may lead to conflict with parents who often relate eating to a measure of health. They may also feel rejected when food they have specially prepared is refused. However, with a welcome break from chemotherapy and a relief from some of its associated side effects, appetites usually improve and teenagers start to enjoy food again, although taste alterations may persist.

Post-operative issues and possible complications

Pain management

The aim of post-operative pain relief is to give comfort to patients, allowing them to breathe, cough and move more easily. Multimodal pain therapy is the most important technique for the treatment of post-operative pain (Kehlet, 1994). This can be achieved by combining NSAIDs and opiates.

An individual's reaction to pain is determined by their past experiences, level of development and health status (McCready et al., 1991). Studies have shown that older children are able to think in more abstract terms and define pain as having both physical and psychological components (McGrath, 1990). This means that they may be more aware of feelings of helplessness, anxiety about how long the pain will last and its significance (Lansdown & Sokel, 1993).

Opiates may be given effectively via a patient-controlled analgesia device or an epidural. Morphine is the drug of choice in PCA, ideally combined with an antiemetic to prevent nausea. This form of analgesia has been well evaluated by teenagers undergoing orthopaedic surgery, as it gives them some choice and control over their relief from pain (Kaufman Rauen & Ho, 1989). Studies have shown that young people use less analgesia post-operatively with PCA than when drugs are given by more conventional routes. The fact that the teenager is active in controlling the pain may enhance the analgesic effect (McGrath, 1990).

Although effective, some teenagers talk about disliking the feeling of being out of control whilst having the opiate and this can make them reluctant to use PCA. There may be some loss of pain control at night when the teenager is asleep if PCA does not have a background infusion. This can be prevented by the use of a long-acting NSAID, such as diclofenac, providing there is not a history of gastritis from chemotherapy.

If surgery has involved the lower limb, the teenager may be offered an epidural infusion as an alternative method of pain control and less opiate may be used compared to intramuscular and intravenous routes (Genge, 1988). This can be very effective and minimise systemic effects, although numbness of the legs makes neurological checks difficult. Special attention needs to be paid to areas which may become sore from pressure, such as the heel, as sensation will be impaired temporarily.

Favaloro (1988) suggests that adolescents may have difficulty expressing pain if they believe that, as young adults, it is not socially acceptable to do so and that consequently they may deny that they have pain. Culture and gender may have an influence on perceptions of pain. In the West males are expected to feel less pain than females, whereas Jews and Italians complain freely (Zborowski, 1952, cited in Parsons, 1992). Good pre-operative preparation should help to balance this, by giving the teenager permission to complain of pain. In addition, time spent giving information, answering questions and helping to allay fears and anxieties should have contributed to the overall effectiveness of pain relief.

Nursing note:

Teenagers respond well to the use of a visual analogue scale, with a numbered scale, as an assessment tool to discuss what is an acceptable level of pain for them and to evaluate how effective the analgesia regime is. Massage can provide not only psychological support through human contact, but can mediate the pain response. The quality of touch is important and this can help in communicating with teenagers who find it difficult to express their feelings. When they are in pain, the hand movements should be lengthened into long, slow strokes which can soothe the sensory nerve endings and block the pain impulse (Day, 1995). A number of teenagers enjoy foot massage and find it particularly relaxing.

Nausea and vomiting

Nausea and vomiting may occur as a routine reaction to anaesthesia, anxiety and surgery, but for the teenager undergoing chemotherapy it holds more emotion as a reminder of his ongoing treatment. Consideration needs to be given to any residual gastritis from chemotherapy and an H_2 antagonistic drug, such as ranitidine, may be indicated to reduce gastric hyperacidity and prevent a stress ulcer occurring, especially if vomiting persists.

Nursing note:

The antiemetic of choice for teenagers is ondansetron as it is less likely than other antiemetics to cause a feeling of light-headedness which for this age group in particular is associated with feeling 'out of control'. For the same reason acupressure wrist bands are often welcomed as an alternative and can be quite effective.

Urinary retention

Urinary retention may occur due to the use of an epidural infusion or intravenous opiates. Routine catheterisation is an issue which is much debated, mainly due to the potential risk of infection. Whether elective or crisis management is in place, the issue of infection is crucially important in limb conservation surgery where an endo-prosthesis has been inserted. Prophylactic antibiotic cover should be given and the opinion of the teenager should be sought and listened to, in relation to this potential problem.

Pressure necrosis

Another potential problem immediately post-operatively following lower limb endoprosthetic replacement surgery is pressure necrosis around the knee. The theatre dressings may include layers of padding and stretch bandages, in the form of a pressure dressing, to provide support and prevent excessive swelling. If the bandages are too restrictive, however, allowing insufficient space for the knee to swell, the blood supply over the knee may be compromised, causing necrosis of the tissue, which, if extensive, may require skin grafting. It is therefore important to check the vascular status of the knee at 24–48 hours post-operatively, by removing the bandages and theatre dressing. If no redness from pressure is apparent, the knee can be re-bandaged to control swelling.

Nursing note:

Excessive pain that is difficult to control may be an indication that over-restriction is present.

Neurological impairment and position of limb

Limb conservation surgery of more advanced tumours may involve sacrificing one of the nerves, especially in the proximal tibia. Careful assessment should be made post-operatively to establish any impairment in sensation and function, and measures should be taken to prevent the associated risks. If foot drop is present then the foot and ankle need to be kept in a neutral position, by use of a pillow or wedge, at the same time ensuring that the heel is kept free from pressure. A drop foot orthosis inside the shoe will be required for long term support when walking.

If surgery has replaced the proximal femur and acetabulum there may be the additional risk of dislocation of the hip. This can be prevented by keeping the leg in abduction, either by suspending it in slings and springs, or using an abduction wedge. A post-operative hip orthosis may be needed when mobilising until the muscles are strong enough to prevent such a dislocation.

Haematoma formation

Another complication which may occur is the formation of a haematoma around the knee. Closed suction wound drainage is usually used to drain excessive blood away from the wound. Established practice in orthopaedic surgery is to remove these drains at 24–48 hours post-operatively. Research has shown that in routine hip replacement surgery minimal drainage occurred after 24 hours and that the continued presence of drainage after that time did not reduce haematoma formation and may introduce skin organisms into the wound (Willett et al., 1988).

Nursing note:

Observations have shown the average amount of drainage from massive replacement surgery involving the knee can be more than double that of hip replacement wounds at 24 hours and ten times more at 48 and 72 hours. This could indicate that wound drains may need to remain in place longer than for the average orthopaedic operation to reduce the possibility of haematoma formation. Another interesting observation is that patients receiving the haemopoietic growth factor, G-CSF, may have increased wound drainage. In order to prevent haematoma formation around the knee and the associated risks of adhesions from delayed flexion and extension and infection from aspiration it may be necessary to review current practice regarding the removal of wound drains at 24–48 hours post-operatively if blood is still being drained.

Reduced mobility

A temporary reduction in mobility is inevitable following surgery, but weight-bearing with support is allowed in all procedures. A canvas splint will keep the knee straight until the quadriceps muscle is strong enough to control the knee and a hip orthosis may need to be worn for a while if muscle was removed during the hip replacement surgery. The physiotherapist has an important role in the multidisciplinary team and every assistance will be given to the young person to achieve optimal function. This level of function is difficult for teenagers to maintain when restarting chemotherapy, as an exercise regime becomes low priority when feeling unwell.

Nursing note:

To maintain motivation during exercise regimes, a structured goal planning approach ensures visually recorded progress which can be acknowledged and encouraged by all the team.

Infection

Routine intravenous antibiotic cover is given at the time of surgery as the possibility of infection will always be the greatest threat to the successful outcome from endoprosthetic procedures. An infection around the prosthesis is difficult to eradicate and may lead to chronic sinus formation and its ultimate removal. The presence of a central venous access device adds to this risk, although good practice and early recognition and treatment of infections will reduce this to a minimum.

Wound healing may be delayed due to devascularisation of the skin following a wide skin incision and bony resection (Hockenberry & Lane, 1988). This may result in large blisters forming around the incision, which need careful management to aid healing and avoid infection. Wound healing should be complete before chemotherapy is resumed.

A reactive hyperpyrexia may be present post-operatively, as well as tachycardia, neither of which are necessarily indicative of an infection unless prolonged.

Nursing note:

Young people need to be aware of the risks of infection to their prosthesis at a later stage, from an untreated sore throat or similar condition. They also need to be aware that the limb with a metal prosthesis in will always feel warmer to touch than the unaffected limb due to the fact that metal conducts heat.

Amputation

A teenager requiring an amputation of whole or part of a limb must be one of the most emotive experiences in orthopaedic surgery. Amputation at any age is distressing, but, although the physical care is similar, the emotional needs differ significantly. Special concerns relate to physical appearance, acceptance by peers and achieving independence (Lasoff, 1985).

During adolescence, teenagers are trying to cope with accepting normal physical changes to their bodies, and to lose part of their body, therefore, is an enormously traumatic experience. Thoughts about boyfriends and girlfriends, going swimming, wearing shorts, looking a freak, being stared at and, particularly, being made fun of at school, are commonly verbalised. These feelings may lead to unpredictable behaviour and bouts of anger which nurses need to be sensitive to and be able to provide emotional support and understanding.

Pre-operative issues

Teenagers expecting to have an amputation of a limb need a great deal of preparation before surgery, both with and separately from their family. The attitudes of nurses, peers, the family and the whole multidisciplinary team will influence the way in which the teenager tries to accept and adapt to the loss and look positively to the future.

The teenagers may ask for the opportunity to visit a limb fitting department to help them visualise how the limb will look, and to discuss the wide range of activities they will be able to do and how the limb will function. Surprise is often expressed at the realistic appearance of the foot and toes and the versatility of the knee. It is also a relief to learn that nearly any style of shoe, trainer or boot can be worn. The staff in these centres are very understanding about the teenager's need to look 'normal' and can allay many fears and anxieties about future appearance.

Sometimes the teenager asks to meet another teenager, who has previously had a similar amputation for cancer and who is willing to share his or her experience. Ideally, the person should be the same sex, as there are usually questions asked about sexuality. Alternatively, the youngster may ask for this meeting during the rehabilitation phase rather than before surgery. Photographs show-ing the appearance of a stump, scars and an artificial limb are useful to have available and pictures of teenage amputees cycling, skiing, playing football and girls looking glamorous, or getting married, all help to promote a positive approach. All visual and educational material is useful, but extreme sensitivity is required to know if, when and how to introduce it. The most welcome information for the teenager is usually that they can learn to drive earlier, at 16 years, and this usually becomes the first goal during rehabilitation.

There have been varying opinions as to whether discussion pre-operatively about phantom limb sensations is likely to increase its incidence, but studies have been unable to demonstrate this (Dernham, 1986). Teenagers should be prepared for the fact that they may still feel their limb when they wake up from surgery and have an idea of the type of sensations that may be associated with this.

Nursing note:

Make sure that the teenager being prepared for an amputation knows the exact level at which the limb is going to be removed, otherwise 'above knee' may mean that literally to them, instead of possibly half the femur, which can cause extreme distress when the dressings are removed. The teenager needs to be aware that he or she will not have an artificial limb straight away and that a plaster cast will have to be taken from the stump, after it has shrunk, before the limb can be made. This will take a few weeks and will be arranged at the local limb fitting centre.

Parents and siblings will find this pre-operative phase very difficult to manage and may take longer than the teenager to adjust. It is particularly important that siblings are involved at every level, as research has shown that the worst experiences healthy siblings had were from lack of information (Craft & Craft, 1989). They also expressed feelings of fear and worry about the ill sibling, especially in relation to the outcome of the illness and strong feelings of loneliness and isolation.

Post-operative issues

Pain management

Three types of pain may be experienced by the young person undergoing an amputation: stump pain, phantom limb pain or sensations and emotional pain. If the teenager is in agreement, the most effective form of pain control for stump pain is via an epidural infusion. It would appear that this has the added advantage of possibly reducing the severity of phantom limb sensations later, especially if commenced prior to surgery, as pain in the limb before amputation is correlated with the incidence and degree of phantom pain afterwards (Spross & Hope, 1985; Rounseville, 1992). Emotional pain and anxiety are inevitably strong factors influencing the experience of pain and must be addressed when trying to achieve its control.

Phantom limb sensations

A phantom limb sensation (PLS) is being able to feel that a part of a limb is still present although it has been amputated (Dernham, 1986). It is important that teenagers are able to distinguish between PLS and stump pain, as opiates are not effective against PLS (Rounseville, 1992). Not all PLS is painful and some may be described as burning, crushing, pins and needles, cramping and itching. The more proximal the amputation, the stronger and more uncomfortable the sensations will be. Stress, anxiety and depression may intensify the sensations but do not cause them (Rounseville, 1992).

Treatment for PLS may include drugs, transcutaneous nerve stimulation (TENS) and the use of deep relaxation and guided imagery. Anticonvulsant drugs, such as carbamazepine and clonazepam, may be used for the sharp, piercing types of pain, to prevent abnormal signals from reaching the brain, and baclofen for the cramping or spasm-like sensations. Tricyclic antidepressants, such as amitryptyline and imipramine, can be used to stop insomnia and these will also help to counteract depression (Rounseville, 1992).

TENS, whereby electrodes are placed on the surface of the skin and a mild electric current is administered, has been shown to be helpful in giving some relief from PLS when applied direct to the stump or to the collateral limb (Bending, 1989). Patients can alter the frequency, pulse widths and duration of the machine and this may help some teenagers to feel more in control and offers an alternative to drugs.

Teenagers generally respond well to the idea of deep relaxation and guided imagery as these are techniques they can learn to help themselves. They can be taught how to relax all the voluntary muscles, to try warm baths and massage and by distracting their thoughts away from the sensations they can gain complete relief. Other teenagers have found that they can gain relief by pretending to massage the painful area where the limb should be, or on the collateral limb. Counselling, hypnosis, focused breathing and keeping a pain diary have also been found to help (Spross & Hope, 1985).

> **Nursing note:**
>
> **NSAIDs appear to give some relief from PLS, if given regularly.**

Unfortunately, it may be necessary to try a variety of different ways to control PLS but, providing adequate time and support are given to exploring them, teenagers are able to achieve long term control without the use of medication. Continuity in care and in nursing staff are important factors in the process.

Care of the stump

Swelling of the stump immediately post-operatively can be controlled by the use of pressure bandaging and elevating the bed. A pillow should not be placed under the stump as this can cause hip or knee flexion contractures.

Painful sensations are usually felt in the stump when the theatre dressings are removed and these are exacerbated by the intense feelings of anxiety at seeing the stump and wound for the first time, and adequate analgesia cover will be required. Ideally, the first dressing should be carried out where there will be minimal interruption and adequate time available to give support and information. The teenager's need for sensitivity and privacy must be respected at all times.

> **Nursing note:**
>
> **A small layer of paraffin gauze over the suture line will prevent adhesion and facilitate the removal of early dressings.**

Spontaneous wound healing and correct stump bandaging are of the utmost importance in ensuring the successful fitting of the artificial limb. The bandages help to mould the shape of the stump by applying even pressure to both sides and when the stump has shrunk sufficiently these are replaced by a firm elasticated sock.

Exercises are required initially for balance, if part of a lower limb has been removed and then to increase muscle tone and power in the remaining muscles, in preparation for walking with the artificial limb. Practising this on the ward is the first stage in adjusting to being seen without a limb by peers. This can be a very positive experience and other teenagers are usually quick to encourage and praise their efforts.

The Van Nes rotationplasty

This surgical procedure was developed to convert an above-knee amputation into a more functional below-knee amputation. It involves the removal of the tumour from the distal femur and the attachment of the proximal tibia after it has been rotated through 180°. The ankle joint functions as the knee joint in the artificial limb. The foot remains, pointing backwards and the toes may be electively removed for cosmetic purposes. The main advantages of this form of amputation, although uncommon in the UK, are a high level of function and lack of PLS. The obvious disadvantage is the unusual appearance of the limb which the teenager would need immense support and guidance in accepting (Pasecki, 1992).

Altered Body Image

Young people need to be able to socialise with friends and anything that prevents this happening will make them stand out from the rest and could affect their own body image and self-esteem. Physical attractiveness is an important factor for acceptance by peers. Race, religion and cultural background have an important influence on a young person's development and the attitude of others will affect their own self-image and self-value (White, 1995).

When teenagers are diagnosed with a malignant bone tumour their identity tends to lose importance as attention is focused on the disease process. They may feel as though they have lost control over their body. As they undergo chemotherapy and surgery they try to adjust to considerable alterations in appearance while trying to maintain a healthy self-esteem (Fedora, 1985). It is crucial that young people are kept fully informed about their illness and are given the opportunity to make decisions about their own future.

Hair loss is the first change to cope with, which can be managed well in the oncology setting where it becomes the 'norm'. If teenagers transfer to a surgical unit for the next phase of treatment, they may be the only young person without hair. At this stage of acceptance it does not appear to be a problem any longer and provides a natural opening for exchanging information about conditions and treatment with peers, especially on a teenage unit.

Regardless of the type of surgery, the teenager's body will never be the same again. Scars and limb shape after surgery are important issues. Spontaneous wound healing will contribute to a neat scar, which will be fairly extensive and need protection from the sun. In time this will be less noticeable and massaging cream into the scar tissue will help to keep it supple. Limb shape following conservation surgery is usually good once the swelling has reduced, concern is sometimes expressed over wasting of muscles but this can be used as motivation to achieve goals in physiotherapy.

When an amputation is performed on a young person, feelings of anger, disgust, mutilation and grief may need to be dealt with and reactions of the family, staff, friends and peers to the new image will be watched closely by the adolescent. Dressing in their own clothes as soon as possible and encouragement and help in looking attractive will have a positive effect. Personal relationships will always be a worry, with lack of acceptance by peers being the greatest fear.

Nursing note:

Teenagers who have survived bone cancer and have had an amputation report that it is easier for males to be involved in an intimate relationship than females, although there appears to be little difference in interaction in the early stages of a relationship. Returning to school or college with an altered body image can present an enormous challenge and lack of confidence may lead to regressive behaviour and a fear of loss of academic performance. Support from teaching staff and possibly the school nurse will be needed to prevent the teenager from becoming isolated. Emphasis will need to be placed on positive attributes rather than focusing on the illness, and a flexible approach may be needed to enable the teenagers to remain with their peers, although they may not have reached the same level of achievement.

A survey looking at the quality of life of young people who had osteosarcoma, at least one year after treatment, showed that the overwhelming psychological problem was a fear of tumour recurrence and the possibility of more treatment (Nirenberg, 1985). However, the survey also showed that many patients had successfully completed their education, had careers and some had started families.

Discharge Planning

Coordinated discharge planning is necessary for young people undergoing surgery for either limb preservation or amputation. It is essential that oncologists are informed of the discharge date to enable them to plan post-operative chemotherapy. Ideally, a few days at home after discharge can be built into the plan, which will help to prepare the teenager and the rest of the family, for the next phase of treatment.

Wound healing should be complete at this stage, but central line care may need to be continued by the community care team. It is useful to discuss with them and the oncology unit any problems associated with the surgical management and any psychosocial issues that may have arisen during treatment.

Similar links should be made between other members of the multidisciplinary teams. Physiotherapists will arrange for continued therapy both in the community and oncology unit. Social workers and counsellors will pass on work that needs to be continued and the medical teams will exchange information relating to future management. Some oncology units have produced shared care folders for recording information such as treatment plans and blood test results.

The hospital school may send a progress report to show what work has been covered, and this is especially important with GCSE course work. They will also link up with the home tutor if appropriate.

Information may need to be given about medication and about precautions that need to be taken to prevent infection of the prosthesis. All young people want to be fully informed about restrictions on activities, both in the short and long term. Amputees should have been linked to a limb fitting centre and a resettlement officer, who can give advice about how when and where to learn to drive and what modifications, if any will need to be made to the car.

Follow-up surgical appointments are usually made to accommodate periods between chemotherapy and neutropenia. Good discharge planning will ensure continuity of care and help to minimise stress for the young person and their family.

Late Effects

Lung metastases

Eighty per cent of young people show no apparent signs of lung metastases at the time of diagnosis, but they may rapidly develop them within the first year in spite of chemotherapy and surgery. This suggests that micrometastases are present at diagnosis and surgery (Schwartz et al., 1993).

Adjuvant chemotherapy can contain or reduce lung metastases, allowing them to be resected. If the lesions are only in one lung, less than six and occur after chemotherapy, then the prognosis is improved after complete resection (Souhami & Tobias, 1986).

Further chemotherapy, using a different drug may be given prior to the metastasectomy. However, not all teenagers will agree to additional chemotherapy and some will opt only for surgery. This decision is usually made when they have just managed to return to normal activities, their hair has grown back and they have started to feel good about themselves, and so feel that they cannot cope with the associated problems of more chemotherapy. Jurgens et al. (1992) state that the value of additional chemotherapy for lung metastases is under debate and that data from trials are not convincing.

Local recurrence

Roberts et al. (1991) found that the incidence of local recurrence, in a review of 133 young patients treated with distal femoral prostheses, was only slightly higher than that recorded for amputation. Although the patients with the recurrence subsequently had an amputation, the results still showed that following the insertion of the prosthesis, 88% of patients would not require an amputation at five years post-operatively.

In the same study, infection was shown to be the major complication, either from surgery, a central line or wound breakdown while on chemotherapy. Two of these cases required amputation for persistent infection.

Loosening and limb inequality

A retrospective study of 1001 prostheses used as replacements for bone tumours showed that aseptic loosening was the main cause of failure of the implant, requiring revision (Unwin et al., 1996). The highest failure group due to aseptic loosening was after distal femoral replacements and could be related to the amount of bone that was removed, the age of the patient and the site of resection. Younger patients, with more than 60% of bone resection in the distal femoral and proximal tibial groups were more at risk from loosening. Interestingly, there were no failures of proximal femoral replacements with more than 60% of bone removed. This could be related to the natural curve of the femur and the quality of bone in the medullary canal, which allowed good fixation with cement.

Younger patients, if they continue to grow rapidly, may have a leg length discrepancy, in spite of the extendable prosthesis and may require an adult size replacement at a later stage. It is possible that only the shaft will need to be changed and that this could be connected to the original replacement knee joint. This problem can also be managed by deliberately damaging a growth plate in the unaffected limb to slow down the rate of growth. Research has shown that, when skeletally mature these adolescents may be above average height for their age (Earl & Souhami, 1990). If this is this case then shortening of the unaffected limb, by removing a wedge of femur, is a realistic alternative.

Restrictions on activities

One of the long term disappointments for some teenagers is the restriction placed on contact sports, especially if they were previously in school or county teams. In some schools great emphasis is placed on sporting ability, which in turn leads to popularity and peer acceptance. Fortunately, other sports such as swimming, cycling and badminton are possible.

Realistic careers are another consideration for teenagers, depending on the type of surgery they have had. Sometimes there has been a delay in education for a year, either as a deliberate decision, or because of treatment complications; but many young people battle on with study and course work, often taking exams between courses of chemotherapy and still managing to achieve good grades. Several of these teenagers are keen to work in the health profession as doctors, nurses or social workers. Difficulties may arise in obtaining health and life insurance at a later stage and this reinforces the uncertainty of their future prognosis, which some young people find difficult to accept.

Infertility

Infertility may be a late complication of treatment and is especially associated with high doses of alkylating agents, which play an important part in the treatment of Ewing's sarcoma. This problem is related to age at time of diagnosis and pre-pubertal children are known to tolerate higher doses of these drugs and may therefore be more at risk (Jurgens et al., 1992). Teenagers have successfully become parents after completion of treatment, in some cases after a hemipelvectomy, and the children have been healthy and normal, following uncomplicated pregnancies and deliveries (Nirenberg, 1985).

Future Trends

Surgery

Studies have shown that limb conservation surgery and, in particular, endoprostheses can be successfully used, reducing the need for amputation (Mertens & Bramwell, 1994). Recent developments in prosthetic design have mainly focused on the extending mechanism to lengthen the shaft with minimal surgical intervention, to achieve greater growth potential; the rotational element of the knee hinge; coating of the prosthesis to prevent tissue reaction to the titanium alloy and the use of calcium hydroxyapatite ceramics (CHA).

Current research is looking at ways of extending an endoprosthesis using a completely non-invasive technique.

CHA are non-toxic substances which are biologically compatible with bone, produce little tissue reaction and can be used in place of bone grafts (Uchida et al., 1990). These substances are being used to coat the end of the prosthesis. X-rays have shown that the host bone is able to grow into the CHA and form a complete union. This is an exciting development which should significantly reduce the incidence of loosening by reducing forces on the cement–bone interface (Unwin et al., 1996). CHA may be further developed for use in conservation surgery, in place of bone graft after tumour excision.

Surgery is also developing the use of external fixators and preservation of the growth plate in limb conservation surgery. Seventy-five per cent of malignant bone tumours in young people occur near the growth cartilage, which has been thought to offer some resistance to the spread of the tumour, but is not impenetrable (Canadell et al., 1994).

It is now possible, in some skeletally immature young people, to excise the tumour from the metaphysis and preserve the epiphysis and knee function, providing there are adequate clearance margins.

This surgery is carried out in three stages:

1. External fixator pins are inserted into the epiphysis and into the diaphysis, or shaft of the bone, with a clearance margin of up to 10 cm below the tumour. An external fixator is then attached to the pins. While the patient is having the first cycles of chemotherapy, a device on the apparatus is turned daily, pulling the shaft of

the bone away from the growth cartilage, a process called distraction. This is continued until the cartilage has lengthened by 2 cm.
2. The entire tumour is resected with clear margins each end and this is confirmed by histopathology.
3. The space left after resection is reconstructed by either bone grafting or bone transportation (Canadell et al., 1994).

This surgery, if successful, would be particularly appropriate in patients with tumours in the proximal tibia.

Results so far have not shown any local recurrence (Canadell et al., 1994). This surgery, if successful, could allow young people with bone tumours near the knee joint, especially in the proximal tibia, to have complete resection of the tumour, avoid a prosthetic replacement and preserve the function of their own knee.

Chemotherapy

Future trends in chemotherapy for bone cancer will be evaluating the data from trials and, in particular, reviewing the impact of high-dose chemotherapy on tumour response and disease-free survival. Results so far have shown difficulties in keeping to schedules, due to thrombocytopenia and the possibility of using a platelet-stimulating factor to improve this may be considered.

Ornadel et al. (1994) have found that chemotherapy given at two-weekly intervals, with the use of G-CSF, instead of at three-weekly intervals without G-CSF, has resulted in reduced renal, cardiac and neurotoxicity, although there was increased mucositis and infections. These authors suggested that G-CSF may therefore be considered for use with the three-weekly regime to allow 100% intensity to be given. These trials are extremely important as tumour necrosis after chemotherapy is an important prognostic factor in determining survival (Pringle, 1987).

Effect of Setting

Teenagers are an age group with their own unique set of needs. When they are diagnosed as having cancer all their developmental tasks are threatened as they try to adjust to major changes in their life (Evans, 1993b). These young people deserve special understanding and need to be cared for by nurses who recognise how problems may affect their mood, behaviour and coping (Taylor & Muller, 1995). Blunden (1989) found that teenagers on adult wards and, to a lesser extent, those on children's wards, were cared for by nurses with little training in their specific needs. Ideally, teenagers with bone tumours should be nursed in teenage units, with nurses specifically trained to care for this age group and speciality (Earl & Souhami, 1990). All teenagers interviewed by Burr (1993), on an adult and a children's ward, stated that they would like to be cared for with their own age group.

The teenage environment is crucial to peer support and interaction. It should be relaxed and friendly, age-appropriate, supportive and flexible with minimal ground rules. Nursing staff should be empathetic, adaptable and have a good sense of humour.

Body image and peer group identification are the developmental tasks that are most affected by having bone cancer (Nirenberg, 1985). Although many of the changes are temporary, it is the 'here and now' that is important to the teenager and especially how their peers accept and treat them. Many young people have reported that having treatment for cancer has made them feel and act differently from their peers, not only because of the changes to their bodies but because it has also made them more mature (Nirenberg, 1985). Fedora (1985) found it very helpful to meet former patients who had completed treatment and who had adjusted to the physical changes. She also felt that staff should encourage and facilitate relationships with other peers, to move the focus away from the individual, towards supporting and encouraging others in their progress. This can be very successful on a mixed surgical unit where not all the young people have cancer, but have many other debilitating and distressing conditions.

Good communication skills are needed by all the team involved in caring for the young person with cancer. Difficulties may arise if adults and teenagers do not identify with each other, and teenagers will be unable to confide in someone with whom they do not have any rapport (Gillies, 1992). Teenagers usually welcome a frank and honest discussion about their condition, and it is important that the environment recognises and facilitates this, encouraging adolescents to be involved in decision making and in planning their own care. Good communication is also required with the parents, who need to come to terms with the fact that, although they have a life-threatening illness, teenagers still need control over their life and need to remain as independent as possible (Taylor & Muller, 1995).

Acute illness and the hospitalisation of a young person puts great strain on all family members, not least on siblings. It is important that brothers and sisters share in the care of the sick sibling, and if the outcome is death, this will help them to adjust to their loss (White, 1995). Issues may include fear and uncertainty as to the outcome of the illness, fear of catching cancer, which may also be expressed by friends, and jealousy, loneliness and resentment due to lack of attention and involvement (Craft, 1993). It is important that the holistic approach to the care of the teenager with bone cancer recognises these potential problems in the healthy sibling and is able to intervene, where appropriate, to prevent or lessen the long term adverse effects.

The teenage environment should try to generate a sense of normality, particularly in relation to leisure and educational needs, offering a wide selection of activities, such as snooker, computer games, televisions, videos, board games and music. The role of education in hospital is an important link with normal life (Wilson, 1993). It can provide stimulation, allow expression of emotions through writing and art, and help to maintain or increase academic progress. Links are made with the teenager's own school to ensure continuity of work and to identify any weak areas which may be helped. The one-to-one tuition available in the larger hospital schools can be invaluable in helping teenagers with learning difficulties. Young people with bone cancer who have opted out of school for a year may enjoy pottery, cookery, art and craft activities and, in particular, work on computers.

Facilities to make drinks and light snacks and their own separate leisure area, are evaluated well by teenagers, as well as a room to go to be quiet and reflect. They will also appreciate being able to spend some private time with friends and visiting needs to be flexible.

Nursing staff on teenage units are in an ideal position to take an active lead in health promotion, however, to be effective, they need to understand the social contexts in which teenagers function (Taylor & Muller, 1995). Displaying leaflets and booklets in a private area such as the toilet will ensure that issues relating to contraception, smoking, sexually transmitted diseases, nutrition, and drug, solvent and alcohol abuse are addressed, and teenagers are empowered to seek out information and help them to understand it. Information leaflets on drugs and contraception are particularly popular and can promote open discussions between teenagers and nurses. These discussions should encourage young people to look at their own practice, talk about their experiences and exchange views. A notice board displaying various helplines, including the teenager cancer support groups, may be appropriate.

Unfortunately, a number of teenagers who have the potential for lung metastases will still make the decision to continue to smoke and this may be difficult for others to understand. A knowledge of the influencing factors, such as personality, peer influence, the media and parental smoking, may help when trying to counsel young people about this problem.

Young people undergoing medical and surgical treatment for primary bone cancer can benefit greatly from being cared for in an age-appropriate environment, by named nurses who understand and appreciate their role in facilitating teenagers to progress with their developmental tasks, especially in relation to psychosocial development. This role can help young people to improve their self-image, achieve and maintain independence and will often develop into long term support and interest, ensuring that their hospitalisation was a positive experience.

These teenagers have a right to open and honest communication, to informed choice and control, privacy, confidentiality and protection, which will lead to a trusting relationship, providing physical and emotional support to the teenagers as they try to cope with the enormous stresses and uncertainties of their illness and treatments.

It is crucial for young people to be able to maintain a sense of normality in their lives and it is important that they spend as little time as possible at the treatment centre. Shared care, between disciplines in specialist units and the community, can therefore be very beneficial to young people, providing there is a similar philosophy of care, as it can offer the optimum quality of life. Effective communication between all key workers is vital to its success.

SECTION FOUR
RADIOTHERAPY

Chapter 20
The nature of radiotherapy

Monica Hopkins

Introduction

Radiotherapy is a poorly understood area of therapeutic medicine. It often strikes fear into people outside the radiotherapy profession, as radiation is primarily linked with harm. Many people perceive that exposure may lead to cancer and death. This is understandable when one is bombarded with media interpretations of the situations in Chernobyl or Hiroshima. Even within this country, functional nuclear power plants remain shrouded in controversy.

When considering the therapeutic effects of this seemingly powerful phenomenon, members of the public appear only to recall that patients undergoing radiotherapy suffer distressing skin reactions and sickness. It is also imagined that many patients become terminally ill after such therapy.

This dark and mysterious image is not assisted by the fact that many radiotherapy departments are situated in hospital basements with a maze of corridors leading to them, with no natural light. The need for staff and patient safety necessitate thick high-density concrete and/or lead-lined walls, large complicated machinery, skin markings that appear to mimic tattoos and an emphasis on complete stillness during treatment. All these situations and unusual images heighten fear and promote misconception. The most valuable help that nurses can provide for children and their families is to demystify some of this and decrease fear by providing knowledge and thus a sense of control. Families require preparation and ongoing support as well as specialised nursing care and observation. It is the aim of this chapter to enhance understanding of this therapy, which though not the most common experience for children with cancer, is still so vital in the battle against this disease.

The literature in this field of study is almost overwhelmingly adult-based (Mandell et al., 1986/87; Brunner et al., 1992; Bucholtz, 1992). Nursing research is extremely limited, especially in the speciality of paediatrics (Baron, 1991; Bucholtz, 1992; Slifer et al., 1994; Slifer, 1996), and is almost exclusively American. Most research being carried out at present is medically based. The available nursing literature is predominantly commentary, with very little research to guide nursing practice. The work that is available for nursing to base its care on often concerns the efficacy of radiotherapy in studied neoplasms, dose-toxicity studies and late biological effects. Descriptions of appropriate nursing care in this chapter are commentaries extrapolated from such work and the experiences of practitioners in the field. Issues such as appropriate mouth care in children are not well-founded in the nursing research literature. Although skin care has become a more popular focus in the adult literature, current research on this topic remains poorly disseminated in practice (Campbell & Lane, 1996). These issues and other pertinent aspects of nursing care will be outlined within this section and include an analysis of the literature concerning patient preparation and family support.

Indications for the Use of Radiation in the Care of Children with Cancer

For some significant part of modern medical history, radiation has been used for imaging to assist investigations to identify a diagnosis. The oldest medical image in this arena is the X-ray, but in recent times radioactive contrast mediums in computerised tomography (CT), bone scans and many modern imaging devices have been used. However, as a therapeutic tool radiation has served modern medicine well and may continue to do so for quite some time, though its form may change.

Radiotherapy may be used as the sole mode of therapy for neoplastic disease or in conjunction with surgery, chemotherapy, or both. Radiotherapy can be used both as a curative intervention and as a palliative measure to control distressing symptoms of advanced disease, such as pain, obstruction, compression and bleeding. Radiotherapy may also be used in the oncological emergency to give temporary relief from a life-threatening complication until full treatment can be commenced, for example superior vena cava syndrome or spinal cord compression. In summary, radiotherapy may be used for:

- Eradication of disease
- Treatment planning
- Emergency intervention
- Imaging
- Symptom control.

The tumours most commonly treated with radiotherapy are medulloblastoma, neuroblastoma, glioma, Ewing's sarcoma, rhabdomyosarcoma, primitive neuroectodermal tumours, Hodgkin's disease, Wilms' tumour and leukaemic infiltration of the central nervous system.

The Nature of Radiation

Since the late nineteenth century, medicine has been aware of the therapeutic potential of radiation (Iwamoto, 1994). However, it was really in the latter half of this century that science began to refine the treatment; to increase its efficacy in curing cancer whilst limiting the damage resulting from this natural but potent power on healthy tissue. To understand how this power is harnessed it is essential that the source of this energy and its characteristics are fully identified and understood.

Radiation energy exists in two main forms: particulate energy and waves of electromagnetic radiation (Hilderley, 1992a, b). Each form of radiation requires an introduction.

Particulate energy

All matter is made up of tiny units called *atoms*. It was thought that these were the smallest material entities, but in recent times it has been discovered that atoms are actually made from a number of different particles (Figure 20.1).

Some of these particles carry their own electrical charge and, through the positive and negative attraction, the particles are bound together, with the help of some uncharged particles (*neutrons*). A number of positively charged particles (*protons*) combine with an approximately equal number of neutrons to form the *nucleus*. Equal numbers of negatively charged particles (*electrons*) orbit the nucleus. This is the situation in a stable atom, and is a common occurrence.

However, occasionally in nature there exist forms of a particular element where the numbers of the individual particles are not so well-balanced and the atom is unstable. This form of specified matter is called an *isotope*. The unstable atom attempts to change its structure and in doing so emits high-energy particles in such a way as to work towards a stable configuration. This change or disintegration is called *radioactive decay* (Iwamoto, 1994).

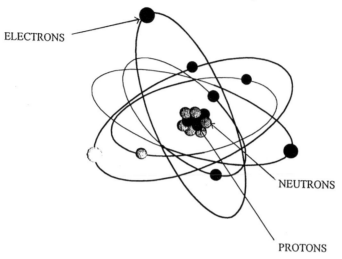

ELECTRONS

NEUTRONS

PROTONS

Figure 20.1: A stable atomic structure

The high-energy particles that are discarded from the unstable configuration within the atom carry their energy with them when they leave the atom. This movement of energy is called *radiation*. Thus, the presence of such an unstable combination of particles in certain elements indicates that the elements are radioactive due to the by-products given off whilst they are decaying.

The radioactivity emitted by these elements can be manifested in a number of forms, commonly, electrons travelling at high speed, or electromagnetic radiation waves, such as gamma rays. This radiation energy is the destructive force used clinically in radiotherapy to damage or destroy diseased cells.

Waves of electromagnetic radiation (wave energy)

As previously noted, radiation is the transference of energy from one point to another. In one of its commonest forms it is thought to move in a wave-like fashion. This is not unlike the energy movement witnessed on a cardiac monitor that visually represents the electrical energy moving across the heart. Waves of energy can be of varying size, and the distance between one point on a wave and its identical position on the wave following is called the *wavelength* (Figure 20.2). Wavelength can be short, and therefore the frequency or number of waves per unit of time is greater, or it may be long, and slower in frequency. The greater the number of waves passing through a distance per unit of time, the greater the amount of energy that is passing through that space.

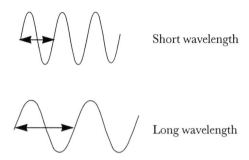

Short wavelength

Long wavelength

Figure 20.2: Short and long wavelengths

A form of electromagnetic wave energy that is extremely familiar is light. Light is made up of radiation energy waves of lots of different lengths, some short, some long, that bundle together to become visible light. Separately, however, they are all different types of radiation wave energy and cover a wide spectrum of wavelengths. The longer wavelength (and therefore lower energy waves) are the infra-red and radio waves. The spectrum continues right through visible light to its other end, where the waves are of the shortest length, the highest frequency and therefore the greatest energy. These are called X-rays and gamma rays. X-rays and gamma rays have energies ranging from a few thousand volts (kilovolts, kV) to several million volts (megavolts, MeV). Energy of this form moves in bundles and a bundle of X-radiation is described as a *photon*. The greater the energy of a photon, the greater its penetration into tissue (Iwamoto, 1994). This is a characteristic that is very important to utilise when planning clinical treatment, as tumour targets are obviously at different depths beneath the skin surface in each individual. Conversely, particulate radiation (i.e. streams of high-speed electrons) can penetrate the skin but have a sharp cut-off point thereafter and so deliver their radiation superficially without reaching structures immediately beneath the cut-off point. Another important characteristic of this energy is that its intensity decreases disproportionately as it travels away from its source (Hilderley, 1992a, b). As a consequence, the distance the radiation beam must travel to its target must be carefully calculated to ensure the required radiation intensity reaches the tumour bed.

Artificial Production of Radiation for Clinical Use

Radiation is often described as either gamma radiation or X-radiation. Gamma radiation is extremely similar to X-radiation in behaviour but it is produced from a different source. X-rays were first discovered by Roentgen in 1895 when he was conducting an experiment applying a high voltage across a discharge tube and moving electrons through a vacuum. Today, X-rays are produced by firing high-speed electrons at a target of densely packed atoms, i.e. matter with a high atomic number, or heavy atoms, such as tungsten. Some of the energy of the fast-moving electrons is converted into waves of energy of the X-ray form, the residue is turned into heat. As a result, all machines that produce X-rays must have effective cooling systems. The actual energy content of the X-ray formed depends on the magnitude of the original voltage and the exact atomic nature of the heavy metal used as the target. In summary, the higher the kV the greater the X-ray energy. The machine used in such production is called a linear accelerator.

Conversely, radiation can be used directly from a decaying isotope. This radiation is concentrated by holding a large quantity of radioactive material in specially constructed machinery that is able to direct the energy as needed. Gamma rays are produced as radioactive isotopes decay and so are a natural by-product of this breakdown of matter.

There are many naturally occurring sources of radioactive elements, such as uranium or radium, but for convenience and safety radiotherapy departments use radiation energy produced artificially, however, they use the same principles as natural atomic decay. Non-radioactive substances or elements are used and their nuclei are destabilised on purpose, resulting in radioactive material. In modern radiotherapy units radium is rarely used. Common radioactive elements artificially produced are the radioactive forms of cobalt (Co) and caesium (Cs) (Co^{60} and Cs^{137}). Caesium produces gamma rays of relatively low energy levels compared to Cobalt which is able to produce gamma rays of very high energy, known as *megavoltage radiation*.

With all materials, the quantity of radioactive atom reduces with time. A term referred to as *half life* or $T^{1/2}$ is used to determine how much radioactivity has decayed. The half life is the time it will take for the intensity of the energy released to decrease to half its original amount (Table 20.1) and is different for each element.

Table 20.1: Half life for some of the more common radioactive materials used in radiotherapy

Radioactive isotope	Half life $(T^{1}/_{2})$
Caesium ^{137}	30 years
Cobalt ^{60}	5.3 years
Gold ^{198}	2.7 days
Iodine ^{131}	8.1 days
Iridium ^{192}	74 days
Strontium ^{85}	64 days
Radium ^{226}	1620 years
Technetium ^{99}	6 hours
Yttrium ^{90}	64.2 hours

Source: Ball and Moore (1980)

This information has implications for the handling, storage and replacement of such materials in a radiotherapy department. All radiotherapy units or oncology wards where radioactive isotopes are used must implement policies that are based on the current Ionising Radiation Regulations (Statutory Instrument Nos 1333 & 778) and Department of Health guidelines on the handling and storage of radioactive matter (Department of Health, 1985a, b).

Radiotherapy departments use a special machine to contain the radioactive material and allow the controlled emission of the radiation beam, i.e. a Cobalt unit. These machines are used in rooms constructed with thick concrete walls.

Due to some of the complex demands of storing such materials safely, and the need to continually replenish stocks, many departments now depend primarily on non-radioactive machines, *linear accelerators*. These machines are able to produce high-energy photons and, if needed, electrons artificially without a radioactive source. Photons, as described earlier, are bundles of short wavelength high-energy wave radiation. Like the high-energy gamma radiation from a Cobalt machine, this radiation can penetrate deeply into the tissue before delivering its full dose.

Until the mid-1980s the radiation unit dose for radiotherapy was the *rad*. However, the international unit of dose is now referred to as a *Gray* (Gy) or one-hundredth of a Gy, the *Centigray* (cGy). One cGy is equal to one rad. The dosages recorded in current clinical trials for childhood tumours are recorded in Gys or cGys, and such standard-isation allows effects from varying dosages to be compared. This is evident in the research to investigate the late effects on cognitive development of children treated with 24 Gy of cranial radiation compared to 18 Gy in children with acute lymphoblastic leukaemia (Moore et al., 1991). The unit of a dose in radioactive isotopes is the *becquerel* (Bq) and refers to the number of disintegrations per second that the element undergoes (Kun & Moulder, 1993).

Effect of Ionising Radiation on Human Tissue

The use of radiation therapy to treat disease began within a year or two of the discovery of the X-ray (Hall, 1986). Radiation was found to destroy the ability of cancer cells to reproduce; this is one of the most disruptive characteristics of such cells, i.e. to continue repro-ducing irrespective of bodily need. Radiation therapy is therefore an extremely useful weapon. This constant tumour growth causes the most significant damage to the body and to impede this process is the most successful way to halt the disease process. Many cells are actu-ally damaged by the X-rays when they cause cell matter to lose essential particles from their molecular structure, i.e. direct ionisa-tion, the loss of orbiting electrons from an atom. The most important method of cell destruction is the ionisation of water where, following radiation interaction, water molecules disassociate and produce hydrogen ions and destructive hydroxyl radicals. These unstable oxygen radicals significantly damage the nucleus of the cell by caus-ing breaks in the DNA. There is almost immediate cell death if the chromosomal damage is irreparable as the cells cannot then form their essential proteins. However, many cells survive this initial onslaught, as the damage at first does not appear to be excessive, but the delayed effect is fatal, as the cell is unable to divide successfully at mitosis (Hilderley, 1992a, b).

In some circumstances, cells become what is often described as *giant cells*, as a result of exposure to sub-lethal doses of radiation. These cells can function satisfactorily initially but cannot divide and although the effect is therefore not seen for some considerable length of time they eventually degenerate and die.

There are cells within the body that are more sensitive to the effects of ionising radiation and these are termed *radiosensitive*. Table 20.2 identifies some of the many factors which contribute to the extent of radiosensitivity a cell might express.

Table 20.2: Factors contributing to cell radiosensitivity
Type of cell
• Phase of the cell cycle the cell is in;   those cells that are resting and not actively producing DNA for cell division are less susceptible to the fatal effects of radiation   • Rate of division of the cell type;   tissues made up of cells that divide more rapidly are likely to have more cells in the dividing phase of their cell cycle and therefore are more radiosensitive, e.g. bone marrow, mucosa of gastrointestinal lining   • Degree of differentiation of the cell type;   poorly differentiated cells are more radiosensitive   • Oxygenation;   the greater the oxygen content of a cell, the more molecules there are to be converted into free radicals which are influential in promoting cell death
Source: Tiffany (1979)

Hazards to Healthy Tissue During Radiotherapy

Non-cancerous cells can be injured by radiation, just as they often are with the use of chemotherapy. However, one of the guiding principles of radiotherapy is to keep the death/damage rate of healthy tissue to a minimum, and so reduce adverse side effects on the body. It is to the body's advantage that healthy non-cancerous cells are able to repair their chromosomal tissue after ionisation far more effectively than malignant cells. Therapy is therefore aimed at the cell death of cancerous tissue with the minimal repairable damage to healthy tissue. Unfortunately, even healthy tissue can only tolerate so much radiation injury without complications, despite the ability to self-repair (Hilderley, 1992a, b).

As previously described, all forms of therapeutic radiation, waves or particles, produce their biological effect by ionisation of important intracellular macromolecules. Damage to DNA directly or through the utilisation of free radicals is most often the case. The adverse effects of such an onslaught on the cell structure and function are delayed in slower-dividing cells (i.e. organ tissue) and radiation injury can actually be repaired over as little as four to six hours in healthy tissue. Consequently, radiotherapy that is given in small frequent doses has a less damaging effect than a single large dose.

This allows the same total dose to be given to the tumour, but by dividing it into fractions, healthy tissue is allowed to survive the whole procedure. The process of breaking up therapeutic radiation into smaller doses, given daily over six to eight weeks, is called *fractionation* (Neal & Hoskin, 1994). In most centres doses are only given Monday to Friday on these regimes to allow patients some extra recovery time each weekend.

Fractionated radiation must be planned to facilitate a favourable therapeutic ratio that allows an efficient repair of sub-lethal radiation damage in healthy tissue compared to an efficient level of death in tumour cells (Steel & Wheldon, 1992). Even when tumour cell death is not immediate, with such small fractions sub-lethal damage eventually accumulates in tumour cells causing overall tumour reduction. Factors which influence the therapeutic ratio are as follows:

- Radiation dosage per fraction
- Total dose of radiotherapy given
- Total treatment time
  (Hilderley, 1992a, b).

Factors which influence the therapeutic ratio are manipulated by experimentation to minimise long and short term toxicity and to maximise local tumour control, based on the tumour type and the tolerance of the tissues surrounding it.

Trials of multiple small daily doses of radiation are based on the knowledge that the ability to repair sub-lethal damage is greater in non-dividing cells (slow-growing healthy tissue) than in rapidly dividing cells (tumour cells, bone marrow, gastrointestinal mucosa and skin). Thus, smaller fractions given over a shorter period, arguably result in more cumulative damage to tumour tissue (Hilderley, 1992a, b). This is of proven benefit in total body irradiation (TBI) (Storb, 1989), but not as yet in the treatment of brain tumours where it had been hoped this would make some considerable difference in reducing treatment neural toxicity (Skowronska-Gardas, 1994).

Chapter 21
Administration of radiotherapy

Monica Hopkins

Introduction

There are three main routes by which radiation can be delivered to tumour cells:

- Externally, in a beam produced by a source external to the body *(teletherapy)*
- Internally, by a radioactive source that has been implanted surgically *(brachytherapy)*
- By attaching a radioactive isotope to a metabolite or even an antigen-specific antibody *(unsealed source)*.

Teletherapy

By far the most common method of delivery is external beam therapy or teletherapy. A beam of radiation energy is produced either in particulate or wave form depending on the machinery chosen. It is then focused for accuracy of target, depth and radiation intensity at a predetermined field of tissue, marked upon the skin. The energy contained within the beam is such that it causes the maximum degree of ionisation in tissues beneath the skin. At this point the radiation energy intensity is such that it is possible for it to be absorbed by the tissue, and so begin ionisation. This ensures minimal skin and superficial tissue damage when the target is, in fact, a deep-seated tumour. However, should skin or superficial tissue be the target the intensity of radiation is altered accordingly, to a level that can be absorbed as soon as it reaches the skin. This may be done by positioning or by placing a barrier between the skin and the machine to decrease the intensity of the beam at that particular site and allow the radiation to act on the identified tissues. This barrier may be made of wax or a similarly dense material (Hilderley, 1992a, b).

The delivery of the external beam needs to be planned in every detail to ensure maximum cell kill of diseased tissue and minimum damage to surrounding areas. For these reasons dose, intensity, direction of beam and target area must be absolutely accurate. Significant time must be spent on planning and ensuring that each fractionated dose enters the tissue with exactly the same accuracy. Hence, positioning, marking and immobility of a child's body are vitally important.

Treatment planning

Integration of radiotherapy into multimodality treatment requires a basic understanding of radiation planning, the influence of fractionation on tumour death and normal cell recovery, and the effect on the body of radiotherapy, including its effects when combined with surgery and chemotherapy.

Treatment planning involves making a number of different decisions on an individual basis. Firstly, there must be accurate tumour imaging to outline the treatment field so that measurements can be collated to calculate the most appropriate form of radiotherapy. The shape and angle of beam (e.g. anterior–posterior, lateral, oblique, rotating arcs) must be ascertained. Secondly, the dose of radiation energy required to reduce or obliterate the tumour load must be determined. This second consideration should be guided primarily by a designated protocol for the child's age and the histology of the tumour, but also by clinical assessment. Thirdly, the type of radiotherapy must be identified; X-rays, gamma rays or particulate radiation will deliver differing voltages, remembering that the energy of the radiotherapy must reflect the depth of penetration required. Kilovoltage (kV) radiation, which is primarily produced from X-rays, has the lowest voltage and is used to treat very superficial lesions. It will, however, deliver significant doses to the skin. Orthovoltage radiation, which can either be in the form of X-rays or gamma rays, has deeper penetration but does deliver quite high doses to the skin and is particularly well absorbed by bone. Megavoltage radiation can be either gamma rays, electrons or photons and allows the deepest penetration. Linear accelerators and Cobalt units are capable of emitting megavoltage radiation (Hilderley, 1992a, b).

The volume of tissue to be treated consists of the tumour plus an area of healthy tissue around it. These clean margins must be identified to account for microscopic tumour extension. There are other considerations to be made, however, before the final area is identified: limitations of imaging investigation, characteristics of the movement and scatter of the form of radiation being used, and slight daily changes in body positioning, might all increase the risk of missing the tumour if they have not been properly considered. Depending on the histology of the tumour, adjacent or regional lymph nodes may also be included in the tissue volume to be treated.

When planning the shape and angle of the beam of radiation it is vital that these factors are simulated with a diagnostic radiographic machine equipped with a fluoroscopic unit. These machines simulate the path of the beam of radiation, but for more complex situations a specialised CT scanner simulation may also be utilised.

The form and energy level of radiotherapy determines the depth of tissue penetration possible and how the radiation will distribute itself throughout the tissues. All of this information is then entered into a computer to be simulated on the CT image.

The planning process can be complicated when a child has had surgery or chemotherapy prior to radiation. In these cases it is often difficult to identify the true position and volume of the original tumour bed and so determine possible areas of microscopic residual disease. To compensate for this possible margin of error, an area larger than that originally identified from the scan may need to be irradiated. For this reason collaboration between surgeons and radio-oncologists before surgery is vital.

After the target tissue volume is set and the field to be irradiated has been identified, thought needs to be given to the total dose of radiation and the number of fractions into which it should be divided, although these considerations may already have been dealt with in a national treatment protocol. There is a considerable effort to be made in balancing the positive and negative effects of prolonging treatment by dividing doses (Cosset et al., 1994).

The larger the dose per fractionation, and the larger the total dose in a shorter period of time, the more significant the risk of late effects, such as fibrosis or necrosis (Thames et al., 1982). These forms of tissue damage are caused by insufficient cell repair between each dose fraction, thereby allowing significant cell damage to occur in healthy tissue (Mandell et al., 1986/87). In addition, fractionation in prolonging total treatment time not only promotes healthy tissue repair but also allows for re-oxygenation of hypoxic tumour tissue, and therefore increases its radiosensitivity (Steel & Wheldon, 1992). This can be useful where the tumour has a hypoxic centre due to its large size outstripping the blood supply. The outer margins of the mass are destroyed by earlier fractions allowing the more resistant central cells to become better oxygenated and therefore more radiosensitive (Steel & Wheldon, 1992). Protracted courses of small doses of radiation may actually allow tumour re-growth, as it does in healthy tissue, because malignant cells have also been allowed time to repair.

Maintaining accuracy of treatment

Once the beams have been planned it is necessary to take steps to ensure that the angles of the beam can be maintained throughout therapy. Radiation energy decreases as it travels over a given distance, obeying the inverse square law: the intensity of radiation at a distance from a point source is inversely proportional to the square of the distance from the source (Hassey-Dow, 1992). This phenomenon must be taken into account when positioning a child for therapy. The actual decrease in energy follows a uniform path, i.e. it is possible by simple calculation, using its energy intensity at source and the distance it is travelling, to calculate the intensity of the radiation at a given point away from the source. This is important for clinical use, as the distance the child is from the radiation source has implications for the intensity of the radiation or dose to which the child's tissue will be exposed. As the dose must be accurately replicated daily, identical body positioning is maintained for, and during each dose. For critical accuracy, such as when treating the brain or head and neck tumours, a shell is made for each individual to immobilise their head. This shell must be an exact fit for each child, so that even the smallest movements are restricted to prevent alterations in the treatment field.

The making of this shell is called mould room preparation. As part of this preparation a cast of the appropriate area is taken using plaster of Paris, which moulds itself to take on an exact shape of the area to be treated (mould rooms in different hospitals may use other techniques and materials to make a cast, therefore the nurse must confirm the exact procedure prior to preparing the child). This dries quickly, taking less than one minute, and is filled with plaster to form a reproduction of the area. The plaster reproduction is then used to make a perspex shell which can be fitted over the area to be treated on the child prior to each treatment fraction. The perspex shell is then checked for comfort and accuracy of fit. Once the shell is deemed to fit well, the rough edges are filed and markings for alignment can then be made. The shell can be clipped to the same position on the table to give pinpoint accuracy for each dose of treatment. The precise treatment field is replicated for each treatment fraction by immobilising the child between the shell and the table.

A shell is not always required. In the treatment of many peripheral areas the radiographers will align the treatment field by means of laser lights on the radiotherapy machine (Hilderley, 1992a, b). This alignment is then checked by anterior and posterior pointers. Radiotherapy only takes a few minutes but much time is often spent beforehand in positioning the child so that the treatment can be given to the exact area required.

The final stage of the planning process, prior to commencement of treatment, is often carried out on a diagnostic X-ray machine, called a *simulator*, which is structured to mimic the geometry of the treatment machine. The simulator uses diagnostic rather than therapeutic doses of radiation to simulate the treatment field in terms of size, shape, angle and volume. The radiographs obtained from this procedure are used to demonstrate adequate coverage of tumour volume and the reproducibility of the treatment field. In order to obtain a satisfactory treatment plan it may be necessary to simulate between two and four treatment fields, approaching the tumour from different positions. Families often worry that during such a delay in starting treatment the tumour may be progressing, therefore constant support and reassurance must be undertaken by the named nurse in preparing the family for these procedures, and full explanations should be given as to their necessity and benefit. The child and the family should be allowed to voice their concerns over delay in treatment but they should be reassured that this period has been anticipated within the treatment plan.

In order that the machinery may be aligned accurately, markings are made around the target treatment field; these are not easily removed. The child's position must then be held throughout the dose of radiation. If a shell is to be used for treatment, the marks will be placed on this. If no shell is required, the child will have the ink marks drawn on to their skin, to define the exact treatment field. This is referred to as *marking up* and special marker pens are used by the radiographers to do this. The marks must remain in place for the duration of treatment. In the event of fading, the radiographers may need to re-draw the lines. The marks should not be washed off during the course of the treatment.

> **Nursing note:**
>
> **Should the marks start to fade whilst on weekend leave, the family should be asked to redraw over the marks with a felt tip pen, which must be a different colour to the one used by the radiographers, so that they can distinguish between the two.**

Planning determines the area to be treated but also those tissues that require extra protection from therapy. Shielding devices may sometimes be used to protect these tissues. These devices are usually made of lead or lead alloy, as this is one of the few materials that can be used to protect healthy surrounding organs and tissues from unnecessary exposure. The lead alloy shapes are 'made to measure' by the mould room staff to the exact measurements of planning images. Body part moulds may incorporate shielding devices as well as wax strips to ensure that a body area or particular tissue mass is protected from irradiation exposure, when positioning precludes its removal from the irradiated field.

Alternatively, lead blocks can be fitted on to the radiotherapy machinery. These may either be regularly shaped pieces of lead, or moulded blocks of lead alloy, mounted on a template, that are placed directly in front of the beam so that a small piece of lead can shield a significant area of tissue.

Parents often voice their concerns and fears that their child will be 'radioactive' after receiving radiotherapy treatment, and fear that their child's skin, clothing, urine and stools may be contaminated following treatment. They may also worry that the treated child may be a danger to other members of the family. During preparation for treatment, it is therefore important to reinforce that the child is not radioactive at any time, and no radiation safety precautions are necessary following teletherapy treatment. Precautions are only required when direct sources are used, such as brachytherapy or [131]ImIBG (metaiodobenzylguanidine) treatment.

Nursing care issues

When considering these issues it can be seen that the true effectiveness of radiotherapy lies in the accuracy of the planning. Nursing care of the child whilst undergoing this experience is critical to ensure that planning is accurate and successful in its goals but also that the child is able to cooperate through understanding and awareness rather than fear and insecurity. The family obviously plays a major part in helping the child to feel safe and protected whilst preparing for therapy. For this experience to be positive and not cause psychological disturbance, the child and the family need to be well-informed of every stage and of its significance. At the same time, they should be involved as partners, planning how best to deal with each experience. It is therefore imperative that nurses have a clear understanding of the planning process itself, in order to be able to prepare the child and family as effectively as possible. Iwamoto (1994) outlines the main teaching priorities in preparing a family for external beam therapy:

- A step-by-step route through all the events that will lead up to treatment, e.g. planning and simulation, moulds and shielding devices, daily treatment schedules, ongoing evaluation through therapy, access to advice and support, follow-up and assessment
- Time factors; length of time in planning, daily visit and treatment, length of course
- The radiotherapy environment, the unit, mould room, treatment room and machinery
- Specific effects and side effects
- What happens, why it happens, when it will happen and how long it will last
- Reassurance must be given that the child is not radioactive
- Explanation of what measures the child and family can take to minimise or even prevent side effects
- Discussion of possible delayed or late effects and the resources available for care, support and advice
- Provision and nature of follow up for the child and family.

These guidelines were developed for the care of adult patients but form a useful framework for use with children. However, the format and educational strategies utilised in dealing with children and their families may need to be tailored to suit individuals. Written information is helpful and there must be time to answer questions. Children require visual and sensory information to understand what is to happen, however, the cognitive ability to utilise abstract information about an unknown subject is not developed until mid-adolescence. Therefore, photographs, models, touching and examining machinery at close quarters, walking around a radiotherapy suite and playing with mould room materials are all vital components of an effective teaching plan.

Play preparation for radiotherapy in children, therefore, is often based upon the concept of *desensitisation* (Slifer et al., 1994) founded upon established methods of reducing children's anxiety

(Warzak et al., 1991) and teaching behavioural control through operant conditioning (Slifer et al., 1993). Desensitisation is a behavioural therapy technique used for decreasing fear and/or anxiety about an identified object or situation (Slifer et al., 1994). The child who is to undergo radiotherapy requires desensitisation to the equipment, staff and routine of planning and treatment prior to its commencement. Children who are too young to be able to identify the source of their fears respond to those of their parents and family, and feel the sense of impending separation. Children can be supported significantly by involving the parents in the desensitisation process (Lew & La Valley, 1995). Desensitisation includes step-by-step rehearsals of the stages of planning and treatment, firstly through experiential play and model equipment and then through exploration of the actual radiotherapy suite. Constant positive reinforcement each time the child manages to touch, hold, manipulate and practise with equipment or a routine is absolutely essential (Slifer et al., 1994). After desensitisation children can go on to learn motion control, again through keeping still for photographs for longer and longer periods, with the use of constant positive feedback (Cooper et al., 1987), gradually resulting in an ability to tolerate therapy without sedation. The role of the play specialist cannot be underestimated in this situation, he or she is perfectly placed to coordinate and lead a team approach to meeting these preparatory needs. The play specialist is highly skilled in strategies and current techniques in play preparation and has the necessary knowledge of development and resources to create a preparation plan to suit any individual. It may also be possible for the play specialist to devote time and experience to accompanying certain children on their first visits to the radiotherapy suite for planning and treatment, until the child and radiotherapy staff have become familiar with each other.

Nursing note:

In preparing the child and the family for planning and therapy, it is essential that the child understands that he will be alone in the machine room for the duration of the treatment fraction. However, this is a short period of time and the child will be observed constantly by staff and the family on a video monitor, and can communicate through the intercom. Favourite toys or blankets may be comforting at these times, in addition to soothing music or an audio story. However, honesty and information often are the most useful ways to decrease the child's fear and anxiety.

Should preparation be unsuccessful due to the child's age, developmental immaturity or extreme psychological distress, then the child can be sedated or even anaesthetised with a short-acting medication, such as ketamine (Edge & Morgan, 1977) or an appropriate alternative under the care of a paediatric anaesthetist. However, the aim of nursing interventions is to avoid this wherever and whenever possible. Bucholtz (1992) and Oski et al. (1990) point out possible concerns about the use of sedation in treating children. Firstly, it is possible that sedation may disrupt a child's daily activity, growth and development. Secondly, it is difficult to guarantee that sedation will always be successful and for how long. Timing sedation to coincide with a tightly timed radiotherapy slot can be problematic and, if unsuccessful, another course of action needs to be considered. It is a significant nursing challenge to negotiate appropriate sedation, time its administration and monitor the child for physical response before, during and after therapy (Bucholtz, 1992). Halperin et al. (1989) suggest that each child should be thoroughly assessed before considering sedation or anaesthesia. Age, developmental level, physical state, previous experience of therapy and anxiety levels should all be taken into account. The ultimate goal is to prevent the child from moving while in the radiotherapy suite but this must be balanced against the possible trauma to the child and the fact that children require close monitoring throughout. Should anaesthesia prove necessary, an anaesthetist must be present to monitor the child. Even when children have been considered suitable for sedation, it is always important to ensure that they are assessed daily for contraindications such as respiratory dysfunction, infection and altered states of consciousness.

It must also be remembered that all children in this country are treated in units that predominantly care for large numbers of adult patients and they have very busy schedules worked around the speed with which adults can be prepared and treated. Children and their required preparation take up an enormous amount of time in these busy departments. The need for sedation or anaesthesia places considerable strain on the department for the extra time and resources to accommodate such a child within a room. If the child is sedated then accuracy of timing cannot be guaranteed and the room may be left waiting for a child that is not quite sedated enough. If anaesthesia is required then extra staff and resources are necessary to prepare, monitor and recover the child in safety. Improved play preparation not only reduces the necessity for sedation and anaesthesia but also means that the child can be helped to cooperate with treatment to such an extent that the radiotherapy rooms are not left unused for large portions of the day whilst staff attempt to assist a child who is experiencing distress and difficulty in maintaining a position for treatment.

Brachytherapy

The use of this method of delivering radiation is quite rare in children, but can often be useful where the employment of surgery or external beam radiotherapy may have devastating consequences for the surrounding tissue. Radioactive material can be placed either interstitially, intracavitarily within an applicator, or placed permanently within selected tissue. Significant local control and fewer late effects make this form of therapy advantageous in paediatrics (Fontanesi et al., 1994). Sealed sources may be used in conjunction with any of the other treatment modalities or on their own. Small quantities of the radioactive forms of caesium (Cs^{137}) or iridium (Ir^{192}) are used. They are housed in a small carriage or applicator and are made to measure for the specific cavity by mould room technicians. To ensure a perfect fit the mould may need to be formed within the cavity with the child possibly under sedation. It therefore follows that preparation by experienced nursing staff is essential for all concerned.

Once it contains the radioactive source, the mould is inserted and perhaps stitched into place under a general anaesthetic. It remains in position for up to 96 hours, and although it is at a much lower dose of energy than even the intravenous materials discussed below, the principles of protective care for both forms of administration are the same.

Nursing care issues

The risk to staff and the family in caring for the child with a sealed radiation source depends upon the dose rate emitted by the source at any given time. Dose rate is the rate at which ionising radiation is delivered to the tissues from its source, and is dependent on the rate of decay of the source (Hassey-Dow, 1992). In many cases the radiation will not penetrate more than the depth of the tissue in which it has been placed and the child should not emit any radiation. However, this is not always the case. This situation should, therefore, always be discussed in advance with the radiation protection adviser within the hospital and care planned accordingly. Should the radiation from the source extend beyond the body, the child should be nursed alone in a cubicle with their own washing and toilet facilities. Nurses and the family should limit contact with the child to approximately 30 minutes per day until the radiation protection officer indicates otherwise or the source is removed.

Information on the care of children in this situation is as that described for the child with an unsealed radiation source.

If the child has had a sealed radiation source placed within a cavity with an external orifice, care must be taken to ensure it is not dislodged. Should this situation occur the source should be retrieved with long-handled forceps and placed in a lead container (Maguire, 1993).

Use of Unsealed Sources (Intravenous Radioactive Materials)

[131]ImIBG (metaiodobenzylguanidine) is a radioactive material currently being retrialled in the UK for the treatment of neuroblastoma Stage 4. Hoefnagel et al. (1994) treated 31 children in this manner with the aim of decreasing the tumour volume to improve the chances of an adequate resection. The idea is to avoid excessive drug therapy which is associated with toxic effects and may induce resistance.

This material contains a specific radioactive isotope of iodine. It is made artificially and then bound to a synthetic form of a chemical called guanethidine that neuroblastoma cells absorb constantly (Plowman & Pinkerton, 1992). Neuroblastoma and other adrenal gland tumours take up [131]ImIBG in a similar way to the transport of noradrenaline in these cells. This affinity for a radioactive chemical allows radiation to be taken directly to tumour cells without damaging surrounding healthy tissue (Gelfand, 1993). The true nature of the success of this form of treatment as a curative measure is yet to be fully proven, as clinical trials are still only at the pilot stage. The radioactive chemical is given intravenously under severely protective conditions and, consequently, patent venous access to prevent extravasation is imperative. Before, during and after administration of this radioactive material, iodine must be given orally. This will prevent uptake of the radioactive form by the thyroid gland, which would lead to its destruction. Saturation of the thyroid gland with non-radioactive iodine is imperative to deflect disastrous long term effects (UKCCSG, 1995). The main acute effect seen in these children is thrombocytopenia (Guerra et al., 1990).

Nursing care issues

As the drug is given intravenously all body tissues become radioactive, and the only exit for this material is through excretion. Therefore, all bodily fluids must be handled as radioactive waste and disposed of in the cubicle (Maguire, 1993). Special facilities are required for the administration of such therapy as the child becomes radioactive and those caring for him as well as other visitors require protection. Visiting should be restricted to adults only and no pregnant women should attend. Nurses and the family should limit contact with the child to approximately 30 minutes per day.

Facilities that allow constant supervision of the child whilst maintaining minimal physical contact are essential. In addition, facilities must allow for all the child's needs to be met within the room as nothing may leave the room until the radioactivity has decreased when isotope decay and excretion occur. As far as possible all material objects required for the duration of the child's stay in the room should be disposable.

During infusion (which lasts approximately 30 minutes to one hour) and for the first four hours afterwards, the child must be monitored closely for signs of an allergic reaction to the radioactive agent. This may necessitate frequent monitoring of vital physical signs, as often as every five minutes. For the safety of the nursing staff the child should be monitored electronically for pulse, respiration and blood pressure, so that the results may be displayed on a monitor outside the room; this would preclude the necessity of continuous direct contact with the child for the first few hours after infusion.

The child will need to be isolated from the family for approximately 10–14 days after the infusion, due to the radioactive emissions from all body tissues. The exact length of stay is dependent on the readings of the emissions assessed daily. When the emissions have decreased considerably the child may leave isolation and return home. Unfortunately, in some cases it may still be some days after this before the child can be in the same building as other children. Siblings may need to be sent to relatives and friends until the radiation protection adviser has released the child. Discharge occurring when the child has been measured at or below 30 Bq for a family with young children at home, or 150 mega bequerels (mBq) if the child is returning to an environment of adults only. Professional contact whilst the child is in isolation, therefore, must also be kept to a maximum of 30 minutes in 24 hours per staff member. This time limit will increase as emissions decrease. Staff that do have contact with the child during this period must carry a radioactivity monitoring device to calculate cumulative doses over the set number of days. It follows from this data that all bodily fluids or matter lost by the child must be carefully collected and disposed of, in keeping with government guidelines on the disposal of radioactive waste (Department of Heath, 1985b) and the ionising radiation regulations (Department of Health, 1985a). These guidelines are actioned by the radiation protection adviser (Gibbs, 1991) within a given institution.

Given the need for such minimal staff contact only the immediate physical needs of the child can be attended to, although they should be monitored visually throughout this period, preferably by use of closed circuit television. This situation would obviously be intolerable for a small anxious child therefore it is often necessary to sedate such children for the entire period of isolation.

Oral sedation is the route of choice for this situation. It is necessary to introduce a nasogastric tube to allow access for topping up the sedation. This port can also be used for the administration of diet and fluids, as well as for the non-radioactive iodine necessary for uptake by the thyroid gland. Administration of ^{131}ImIBG may cause considerable feelings of nausea and at times vomiting may ensue; this vomit is potentially very dangerous radioactive material and in the sedated child there is also the risk of aspiration. It is recommended that thought be given to the administration of effective anti-emetic cover during the first 2–3 days.

The room in which the child is nursed should be designed for the use of radioactive materials and, indeed, some pilot sites have had such a room specially constructed with protective walls. Where this is not the case the child must be nursed in an isolated cubicle with a barrier marked out on the floor around all four sides of the room. This barrier should be placed at a measured distance, confirmed as a safe limit for such radioactive decay by the radiation protection adviser. All health personnel not caring for the child, other patients and their families, should remain behind this barrier at all times. This is not entirely satisfactory and can cause some considerable disruption on a unit.

A Geiger counter should be kept within the designated cubicle to monitor the emissions from the treated child. Their decrease in magnitude must be recorded accurately and, indeed, all items of equipment and materials required in the child's care must be assessed before disposal or removal from the room once treatment has commenced. All this equipment may be anxiety-provoking for both the child and the family; it is therefore essential that the family be prepared for these measures with clear and accurate information and ongoing support and advice throughout the treatment.

Nursing note:

The parents and members of the child's family find the separation and possible sedation of the child extremely distressing. It can be anxiety-provoking to think of one's own child being so dangerously radioactive that such extreme safety measures are needed. As a consequence, nursing care must respond to the need for information, reassurance and support throughout this difficult time. Encouraging the parents to make up feeds or fluids, choose clothing or advise on positioning for the sedated child promotes a sense of protection. For the child who is awake during this time, telephone and video links are invaluable. Choosing games or videos, and preparing favourite foods also help to maintain caring contact, essential to the child and the parents or siblings.

Administration of Alternative Radiotherapy Techniques

Stereotactic radiation

Stereotactic radiotherapy merges stereotactic surgery with conventional fractionated radiotherapy (Lew & LaValley, 1995). This method of radiation delivery is utilised when a small intracranial area of cancerous tissue requires radiotherapy. It allows the delivery of maximum tumourcidal doses of radiation whilst limiting the damaging dose to surrounding tissue. A three-dimensional approach is taken to locate and fix the target for therapy and, indeed, for the guidance of therapy (Dunbar & Loeffler, 1994). A stereotactic frame is constructed to the exact measurements of the child's skull. It does not require surgical fixation to the skull as it is constructed with a fixed bite block so that when this is in the correct position within the mouth all other points are identically located on the skull. This frame is used to guide an external beam of radiation to the precise point of the disease. The frame should be non-invasive, relocatable and immobilising to assure accurate reproducible positioning throughout planning and treatment (Kooy, 1993). The radiotherapy is then given in fractionated doses to attain the most effective tumour control with minimal late effects (Sheline et al., 1980). In the case of stereotactic radiosurgery, often referred to as the 'gamma knife', a large dose of Cobalt^{60} radiation is given in a single fraction. The dosage is usually sufficiently high to cause immediate cell death to the targeted tumour bed, almost mirroring radical surgical removal (Kooy, 1993).

According to Lew and LaValley (1995), the role of stereotactic radiotherapy in malignant brain tumours is strengthened by the possible avoidance of certain long term sequelae of cranial irradiation.

Total body irradiation in the treatment of leukaemia

As leukaemic cells are well-oxygenated and highly proliferative, they are extremely radiosensitive. However, they are difficult to locate and identify for therapy. Total body irradiation (TBI) is a procedure in which the entire body is exposed at one time to gamma radiation (Dreifke & DeMeyer, 1992).

The goals of TBI are to eradicate the leukaemic cell count, in addition to immunosuppressing the child so that they can receive a donor marrow without mounting an immune response. In summary, the goals of TBI are:

- To attain sufficient immunosuppression to allow engraftment of a foreign donor marrow for allogeneic bone marrow transplant
- To remove or reduce residual disease
- To provide sufficient space for the new donor marrow to grow (Silverman & Goldberg, 1996).

This removal of the child's immune system and circulating leukaemic cells involves giving a homogeneous dose of radiation to all body tissues. The radiation given is of a lower dose and intensity than a beam directed at a localised area (Iwamoto, 1994). The dose is usually within the 8–14 Gy range (depending on fractionation), although it can be given as a single dose. This does, however, cause far more side effects.

This form of preparation for transplant was first attempted in 1925, although the concept had first been discussed almost 20 years earlier (Dudjak, 1992). Until 1979 most regimes of TBI were single-fraction (Dudjak, 1992), fractionated doses were then introduced in an attempt to decrease late-onset toxicity without adverse effect on efficacy (Goolden et al., 1983). It was then found that fractionation worked more efficiently even when given in very small doses (Storb, 1989). The total dose given is sufficient to be lethal to the bone marrow tissue. Stem cells within the marrow are destroyed and so regrowth is impeded. A hyper-fractionated regime (twice daily) is followed over three to five days to allow healthy tissue throughout the body to repair itself. Complex calculations need to be made to ensure effective yet safe doses are given equally throughout the varied tissues of the body. Positioning of the child may need to be altered during a fractionated dose to facilitate this. A lower dose of radiation is aimed at the lungs to offset unnecessary fibrosis; this is accomplished by using the arms as a shield for each lung or use shields made from pieces of radiation-blocking material.

TBI can only be carried out with the child positioned quite some considerable distance from the radiation source, so as to ensure small doses are given accurately to all sections of the body. Although small doses are recommended when treating the whole body, care must be taken as too low a dose rate can allow only sub-lethal damage to occur. This may result in leukaemic cells surviving TBI, as well as the child's own immune system, which could then attack the donor marrow. In contrast, too high a dose rate can cause irreversible organ damage, for example, to the tissue of the lungs. Positioning is therefore an extremely important variable in TBI. It can be manipulated to control the energy of the beam when it enters the child, the homogeneity of the dose and the protection of critical organs. Dose rate fractions and treatment distance also vary considerably. However, Dudjak (1992) outlines some more common elements from the literature:

- The regime usually lasts 3–4 days, often on a hyper-fractionated or twice-daily schedule
- It is a small daily dose of 1.5–2 Gy split between the two fractions
- Children and adolescents should lie on their side, turning half-way through each fraction to maintain homogeneity.

This form of conditioning regime can cause many acute and chronic side effects, many more than a chemotherapy only regime, and therefore these children require intensive preparation and support throughout their treatment. Although TBI is given in fractionated doses to reduce some of these toxicities, they may still cause considerable problems to children treated in this manner. The possible side effects of TBI are summarised in Table 21.1.

Locatelli et al. (1993) highlight that the majority of late effects from bone marrow transplant are due to this conditioning regime, although hypothyroidism is usually only seen with single-fraction doses. Cataracts (Calissendorff et al., 1991), lachrymal gland dysfunction and endocrine dysfunction are particularly worrying side effects which may account for the interest in alternative conditioning regimes over the years.

Table 21.1: Possible side effects of TBI

System	Side effect	Time from TBI to symptoms
Gastrointestinal	Nausea and vomiting	Immediately to 24 hours
	Stomatitis	Within a few days
	Diarrhoea	Immediately to a few days
	Loss of appetite	Immediately to a few days
	Pain or swelling in salivary glands	Immediately to 24 hours
	Dry mouth	Immediately to a few days
	Thick saliva	Immediately to a few days
Skin	Redness	Within a few hours
	Itching/tingling	Within a few hours
	Darkening of skin	2–3 weeks
	Hair loss (all of body)	7–10 days
Reproductive	Sterility	Immediately
	Premature menopausal symptoms	Months to years
Miscellaneous	Cataracts	1.5–5 years
	Fatigue	Sudden or gradual
	Fever	Within a few hours
	Bone marrow failure	7–10 days
	Abnormal growth	Months to years

Source: Dreifke & DeMeyer (1993)

Radioactive isotopes bound to tumour-specific antibodies

This is a relatively new and extremely experimental form of radiation therapy. Antibodies are identified that are specific to the surface antigens being presented on the tumour cell surface. These are then bound to radioactive particles of relatively low energy and given intravenously to the patient. This is an extremely complicated procedure as tumour antigens must be identified, monoclonal or polyclonal antibodies must then be developed and produced in sufficient quantities (usually in mice or rabbits), and then they must be successfully combined with a radioactive source. Although the radioactive load in this therapy is much lower than [131]ImIBG therapy, protective care of the children involved should follow the same government guidelines until their emitted radioactivity is below safe contact levels. This timeframe will depend entirely on the half life of the radioactive isotope attached to the antibody (Coons, 1995).

This technique has been used for some time to image the tumour more clearly and define the tumour volume more accurately, but its use as a viable treatment option in paediatric tumours is still in its infancy. Pizer et al. (1991) carried out a pilot study to investigate both the toxicity and therapeutic effect of intrathecal radiolabelled monoclonal antibodies for the treatment of children with ALL that had seeded into the meninges. Using I^{131} (Iodine), the radioactive antibodies were given via a lumbar puncture or directly into an Omaya reservoir. Temporary remission was achieved in five of the six children. The main side effects experienced by these children were headache, nausea and vomiting and some transient myelosuppression. The initial three symptoms were absent after three days.

Plowman and Pinkerton (1992) also report some degree of response in craniopharingiomas using radioactive Yttrium (Yttrium^{90}), administered directly into the cystic mass to attack the secretory epithelium. Unfortunately, nursing care for these children and their families has not been published to date, therefore care must be negotiated with the radiation protection officer.

Chapter 22
Tumours and radiotherapy treatment

Monica Hopkins

Brain Tumours

The main radiosensitive brain tumours are:

- Germ cell tumour
- Glioma
- Ependymoma
- Pinealblastoma
- Medulloblastoma
- Primitive neuroectodermal tumour
- Astrocytoma
- Craniopharyngioma.

Tumours that are considered low-grade, and where at least 95% of the mass can be removed, may in some instances require no further therapy. These children will be followed up closely by imaging surveillance and clinical examination. Where the tumour is high-grade or anaplastic and fast-growing, it is considered malignant and always requires further therapy after surgery (Shiminski-Maher & Wisoff, 1995).

In the last decade the use of chemotherapy in addition to, or even replacing, the more traditional radiotherapy has increased greatly the hope of increasing the survival rate of these children (Shiminski-Maher, 1990; Wisoff & Epstein, 1994). The status of benign or malignant does not always equate with survival in brain tumours (Shiminski-Maher, 1993) and so often causes confusion in children and their parents; individual tumour growth, position and clinical consequences must be explained when discussing the possible future morbidity and prognosis, with the family.

Some tumours, such as the germ cell tumours, brain stem gliomas, PNETs and medulloblastomas are currently being researched in clinical trials to estimate the efficacy of radiotherapy in their treatment. For all tumours, the decision on the most appropriate therapy must be made on radiobiological data. The decision to treat the neoplasm by use of radiotherapy alone, is usually reserved for tumours that do not metastasise outside the brain or seed the CSF. Combined modality of chemotherapy and radiotherapy may be efficacious in these cases.

Tumours with potential for neuroaxis spread or already metastasises at diagnosis

The constant debate within the research field about the treatment of such tumours concerns the relative efficacy of craniospinal radiotherapy alone compared with localised radiotherapy with adjuvant chemotherapy. Combined-modality therapy is a significantly more prolonged regime and will require many visits to the radiotherapy centre. This has social and financial implications for the family and emotional implications for the child.

In recent years chemotherapy for these tumours has included extremely myelosuppressive regimes which often precede local radiotherapy. Therefore there may possibly be delays to radiotherapy schedules whilst bone marrow recovery is observed, especially if the child has an infection.

Future developments in this field include the use of stereotactic radiotherapy and targeted radiotherapy using monoclonal antibodies (Pizer et al., 1991).

Adverse Effects of Radiotherapy in the Treatment of Brain Tumours

Localised radiation to the brain may cause significant morbidity to surrounding tissue. The immediate acute side effects of this form of radiotherapy are documented in Table 23.1 (see Chapter 23).

As a result of these problems, the parents and the child will require honest informative preparation to allow them to feel that they have made an active informed decision. The acute symptoms may be extremely distressing, in addition to the experience of therapy every day. The nursing role is undoubtedly one of preparation and support throughout therapy. In addition, it is imperative that there is sensitive assessment for alterations in neurological status, discomfort due to pain, fatigue or nausea, fear and anxiety, and altered nutritional status. Diligent skin care must be performed at the entry site and daily assessment of tissue viability made.

Nursing note:

In some treatment protocols up to three fields will be irradiated together, it is therefore essential to monitor children closely for any evidence of skin injury, especially if the fields have overlapped at any time. The occurrence of such overlap may precipitate small areas of skin erythema or even desquamation, as well as that which may arise from the point of the localised beam to the tumour bed. It must also be a priority to observe the child's original surgical wound site for signs of tissue damage. Radiotherapy to the brain requires the use of immobilisation devices, i.e. wearing a mask or mould; some children may even need to lie in a prone position for access to the spinal fields. These positions and immobilisation devices may cause distress and anxiety in some children and their preparation should reflect such an awareness. Should sedation prove unavoidable, it must be highlighted that radiotherapy schedules may be quite prolonged and it may prove problematic to sedate the child every day; short-acting anaesthesia must be a consideration.

Finally, the somnolence often associated with radiation to the cranial region may make it necessary to re-assess the child's need for sedation, at approximately three weeks into treatment.

Acute Lymphoblastic Leukaemia with CNS Involvement

Craniospinal radiation can precipitate a wide variety of acute adverse effects, these are summarised in Table 23.1 (see Chapter 23).

Tumours of the Head and Neck

Post-nasal space and parameningeal sites of soft tissue sarcomas (including rhabdomyosarcomas), require irradiation to the head and neck regions which presents a host of nursing challenges due to the severe acute side effects observed with these treatments. Hyperfractionated doses of radiation to the head and neck may be utilised in some children, therefore sedation or perhaps anaesthesia may become necessary twice a day. Health professionals must endeavour to minimise this wherever possible through play preparation, although this may be difficult in the young child with parameningeal disease.

Nursing note:

Children presenting with established CNS disease are rare and those with high white cell counts are often transferred to a high-risk protocol with the possibility of transplant. Therefore it may be that very few nurses will care for a child with ALL who requires craniospinal radiation. When this does occur the family is often extremely vulnerable as they are aware that they have been placed in a poorer prognosis grouping, i.e. a high white cell count or established progressive disease. They have also learned that their child could potentially suffer many more late effects than any other child with leukaemia. Paediatric nurses caring for the child and the family must ensure that the interdisciplinary plan of care that they coordinate reflects the needs of the whole family. Craniospinal radiotherapy may result in many unpleasant immediate effects, including stomatitis, myelosuppression and some degree of somnolence. This combination of effects can cause the child to be severely compromised nutritionally and to suffer considerable discomfort as it is often difficult to assess oral cavity status and the need for pain relief in a somnolent child. Nursing care should reflect this awareness in child and family preparation, and in oral cavity care.

The possibility of a prolonged treatment period in children with Stage 4 mesenchymal disease may also lead to an increased risk of mucosal and skin breakdown if sufficient respite is not allowed for these tissues to repair themselves. There must be a break in therapy if larger doses of radiation are planned.

Radiotherapy treatment of post-nasal space tumours may cause considerable mucosal damage within the nasal passages, buccal cavity and pharynx. Tissue breakdown here, as well as causing discomfort and pain, may be a significant cause of systemic infection. The salivary glands may also be damaged and therefore unable to produce saliva for lubrication, host defence and preliminary digestion. An aspect of care which may be overlooked is that of nutritional status. Prolonged radiotherapy to this area plus the time that recovery of such an area requires, may cause the child's nutritional status to be compromised for some time. Many children have their nutritional requirements met nasogastrically throughout radiotherapy treatment but this may be difficult with nasopharyngeal tumours. There is therefore increasing interest and exploration into the use of percutaneous gastrostomies.

Tumours of the Eye

Weiss et al. (1994) identified that radiation therapy played an important role in the control of multifocal tumours and tumours situated near the optic nerve or macula. In the treatment of retinoblastoma the two goals of inclusion of the entire retina in the beam and protection of the lens have always represented a challenge to the radiation oncologist. Early external beam radiotherapy treated the whole eye, which had the advantage of treating the whole retina and vitreous humour without involving the other eye in a significant dose, thereby enabling each eye to be treated independently. In recent years, the advent of the lens-sparing technique of radiotherapy enabled the whole retina to be treated without irreparable damage to the retina so maintaining useful vision (Hungerford et al., 1995).

Education for the child and the family includes good skin care. Discussion about late effects must include information about possible bone deformities and muscle changes around the orbit.

As chemotherapy for retinoblastoma has become so successful, fewer children are receiving radiotherapy.

T-cell Non-Hodgkin's Lymphoma

Radiotherapy is utilised in three sites in the treatment of this malignancy: the cranium, testes and mediastinum. Cranial irradiation is employed in the treatment of this neoplasm for those children who present with evidence of CNS disease or disease in the CSF. In the case of an isolated testicular relapse, the child or adolescent can receive radiotherapy locally to the scrotum, testes and spermatic cords up to the inguinal ring. Children who are found to have residual mediastinal disease, as proven by biopsy, receive radiotherapy to the area with all fields treated daily.

Hodgkin's Lymphoma

Radiotherapy is confined in its use to Stage 1 of this childhood malignancy, and for recurrence of disease in more advanced stages. Radiotherapy is administered bilaterally to the nodal region to ensure symmetry of tissue growth. The most common area of treatment is to the cervical and submandibular nodes, although other regions may be irradiated depending on the position of the primary disease or recurrence.

Where disease is situated in the cervical or mandibular regions, radiotherapy fields must be planned with care to minimise adverse reactions. The mandibles and clavicles are shielded where possible to prevent serious growth retardation in these bones which, in turn, leads to severe deformity and body image difficulties. Thyroid function is an area of concern after associated radiotherapy field treatment and must be monitored. There are no criteria for the routine use of radiotherapy to treat mediastinal masses in these children in any of the protocols used at present.

Nursing note:

The possible adverse effects of radiotherapy to the cervical region and pharyngeal area have been highlighted elsewhere. However, skin changes which may cause discoloration following erythema, in conjunction with weight loss due to nutritional deficits may result in significant alterations to a teenager's body image; these must be addressed in an ongoing and supportive manner. It is also imperative, in view of possible thyroid dysfunction, that investigation of hormonal function is carried out regularly and that the family is kept informed of the significance of such results. Thyroxine replacement therapy should be instituted promptly, if required, as it is essential for continued growth and development. Teenagers are one of the main age groups affected with this particular malignancy and their preparation needs may be different from younger children but no less demanding. These young men and women may already have established views on the advantages and disadvantages of nuclear radiation, as well as many concerns about bodily insult and the effects on the hormonal system so important to their burgeoning sexuality.

Radiotherapy for Abdominal Tumours

This field of treatment is often used for the irradition of hepatoblastoma, Wilms' tumour and neuroblastoma. Full abdominal radiation is almost unheard of in the treatment of children. Flank radiotherapy is a more commonly desired field.

When caring for children undergoing therapy for these forms of cancer there will be a considerable number of very young children undergoing radiotherapy. There is therefore a need for effective preparation to elicit some degree of cooperation and, more importantly, to decrease fear and anxiety.

Malignant mesenchymal tumours such as rhabdomyosarcoma

For treatment purposes children with mesenchymal tumours are often assessed on the extent of their disease, the position of the tumour and histology. They are then placed in one of three risk groups: low, medium or high. In general, children with low-risk disease are not randomised to receive radiotherapy, whereas children with high-risk non-metastatic disease require localised therapy. The most common tumours in this group treated in paediatric units are rhabdomyosarcomas and these are treated on a number of different protocols, depending on their site, stage and histological subtype. Non-rhabdoid tumours are treated on the basis of their histology, chemosensitivity and post-surgical stage.

Nursing note:

Decisions about radiotherapy may be taken following rigorous periods of chemotherapy, surgery and anxiety-provoking re-assessment scans. Preparation for radiotherapy must be sensitive to the fact that the child and the family may have recently received information that there remains residual disease after initial therapy, and they may therefore be extremely distressed. Radiotherapy, post-surgery, requires acute nursing observation for (and a research-based response to) possible tissue injury at the wound site.

Radiotherapy is offered as a treatment option for many children with tumours of Stage 4 classification. Treatment may be extensive and a short rest may be needed during the treatment episode to allow for mucosal regeneration at any point along the gastro-intestinal tract. In situations where the child has metastatic disease, both primary and metastatic sites, these can be treated simultaneously. Treating multiple sites highlights the need for pro-active care to minimise side effects. This must be discussed thoroughly with the family at treatment planning and be considered by nursing staff when they are observing the child for adverse responses.

Wilms' tumour

In the child with Stage 3 disease, radiotherapy may be given to the flank of the body in dosages and fractions dependent on the histology. Tumours found to have favourable histology receive about a 30% lower dose than those with unfavourable histology. Treatment fields will extend medially to include the full width of the spinal column to ensure symmetrical growth retardation in this area. In the case of lung metastases, radiotherapy is also included for disease containment. The lungs can be irradiated from the apex to T11/T12.

As children are given chemotherapy in addition to radiotherapy, it must be considered that drugs such as dactinomycin and doxorubicin may enhance skin and lung injury in some children.

> **Nursing note:**
>
> Although the spinal column is always included in the radiation field to ensure symmetry of growth, unilateral exposure of ribs and flank muscles can cause some degree of atrophy on the affected side. This, in turn, presents the child with the potential for quite severe body image difficulties later in life. The family of such a child must be informed of this risk so that they can prepare their child in later life. Lung irradiation, with its attendant morbidity, must be fully explained to the parents and the child so that their experiences post-radiotherapy will not leave them feeling bewildered at the degree of morbidity the child may experience.

Neuroblastoma

In the treatment of neuroblastoma all three modalities of therapy may be utilised. Because of this, wound healing and skin care require consideration, depending on the sequencing of events and the time between surgery and radiotherapy.

> **Nursing note:**
>
> Pre- and post-operative care of the child who has recently received radiotherapy presents challenges for the promotion of tissue viability. The surrounding skin may be excessively dry or even broken so pro-active skin care must be undertaken prior to surgery to ensure that the skin is unbroken and there is no evidence of dry desquamation. Planning, using CT scans and radiation simulators takes time and patience with young children, especially when this planning may have to begin very soon after surgery in order to begin treatment on schedule. Finally, residual tumour plus associated nodes and a 2 cm margin may constitute a fairly large area to be treated. This extensive field may include vital structures, especially bone, with attendant growth failure risks. The family should receive all possible information before treatment so that active participation in long term decisions can be maintained.

Systemic radiotherapy for neuroblastoma Stage 4

A current protocol (commenced in 1995) is aimed at testing the efficacy of using a radioactive isotope in a therapeutic manner as first-line treatment prior to conventional chemotherapy in children with advanced disease. There are a number of criteria for inclusion to the study:

- The children must have mIBG positive disease
- They must also have skeletal disease detected by bone scan
- Their GFR must be at least 50 ml/min/1.73 m^2 in order to clear the isotope effectively

  Myelosuppression is the main criterion for dose-limiting toxicity.

Pelvic irradiation

Rhabdomyosarcoma and other soft tissue sarcomas may also be found in the lower abdomen and pelvis. Irradiation of this area of the body results in many acute and distressing side effects (see Table 23.1). Localised tissue changes may produce pain and disruption to elimination of faecal matter and urine if the area includes the bladder or the bowel. The parents and the child should be fully aware of potential problems that may arise after such therapy, although they may not occur in all children. This will serve to reduce anxiety and distress should symptoms present. The parents should have sufficient knowledge to recognise symptoms at home during and after treatment so that they can contact the unit and not become distressed at the thought that the symptoms may be due to advancing disease.

Nursing note:

Extensive radiotherapy to the pelvic area may lead to particular problems in maintaining skin integrity due to the difficulty in keeping clothing loose and reducing shearing forces in undergarments. In addition, areas of irradiated skin may rub against one another as the child moves, causing pain and further skin trauma. This discomfort may discourage the child from moving about and so decrease their self-care abilities. Older children and teenagers may find the position of the radiation injury a source of considerable embarrassment when skin integrity assessment is carried out by nursing staff or when extensive skin care interventions are necessary. This embarrassment may lead to a reluctance to permit observation and so skin care may not be instigated as appropriately as necessary. Careful discussion and negotiation must be undertaken by nursing staff with the child, to determine levels of observation and physical contact that are both psychologically comfortable for the child, and appropriate for the safe maintainance of skin integrity and prevention of tissue breakdown.

Extremity Radiation

These areas are commonly used for bone tumours and rhabdomyosarcomas of skeletal muscle. Associated acute effects are relatively less distressing than in many other radiation fields (see Table 23.1), but may cause restrictions in activities that may have social implications.

Nursing note:

All children who receive radiotherapy to their limbs must be protected from unnecessary trauma to the bone until the tissue is healed. This means that health education about avoiding traumatic contact that may damage the bone must be stressed, for example, some sports or social interests. It may also be the case that the child undergoes surgery either before or after radiotherapy; tissue viability must be a primary concern in these situations.

Chapter 23
Acute and subacute side effects of radiotherapy

Monica Hopkins, Jane Pownall and Linda Scott

Introduction

The dose of radiotherapy is limited by normal tissue toxicity (Emami et al., 1991). The aim of treatment is to deliver a therapeutic dose of radiation to tumour cells whilst sparing healthy tissues. In order to be pro-active in preventing unnecessary trauma, it is essential to understand how different tissues within the body react to radiation. The reactions to radiation in healthy tissues can be described as *acute* (occurring during or immediately after therapy), *subacute* (3–6 months after therapy) and *late* (more than 6 months after therapy) (Kun & Moulder, 1993).

Healthy tissues can be divided into two types for the purposes of anticipating reactions to ionising radiation. There are those which proliferate rapidly, for example skin, gut, bone marrow and hair follicles. These are known as acute reacting tissues. Then there are tissues that proliferate slowly, if at all, and these include lungs, brain and kidneys. These tissues express radiation damage at a later stage. In each case cellular injury occurs by the same process but is not expressed until the cell attempts division. The severity of damage is influenced by a number of factors:

- The treatment field
- Radiation fraction interval
- Dose per radiation fraction
- Duration of treatment
- Radiosensitivity of the tissue

433

Table 23.1: Acute side effects of radiotherapy

Site of radiotherapy	Tumour group	Side effect	Nursing care
Brain	CNS prophylaxis for ALL Brain tumours (astrocytoma, glioma, craniopharyngioma) Brain metastases	Cranial-meningeal irritation Nausea and vomiting Headache Skin sensitivity Alopecia Somnolence Fatigue Cerebral oedema	Assess for symptoms of meningitis and neurological dysfunction Pain control Antiemetic cover and possible need for i.v. fluids Skin care teaching Preparation for somnolence Encourage rest and adequate nutrition Monitor for signs of raised intracranial pressure Preparation for alopecia
Spinal	Medulloblastoma Primitive neuroectodermal tumour (PNET) CNS prophylaxis for ALL	Nausea and vomiting Headache Alopecia Fatigue Somnolence Tracheal irritation Oesophagitis Myelosuppression Skin sensitivity	Antiemetic cover Pain control and rest Monitor blood counts — assess for signs of infection, anaemia and bleeding Pain control and fluids for oesophagitis Skin care teaching and nutritional advice

(contd)

Table 23.1: (contd)

Site of radiotherapy	Tumour group	Side effect	Nursing care
Head and neck	Nasopharyngeal sarcomas Parameningeal mesenchymal tumours Hodgkin's disease	Skin — chemotherapy recall reactions Mucositis Orbital inflammation Taste alteration Xerostomia Oesophagitis	Rigorous oral assessment and mouth care Clean nares with warm water and saline nose drops Soft, non-irritant foods, encourage fluids Pain control and saline eye care Baseline dental and ENT assessments Skin care teaching
Eye	Retinoblastoma	Conjunctivitis Skin sensitivity Reduced tear production Minimal alopecia	Saline eye care Skin care as per protocol Artificial tears Preparation for hair loss
Chest	Neuroblastoma Lymphoma Pulmonary metastases PNET	Pneumonitis Myelosuppression Oesophagitis	Monitor respiratory status closely Soft diet and encourage fluids Pain control Monitor for signs of bone marrow suppression Infection control education Nutritional assessment

(contd)

Table 23.1: (contd)

Site of radiotherapy	Tumour group	Side effect	Nursing care
Abdomen (including para-aortic nodal fields)	Hepatoblastoma Neuroblastoma Wilms' tumour Rhabdomyosarcoma Soft tissue sarcomas PNET	Abdominal cramping Nausea and vomiting Diarrhoea Myelosuppression Skin sensitivity Infertility — girls Mucositis Anorexia	Pain control in addition to antispasmodics and antidiarrhoeals Antiemetic cover Oral assessment and mouth care Monitor blood counts and administer blood product support Nutritional support — low-residue diet Skin care education Possible oöphoropexy for girls Personal assessment and care
Pelvis	PNET Rhabdomyosarcoma	Infertility Abdominal cramping Diarrhoea Cystitis Mucositis Proctitis Alopecia Skin recall reactions	Counselling prior to therapy re sexuality and fertility Antispasmodics and antidiarrhoeal medication Nutritional support and encourage fluids Monitor gastro/urinary discomfort and monitor for signs of infection — pain control Topical pain relief for anal discomfort Skin assessment and prompt skin care Personal hygiene education

(contd)

Table 23.1: (contd)

Site of radiotherapy	Tumour group	Side effect	Nursing care
Extremities	Ewing's sarcoma Rhabdomyosarcoma	Functional limitation Skin recall reactions Increased susceptibility to fracture	Monitor skin condition and treat appropriately Loose comfortable clothing, passive exercises with physiotherapy supervision Health education on avoidance of trauma

- Type of machine and energy of the radiation
  (Kun & Moulder, 1993; Dunne-Daly, 1994).

In contrast, subacute and late reactions depend on time, dose factors and total dose (Kun & Moulder, 1993).

Acute Reactions in Healthy Tissue

Both healthy and malignant cells attempt to repair themselves within three to four hours after exposure to radiation (Hilderley, 1992a, b). However, malignant cells are far less effective in their attempt to recover (Hilderley, 1992a, b). Healthy tissues which proliferate rapidly, unfortunately, can still sustain damage which though often repairable does temporarily affect function. The more proliferative tissues, such as skin, gastrointestinal mucosa, bone marrow, and hair follicles, will demonstrate the adverse effects of radiation quite rapidly, usually during the course of treatment. In addition, some of the less proliferative tissues in the body express acute trauma when directly targeted in radiotherapy. Acute reacting tissues may, as a result of their injury, proceed to demonstrate chronic and long term dysfunction.

Skin

It takes approximately two to three weeks for cells in the epidermis to complete their life cycle. Skin reactions therefore often begin around this time, following the commencement of radiotherapy, and continue for a similar period of time after completion of treatment. Clinical signs that may be observed are:

- *Initial redness or erythema.* This is usually seen within seven days of the onset of radiotherapy. The characteristic redness is due to dilation of the capillaries in response to radiation damage (Lawton & Twoomey, 1991). As erythema progresses, increased vascularity and obstruction of the capillaries develops.
- *Dry desquamation.* This is caused when there is cell death in the upper layers of skin. The decreased ability of the epidermis basal cells to replace the surface cells leads to desquamation. The sweat and sebaceous glands are also damaged and are dysfunctional, causing extreme dryness (Dunne-Daly, 1994). This often begins approximately 2–4 weeks after therapy commences.
- *Moist desquamation.* This clinical presentation is seen as doses approach the limits of skin tolerance. Moist desquamation is a result of extreme damage to the epidermis allowing the dermis to

be exposed and serous fluid to leak from the tissue (Lawton & Twoomey, 1991). The area is now at risk of infection and, in cases of widespread damage, fluid loss (McDonald, 1992). This is a potentially serious situation that may even lead to a break in therapy to allow the tissue to heal.

At the end of treatment the remaining basal cells will repopulate the tissue. However, if the tolerance dose has been exceeded, the basal cells will have been killed, resulting in ulceration (McDonald, 1992) and possibly leading to tissue necrosis (Barkham, 1993).

Adverse reactions to radiotherapy in healthy tissue are often graded as to their severity as part of an overall toleration assessment. Grading is normally based on how severely the radiotherapy damage affects quality of life. There are few recognised tools or assessment frameworks for acute reactions, except in stomatitis, which are co-used in the assessment of chemotherapy effects (Dudjak, 1987). In the past, the use of varied systems for recording integumentary system damage were confusing as they often combined different manifestations of injury in the same tissue. Sittom (1992) maintains that adherence to skin management regimes, as well as innate individual differences may account for varying skin responses to radiotherapy. Campbell and Lane (1996) maintain that as skin cannot repair itself until radiotherapy is completed, nursing care must focus upon the relief of discomfort and the promotion of a good healing environment. At all times the priority should be to minimise the injury caused to the skin by prevention of the excessive dryness that follows erythema, as this can lead to skin breakdown. Doing so prevents further trauma and, at the same time, treating the skin gently at all times decreases friction and erosion of epidermal cells. It should also be stressed that no skin agent other than moisturisers should be used on wounds unless a substantial case can be made as to its contribution to wound healing.

Nursing care varies around the country and yet practice needs to be confirmed through research (Barkham, 1993). A survey by Barkham (1993) of 42 radiotherapy units in the UK revealed a remarkable variety of practices for radiotherapy-induced skin trauma. There was evidence of confusion over identification of the levels of skin injury. Topical agents ranged from simple moisturisers to steroid preparations, zinc oxide cream, powders and silicon compounds and myriad dressings were utilised in practice with little rationale as to the choice of each.

The literature in the UK has little to offer in terms of research-based interventions, but examination of practice and wound care research from other areas of practice has contributed to a growing knowledge base. Core principles now seem to be consistent in many commentaries on radiotherapy care. The aim of care should be to relieve discomfort and symptoms until radiotherapy has taken its full effect. In this way, nurses are able to prevent further trauma and infection and so promote healing after therapy is complete. These core principles have been brought together in a skin care policy developed by Campbell and Lane (1996) (Table 23.2).

Table 23.2: Cookridge Hospital skin care policy

General practice guidelines
  Information and advice given to patients will be consistent and follow the practice guidelines, irrespective of who is giving the advice

General advice
  All patients receiving radical radiotherapy to superficial tissues will receive moisturising or aqueous cream to be applied at least twice daily to their treatment area from the start of treatment; the frequency may be increased as the skin becomes drier
  Rationale: to ensure that the skin is in optimum condition during radiotherapy treatment and to avoid dry desquamation

Hygiene
  All patients must be given advice about washing the skin during treatment. The treatment area can be washed carefully according to the patient's wishes. Stress that the skin should be patted not rubbed dry. If the patient has marks which need to be preserved, this must be explained. Patients may still wash with their usual soap and water, unless this stings, in which case they should be advised to use a milder brand of soap. Hair can be washed gently according to the patient's usual regime, using the usual shampoo, even if it is within the treatment field. For patients who have treatment marks on the scalp, hair washing should be discussed on an individual basis. An electric razor should be suggested if the patient wishes to continue shaving an area within the treatment field
  Rationale: to enhance individual feelings of well-being and overall quality of life; to prevent increased irritation of the epithelium and the build-up of bacteria; to avoid physical trauma to the skin causing exaggerated skin reactions

Clothing
  Clothing covering the treatment field should not cause a shearing force (e.g. bras and belts)
  Rationale: to prevent friction and trauma in the treatment area caused by tight-fitting garments which may increase the damage to the skin

Special guidelines for radiation-damaged skin
  All patients should be assessed individually by a nurse who will select the most appropriate dressing

(contd)

Table 23.2: (contd)
Special guidelines for radiation-damaged skin (contd) **Pruritus:** For patients with intractable pruritus, 1% hydrocortisone can be used twice daily; it should be used sparingly after the moisturiser **Erythema:** Continue to apply the moisturising cream generously as frequently as the patient wishes until the skin returns to its normal state **Moist desquamation:** For slightly exuding moist desquamation continue to use moisturising cream and cover with a non-adherent dressing; other dressings to consider are jelonet, with a non-adherent dressing, or granuflex **Heavy exuding wounds:** Dress with allevyn and change only when 'strike through' occurs; no creams should be used with this dressing *Rationale:* Allevyn is a highly absorbent, hydrophilic foam pad which can provide an optimum healing environment
Source: Campbell & Lane (1996)

A formal assessment tool for assessing skin integrity before instigating care is not yet available in the UK literature. However, from work undertaken in the USA and the preliminary commentary on experience by specialist nurses in this country, recommendations for assessment methodology can be proposed. Issues to consider in daily skin observation are:

- The total radiation field must be fully described and identified on the child's care plan. It is imperative that the nurse caring for the child is fully aware of the treatment angles in order to be cognisant of the exact treatment field. It is possible to have a significant skin reaction at the exit site of the treatment field, therefore this area also requires close observation.
- Preventative measures should be instigated from the day of treatment to keep the affected area of skin well moisturised.
- Daily assessment should be made in conjunction with the child and the family for the presence and severity of erythema, moisture level of skin, and evidence of breaks in skin integrity. It must be remembered that radiation skin injury is cumulative and will extend for some weeks after therapy ends.
- All areas of erythema and desquamation must be documented and preferably drawn, with accurate dimensions, in the child's assessment documentation and care plan.

- All teaching and guidance given, in addition to actual intervention, must be documented in detail and adhere to the recognised policy of the unit to prevent confusion and inconsistency of care.

Nursing note:

It is recommended that to aid consistency of approach in grading skin damage, of the four stages of tissue injury visual aids are preferable to written description alone. Clear colour photographs of each stage can promote increased staff awareness and expertise in recognition of each stage. This can only aid consistency of approach in care and family education. These photographs may be displayed in teaching rooms within the unit, or in a learning package within the treatment area for ease of referral for assessment of a child.

Once the skin area has been assessed a pro-active plan of care needs to be negotiated to assist the child in caring for their skin, and to prevent further trauma. Nurses must also be aware of the most effective measures for dealing with skin breakdown should it occur during or after therapy. The basic principles of skin care for radiotherapy injury are summarised in the policy of Campbell and Lane (1996) (Table 23.2 above). Each aspect: hygiene, moisturisation, wound healing and health promotion, is now considered in more detail.

Hygiene and general skin care

Throughout treatment and afterwards, warm rather than hot water is recommended for daily hygiene. In addition, it is advocated that rubbing the skin should be avoided, instead it should be gently patted dry with a soft towel. Rubbing the area dry will traumatise the skin, but areas left damp may encourage infection. The use of unperfumed soap and talcum powder is recommended if such products are desired by the family (Campbell & Illingworth, 1992). Perfumes should be avoided before and during radiotherapy as they can cause increased tissue sensitivity. In addition, many perfumed products contain metallic elements which can cause scattering of the radiation beams during therapy. This may increase the dose to the skin. Teenage males should be encouraged not to wet shave, as cuts on irradiated skin may be slow to heal and may be prone to infection. The same applies to females who shave their legs or pubic area (should these areas be included in the radiation field).

Preventing dehydration of the epithelium

Moisturising the skin has four main contributions to make to maintaining skin integrity (Spencer, 1988):

- Ensures that the skin has access to a large quantity of water for hydration.
- Prevents water loss by forming a barrier over the skin area.
- Provides the skin with humicants which assist its capacity to retain water and therefore increases pliability and flexibility. It also reduces the desire to scratch.
- Lubricates, and therefore reduces friction and so decreases the epidermal cells, potential for erosion.

Radiotherapy also sensitises the skin to the effects of ultraviolet radiation (Sittom, 1992), making sun exposure hazardous. When children are out in the sun it is essential that they keep the treated area covered, especially the head. If this is not possible, an unperfumed total sun block must be used. Covering skin previously exposed to radiation when in the sun is advised for at least a year after treatment but if possible this should be a life-long recommendation.

Children should be advised to wear loose cotton clothing to avoid friction and further irritation. The skin must be re-assessed on a daily basis as radiation damage to the skin is cumulative.

Care in the event of a breach of skin integrity

In the event of skin integrity not being maintained, intervention should be based upon two fundamental principles of wound care.

Firstly, a moist environment promotes wound healing (Thomas, 1990). The exudate from a clean wound contains essential nutrients and components of the immune system that are required for epithelial growth. Ensuring the wound is maintained at approximately body temperature also facilitates cell reproduction and tissue growth (Quick, 1994).

The breakdown of skin integrity during or immediately following treatment (a more significant form of moist desquamation) can be extremely difficult to treat. In these circumstances it is important to take advice from a specialist nurse not only in tissue viability but also radiotherapy. Many products that are effective in healing tissue damage not caused by radiotherapy may be contraindicated in these cases.

Secondly, a radiotherapy wound should not be treated as a burn or surgical wound. It must be nursed open and dry wherever possible. Sulcrafate has been suggested in the American literature as a topical product to prevent radiotherapy damage actually occurring to the skin on entry of the beam (Maiche et al., 1994). Sulcrafate has recognised anti-inflammatory properties, seen in its ulcer-healing application, and is also known to activate cell proliferation. Clinical trials with breast cancer patients indicate that initial radiation damage to the skin is significantly less when the product is used topically to the treatment field (Maiche et al., 1994). The healing of damaged skin is reported to be significantly enhanced with its use. Unfortunately no further research has been published to date to support these useful findings.

All dressings must be removed before each radiotherapy session, but if gentian violet paint (which has both antifungal and antibacterial properties) is used it will obviously remain on the skin during each treatment fraction. Gentian violet has been recognised in the past as one of the most useful preparations for infected wounds. In recent years, work has been published on the use of this particular preparation and its potential carcinogenic effect in mice when ingested in large quantities (Hewitt & Gaylor, 1985). It is now not recommended for prolonged use on open wounds or mucous membranes by the Department of Health (1987). However, on occasions, it may be necessary to weigh up the benefits against the risks in the treatment of a wound in a radiotherapy field. If treatment has to be withheld because of problems at the wound site, the child is placed at risk of incomplete treatment. In these rare instances, therefore, it is extremely important to use a preparation which the radiotherapist knows will work, so that therapy can continue.

Nursing note:

One per cent hydrocortisone cream appears to be a popular and, at times, effective treatment for skin erythema. However, it should only be applied once the skin becomes reddened, and within the treatment field only. If used, it should be applied sparingly, twice a day. Campbell and Lane (1996) warn that over-use of this product thins the skin, and due to its anti-inflammatory effect, inhibits healing. Aqueous cream can also be used, but this is a product best-suited to the alleviation of dryness. This not only promotes healing but also helps to reduce further trauma both from friction on dry skin and by preventing cracking. For protection from further ultraviolet damage from the sun, sun blocks advertised for infant use are often the most appropriate. In addition the wearing of T-shirts over swimwear should be recommended for a minimum of one year but ideally for life.

Around the country many different approaches are taken to the use of dressings. The policy launched at Cookridge Hospital in Leeds (Campbell & Lane, 1996) (Table 23.2) suggests beginning with non-adherent dressings such as granuflex for more severe radiotherapy injury, and progressing to allevyn (synthetic skin dressings) with heavy moist desquamation.

In addition to the physical nursing care of skin injury, the psychological consequences must also be considered. Skin injury is an outwardly visible reminder of the disease and its treatment, a constant reflection of the loss of body integrity during treatment. Children and teenagers may find this very distressing and suffer with body image difficulties at this time and thereafter. It is vitally important to generate an awareness of these difficulties with relevant personnel and seek to allow expression of feelings and emotions around this subject without platitudes and dismissals. Concerns about tissue integrity must be dealt with promptly, honestly and with appreciation of the social implications of body image to the child.

The gastrointestinal tract

The replacement time of cells in the gastrointestinal tract is approximately three to six days. Cell loss and denuding of the mucosa can, therefore, occur within a few days of starting treatment. Damage to the mucosa of the oropharynx is a significant management issue in caring for children receiving radiotherapy to the head and neck area. These treatments can have a variety of effects on the involved mucosa, from mild inflammation to ulcerated, bleeding tissues (Holmes, 1986). Semba et al. (1994) advocate that significantly more work is directed at the recognition, diagnosis and treatment of oral radiotherapy injury in patients receiving head and neck radiotherapy. There is at present no paediatric literature specifically related to this issue. In general, nursing research has focused on the child receiving chemotherapy or combined modality therapy.

Mouth

Greifzu (1990) discusses the effect of radiation on the oral cavity. Radiation stomatitis is the injury that occurs when the rate of mucosal cell death exceeds the rate of tissue repair, resulting in the mucosa becoming thin and inflamed. Stomatitis is an early sign of radiation damage and occurs within 7–14 days of the onset of treatment (Iwamoto, 1992) when the oral cavity is within the treatment field, for example when receiving craniospinal radiation. Stomatitis may last up to three weeks after the end of treatment and, in severe cases, can last for much longer after therapy completion. When receiving TBI the oral cavity will be within the treatment field and here, too, mucosal damage is significant. Zerbe et al. (1992) argue that those patients who receive TBI as part of their conditioning regime for transplant have significantly more severe stomatitis than those transplant patients who do not.

Radiation stomatitis can be a serious problem. Actively proliferating cells of the mucosa are killed and regeneration is suppressed throughout treatment. In addition, salivary glands may also be irradiated and damage can occur to such an extent that secretion of saliva is precluded. This is usually a temporary effect but can be permanent (Iwamoto, 1994). As a result of this tissue trauma, inflammation causing pain and distress is often prevalent. Erythema develops as dead mucosal cells are desloughed with cleansing, leading to mucosal tenderness, altered taste sensations and some degree of dryness (Little, 1996). As erythema increases in severity, so does the associated sensation of pain and an understandable decrease in motivation to eat, to maintain oral hygiene and even to communicate. The damage to the mucosa will continue to progress throughout the treatment period and will often appear to be most severe after the completion of therapy, at which time the slightest trauma to the mucosa will result in bleeding, ulceration and extreme pain (Holmes, 1986).

If infection of this damaged tissue can be prevented or minimised, and the child receives adequate nutrition to produce new tissue, then these acute effects will heal quickly (Little, 1996). These two conditions are pivotal nursing aims that can only be addressed if the child is pain free and is adequately supported psychologically throughout this emotionally debilitating period.

Radiotherapy for nasopharyngeal tumours presents some of the best examples of severe stomatitis in paediatric oncology. However, in the past preventitive measures have been considered to compromise local control and the decision still lies with the radiation oncologist. It has been suggested in adults that the use of mucosa-sparing blocks placed in the mid-line of the head and neck field can decrease the amount of severe toxicity experienced in the buccal cavity without compromising tumour control in these tumours (Perch et al., 1995).

Radiotherapy damage to the salivary glands is due to an alteration in their vascular supply brought about by irradiation. Ductal and acinar cells of the glands, which produce the required combination of enzymes and bactericidal serous fluid, respectively, subsequently degenerate and so salivary output is both decreased in volume and altered in composition (Little, 1996). Initially, saliva becomes more viscous and so lubrication is decreased; as the salivary gland damage progresses the mouth becomes increasingly dry so that chewing and swallowing become difficult. In addition to the acutely painful stomatitis and consequent psychological distress such symptoms can sometimes elicit it must be remembered that certain analgesics and antidepressants can also dehydrate the oral mucosa (Fox et al., 1986). Therefore, it may be necessary to increase fluid intake with these pharmacological agents.

Saliva has the function of controlling bacterial growth by the lubrication of the buccal cavity with bacteriostatic enzymes and so aids the motility of food and debris out of the cavity and into the gut (Carl, 1983). McDonald and Marino (1992) state that saliva also prevents the cavity being subjected to extremes of temperature when food and fluid are being ingested, in addition to the re-mineralisation of teeth with calcium, and the facilitation of taste by presenting the buds with particulate matter in fluid. Should saliva production be reduced, dental decay and an increased potential oral infection will ensue.

Oral candida is the most significant infective agent associated with severe stomatitis. However, other infective agents may be found if saliva production has decreased or is absent due to direct radiation damage to the salivary glands. Where this is the case, food debris adheres to the tissue surfaces by becoming trapped around teeth, and then decomposes. Tooth decay can be enhanced by this situation as well as demineralisation of the tooth enamel (Little, 1996). All these conditions can cause the breath to become foul smelling which is embarrassing and emotionally distressing for all age groups.

Knowledge of all these potential problems has assisted oncology nurses in identifying the primary objectives of mouth care for the child receiving radiotherapy to the oral cavity (Feber, 1995):

- Relief of the pain and discomfort of mucosal and salivary injury
- Removal of food debris from the teeth and oral cavity before decomposition occurs
- Facilitation of the maintenance of nutritional and fluid intake, as well as communication
- Prevention of oral infection (although some children will not be immunocompromised).

All four objectives will help to promote the rapid healing of mucosal and salivary injury whilst optimising comfort and psychological well-being. These objectives should be addressed simultaneously, and within an assessment/evaluation framework, for consistent and effective care.

Oral hygiene and the prevention of infection

The removal of food debris from the mouth is essential to prevent further tissue damage and infection. Watson (1989) proposes that a small, soft toothbrush is the essential tool for this purpose. Holmes (1991) also suggests that brushing the teeth is the most effective way of maintaining oral hygiene, but this is extremely difficult for the child when his mouth is already sore. Indeed, there is no research to clarify the possible negative effects of brushing, such as trauma and the potential for infection. Foam sticks are often used but they are not as effective at removing debris as a brush, although they are better tolerated by children and they will at least clean soft tissues (Holmes, 1991).

A meticulous mouth care regime is therefore vital for these children (Watson, 1989). Corsodyl and nystatin are two commonly used preparations for the maintenance of oral hygiene. Fluconazole may be used if the child is unable to tolerate nystatin; however, children who have received head and neck radiotherapy may not, in fact, be immunocompromised unless they are receiving adjuvant chemotherapy, therefore antifungals may not be required. Strong commercial mouthwashes are not advised as they can cause dryness and irritation (Campbell, 1987). Consequently, alternative regimes may be utilised to relieve the discomfort caused by the mucosal damage and clean the buccal cavity. Gentle syringing of water or normal saline can be used to remove food debris when stomatitis is particularly severe (Campbell, 1987). Effervescent soda water is also recommended in the literature for loosening food debris without irritating the mucosa (Little, 1996). Sodium bicarbonate mouthwashes can be extremely effective in cleansing the mouth of debris without causing distress, although no research exists to support this practice. However, Feber (1995) suggests these may be perceived as irritating by patients and so cause some distress. Sodium bicarbonate is a mild alkali and therefore has the ability to neutralise the potentially damaging acidic environment produced by bacteria in the mouth, but only when diluted correctly; if the pH becomes too alkaline, it may have adverse effects on the mucosa.

Some units use normal saline washes four-hourly as a means of removing debris from the buccal cavity and in the presence of decreased salivary output to moisten the mucosa and so decrease friction and mucosal trauma (Iwamoto, 1994). Feber (1995) argues that normal saline is non-irritating, palatable and does not cause injury to the new epithelial cells, and is therefore the solution of choice when a toothbrush is no longer tolerable (Campbell, 1987).

> **Nursing note:**
>
> **Where bicarbonate solution is utilised a solution of 8.4% is recommended for oral use. Care should be taken with the use of normal saline and sodium bicarbonate as the child may swallow them, causing thirst and even vomiting which may negate the intervention. They may also be perceived to have an unpleasant taste to some children. It may be better in some cases to use water which will be just as effective if moisture is required. Glycerine and lemon should not be used as they cause drying of the mucosa.**

Prostaglandin E_2 has been used in the treatment of radiotherapy-induced stomatitis in adults (Matejka et al., 1990). The product reportedly reduces cell breakdown by protecting the DNA in the mucosal cells. It is administered topically to reduce the risk of systemic effects and is claimed to reduce desquamation, pain and inflammation within 15 days (Coleman, 1995).

Other possibly effective products, cited only in the adult literature, are allopurinol mouthwashes (Porta et al., 1994) and topical vitamin E (Wadleigh et al., 1992). However, their mechanisms of action are unclear and their results have not been widely demonstrated.

It is a widely held tenet (Coleman, 1995; Feber 1995) that the single most important variable in the healing of mucosal damage, irrespective of the methods used, is the frequency of mouth care, resulting in improved oral hygiene. Removing food debris and moisturising the mucosal tissue are the most important issues as only then can nutritional intake have its effect on mucosal regeneration. Therefore, as radiation stomatitis becomes more severe, mouth care must increase in frequency. It is also essential that there is concomitant pain relief to facilitate this.

It is essential that children have a full dental assessment, as well as ongoing dental support, prior to head and neck radiotherapy (Bentzen & Overgaard, 1995). Radiation-induced dental decay has long been a recognised hazard of treatment to the head and neck

(Trowbridge & Carl, 1975). This is due to the increased risk of caries following treatment to this area. It is therefore important that children are told of the importance of taking great care of their teeth for the rest of their lives. Significant dental problems are caused by a combination of decreased salivary fluid, alterations in oral microflora, decreased buccal lubrication and changes in the salivary pH. Should children complain of tooth pain or report changes in tooth appearance, further consultation with a dentist should be sought immediately.

Promotion of nutritional intake

Nutrition can often pose a major problem for children and in particular for those children receiving treatment for head and neck cancers. Good nutrition is vital for cell repair and will increase the child's ability to tolerate therapy (Iwamoto, 1992). Those children who receive therapy to the head and neck region may suffer severe damage to many areas involved in the ingestion of nutritional food and drink. In addition to the damage caused, enjoyment of their food may also be compromised. The pain and discomfort of stomatitis is in addition to the damage caused to the salivary glands, the cause of mucosal dryness. This lack of fluid prevents lubrication of food, making it extremely difficult to swallow. The salivary glands may recover to an extent after completion of treatment, but it is important to inform the parents and the child that it could continue to be a problem for the rest of his life.

Alteration in taste may also be experienced, which can result in dislike of many common, and previously favourite foods, and may, in some cases, even lead to anorexia. The irradiation of the buccal cavity damages the child's taste cells, taste buds simply atrophy and die (Young, 1988). Taste sensation can be lost temporarily which decreases the child's motivation to eat. This effect can last for many months post-treatment and in some cases it is permanent (Young, 1988). The child may also experience dysphagia if the oesophagus is in the treatment field. This may mean communication is impaired, which leads to a sense of isolation and may precipitate further emotional distress.

The importance of adequate nutrition cannot be underestimated when caring for the child undergoing radiotherapy. Young (1988) points out that a balanced nutritional intake of appropriate proportions of basic food elements reduces the risk of infection and tissue breakdown, and so assists in the repair of injured tissue.

Weight should be closely monitored throughout therapy and calorie supplements should be utilised earlier rather than later. This is extremely important, as the child may be able to tolerate only water towards the end of treatment, and for about two weeks afterwards, when the mouth is at its most painful.

A diet that is visually attractive, with enticing aromas and tastes to the individual, should be a primary objective. However, food must also be nutritionally appropriate, with additional calories and protein to ensure adequate resources for cell repair. Small, frequent meals are often more acceptable to a child with a diminished appetite. The child should be allowed as much time as possible to eat meals, as discomfort, altered taste sensation and decreased salivary output may make chewing and swallowing difficult. Extra fluids should be encouraged, particularly with meals and snacks (sauces and gravies are often useful). In addition, it may be necessary to inform the child and the family that spicy and citrus foods can cause considerable pain. This may be an area of concern for the family whose daily diet contains high proportions of these ingredients, and in this case, dietetic support can be invaluable.

Where oral intake is no longer possible and the condition of the nasopharygeal mucosa does not permit nasogastric feeding there is now a new approach to enteral feeding. The use of percutaneous endoscopically guided gastrostomy tubes (PEG) in patients receiving radiation therapy to a tumour of the head and neck area is a relatively new concept that is gaining in popularity in children's units across the country. Saunders et al. (1991) report from a study of 126 adult patients that results have been very positive. The patients were able to maintain full nutritional intake throughout radiotherapy without any additional inpatient episodes for nutritional support. Only 1% of the sample experienced a localised wound infection and no other placement complications were witnessed. Flietkau et al. (1991) have also experimented with this device in patients who were quite severely nutritionally compromised prior to therapy. They suggest that nutritional status can actually be improved during therapy by the use of this gastrointestinal access. There is no paediatric literature related to this subject as yet, but individual units are attempting to use PEGs in children with nasopharyngeal tumours. Additional nursing care would include care of the entry site and prevention of infection. Education and preparation for children and their families would be required in order that the device could be used safely and effectively at home. Vigilance for signs and symptoms of wound infection would have to be maintained in hospital and at home; paediatric oncology outreach nurse specialists and community children's nurses could help to facilitate this.

Oral cavity assessment to plan effective care

Hatton-Smith (1994) argues strenuously that an oral assessment guide is vital to ensure appropriate and consistent care for patients with radiation stomatitis. Hatton-Smith (1994) also maintains that for these tools to be truly effective all staff need to raise their knowledge base about the causes and consequences of such tissue trauma. Kenny (1990) and Graham et al. (1993) have shown that the use of a consistent assessment tool resulted in improvements in nursing care and better patient education. Feber (1995) has adapted the tool used by Eilers et al. (1988) to produce a clear and easy-to-follow assessment document. This could, however, be enhanced by clear colour photographic examples of mucosal damage (Table 23.3). It is essential that as assessments progress, changes in the scores of individual categories are responded to, in addition to the overall cavity score.

Pain control

Protocols for oral pain control must be based upon a consistent oral assessment. The child's perception of their oral pain should be assessed on a regular and frequent basis alongside that of their mucosa so that appropriate analgesics can be maintained and so mouth care and nutritional intake are facilitated. Opiates are most often the drugs of choice with severe stomatitis pain. However, experience in this area has also led to the use of certain topical agents.

Nursing note:

Pain control should be dealt with promptly and where possible prophylactically, as once the child has made the link between pain and eating it is exceptionally hard to break this association. Medications should be offered which will help to soothe the pain experienced in the mouth and throat, in particular, prior to mealtimes. This should help to facilitate eating as far as possible. Mist. paracetamol is one of the most beneficial products to use (this is a preparation from the Christie Hospital in Manchester), however, children sometimes have problems because of its lack of palatability. Gels containing local anaesthetics, such as mucaine or lignocaine, can also be extremely useful (Little, 1996). Alternatives may be found within the range of soluble aspirin compounds. However, these must be used with caution in children aged under 12 years, and then never in the presence of a low platelet count. Finally, there are local anaesthetic sprays and rinses, such as Difflam, but care needs to be taken as many of these are drying to the mucosa (Fox et al., 1986). Artificial saliva sometimes helps to relieve dryness, but many children find the available preparations unpalatable.

Table 23.3: Oral assessment guide

	Nursing issues to consider
Voice	
1 = normal for child	Pain control
2 = deeper/raspy	Frequent fluids
3 = difficult/painful speech	Artificial saliva
Swallow	
1 = normal for child	Pain control
2 = painful	Frequent fluids
3 = unable to swallow	Artificial saliva
Lips	
1 = smooth, pink, moist	Lubrication ointments or soft paraffin
2 = dry/cracked	Pain control
3 = ulcerated/bleeding	
Tongue	
1 = pink, moist, papillae present	Increase frequency of mouth care
2 = coated or loss of papillae	Pain control
3 = blistered/cracked	
Mucous membranes	
1 = pink and moist	Increase frequency of mouth care
2 = reddened/coated	Suspend brushing
3 = ulceration/bleeding	
Gums	
1 = pink and firm	Cool solutions, pain control
2= oedematous/red	Suspend brushing
3 = spontaneous bleeding	
Teeth	
1 = clean, no debris	Re-assess brushing technique
2 = localised plaque/debris	Increase frequency of mouth care
3 = generalised plaque/debris	
Candida	
0 = no	Antifungal preparations should be
1 = yes	instigated
Oral cavity score	21 = very poor oral condition

Small intestine

The gastrointestinal tract has a tolerance for treatment lower than that of the skin. Abdominal discomfort and diarrhoea may therefore occur with abdominal radiotherapy as a result of a widespread inflammatory response to tissue destruction in the bowel.

Husebye et al. (1994) identified that enteropathy was a serious and acute side effect of abdominal radiotherapy that is poorly diagnosed and treated. These authors argue that in severe cases it can present with symptoms of malnutrition, poor small bowel motility or intestinal obstruction. Work by Meric et al. (1994) at the Children's Hospital of Philadelphia, has sought to prevent the problem altogether. This team has experimented with an absorbable pelvic mesh sling, to pull the small bowel out of the field of aggressive pelvic radiotherapy. They reported no significant complications in seven children; however, one child experienced a post-operative ileus, and a further child had a temporary small bowel obstruction. Although the team succeeded in preventing radiation enteritis, significant surgical care was necessary to overcome complications. Pelvic radiotherapy can also have devastating consequences for the large bowel (Sedgewick et al., 1994), and the rectum may be particularly affected. Excessive diarrhoea is often experienced, with pain on defecation and incontinence in severe cases.

Although abdominal radiation is rare in treatment for children in the UK, possible side effects must be borne in mind for the occasional situation where a paediatric oncology nurse is called upon to care for such a child. The child may be particularly weakened by side effects, and with acute enteritis, this may be enough to temporarily prevent continuation of therapy. Children require close observation throughout these episodes, as dehydration and acute electrolyte imbalances may occur very quickly. These children may be in considerable distress due to the pain associated with the inflammatory process, and may require intensive pain management with opiates. As the wall of the bowel may become ulcerated at any point, extreme care must be taken in assessing all symptoms to ensure that any breach in the bowel wall is quickly identified. Close observation of vital signs, including changes in abdominal appearance, and the loss of bowel sound, is required, in addition to the monitoring of fluid and electrolyte status. A high standard of perianal care is also needed, as profuse diarrhoea is likely to cause anal excoriation and possibly fissures, which can then become a focus for infection. If the radiation field extends to include the perianal area, as in extensive pelvic tumours, the skin may already be friable from radiation erythema and therefore even more susceptible to breakdown.

Children with profuse and often distressing diarrhoea require a low residue diet, antispasmodics and occasionally medication to thicken the stools. All stools should be observed for evidence of bleeding within the bowel from ulceration and documented accordingly. Hygiene and pain control are the primary caring objectives in addition to maintenance of homeostasis.

In the long term, such manifestations of inflammation may lead to adhesions within the pelvic or abdominal cavity and these must be considered when symptoms are prolonged.

Nausea and/or vomiting may also be induced if the lining of the stomach or brain is involved in the treatment field. The effect to either site can cause irritation of the chemoreceptor trigger zone, and so the vomiting centre, by 5HT binding to receptor sites within the vagus nerve (Pervan, 1993). In addition, raised intracranial pressure due to cerebral oedema following brain irradiation can also precipitate extreme nausea (Dunne-Daly, 1994). On assessment it may be necessary to give antiemetic medication before therapy. In children who receive spinal and/or abdominal radiotherapy, sickness can be a refractory problem. Giving a $5HT_3$ receptor antagonist half an hour prior to treatment has been found to be effective (Sullivan et al., 1992; Zoubek et al., 1993). Dexamethasone may also be added to the $5HT_3$ antagonist to enhance its effect, although this practice is not as yet research-based. Metoclopramide, which promotes gastric emptying, is often tried initially as it is effective in many cases (Priestman, 1990). TBI can cause severe nausea and vomiting, especially following emetogenic chemotherapy (Pervan, 1993), however, it has been treated to good effect with ondansetron.

Bone marrow

Normal bone marrow is essential for life, since the cells it produces are responsible for the transportation of oxygen and carbon dioxide, for homeostasis and for the maintenance of the body's defence system. This bodily system, with its rapidly proliferating cell population, is extremely radiosensitive (McDonald, 1992). Destruction of the bone marrow will therefore have significant and far-reaching effects on the whole body.

Treatment fields involving small areas of bone marrow will not have a significant effect on blood counts. Abdominal or thoracic irradiation includes 15–25% of the active bone marrow in children and therefore a drop in blood counts will be obvious. More than 25–30% of a child's active bone marrow is located in the extremities, and this then concentrates in the central bones at adolescence (Plowman, 1983). Irradiation of these sites should be considered myelosuppressive. Bone marrow failure is complete after total body doses of 5–10 Gy (Kun & Moulder, 1993). Consequently, if large areas of the bone marrow are involved in the treatment field, haematopoiesis will be affected and peripheral blood counts will need careful monitoring during and after treatment. Poor red cell production can often be sustainable without intervention for several weeks, due to the long lifespan of the red blood cell in the peripheral system (120 days). However, the radiotherapist will aim to maintain haemoglobin levels above 9 gm/l, as it is considered that therapy may not be as effective if it is given when the haemoglobin is below this level. Ionising radiation, as previously noted, is potentiated in its clinical effect by the availability of oxygen, aiding the production of free radicals to cause cell damage. Radiotherapy is far more effective if tissues are well-oxygenated. Low haemoglobin levels, therefore, can compromise the efficacy of therapy.

Since leukocytes play a major role in the body's resistance to infection, a decreased white cell count significantly increases the risk of infection. A fall in the white blood cell count can occur within the first week of radiotherapy treatment (Plowman, 1983). This is due primarily to the fact that the large marrow reserve of already differentiated cells, compensates for the initial loss of proliferating cells. In addition, white blood cells generally spend a much shorter part of their lifespan in the peripheral system. Neutropenia may then follow which leaves the child at an increased risk of systemic infection, which is no less serious than that caused by chemotherapy (Kun & Moulder, 1993). Lymphopenia occurs most frequently in patients receiving craniospinal radiotherapy or widespread nodal therapy (Kun & Moulder, 1993), due to a large area of the marrow and lymphatic system being treated. The lymphocytes are affected more quickly than the neutrophils as they are more radiosensitive (Plowman, 1983). If the child does become lymphopenic, they should receive prophylaxis against opportunistic infections, particularly pneumocystis infections, which can prove fatal. Repopulation of the marrow in the treated areas may take several weeks and it may be necessary to continue to monitor blood counts closely and for some time after therapy has been completed.

Nursing intervention to prepare and educate the child and the family about how to recognise and avoid infection are comparable to those implemented for myelosuppression caused by chemotherapy. The cell turnover of platelets is particularly rapid in the peripheral system when prevention of bleeding is required or when they reach the end of their normal lifespan. They are extremely vulnerable to ionising radiation and thrombocytopenia may be the first sign of bone marrow suppression (Kun & Moulder, 1993). A fall in the platelet count can occur within seven days of starting treatment. Again, the large marrow reserve compensates for the initial loss of proliferating cells, but as the platelets themselves survive in the blood for only approximately nine days, this reserve is soon depleted. Blood product support is fundamental to the care of the child, but perhaps more important is the advice and support given to the family to facilitate their avoidance of trauma and prompt identification of petechiae and bruising. Cytomegalovirus precautions will be necessary in potential bone marrow transplant recipients.

Craniospinal radiotherapy affects a large area of bone that contains functional marrow. During this form of treatment, in particular, the blood counts will need to be closely monitored. It may be possible to check the blood counts twice a week initially, but as the blood counts begin to fall it is necessary to check them on occasion as frequently as daily. It is also necessary to check them prior to the radiotherapy treatment, as the treatment may be delayed if the patient is neutropenic, or if the platelet count is too low (less than 30 000/ml). This may be the case where the child has previously received chemotherapy.

Hair follicles

Hair follicles renew themselves rapidly and are therefore easily susceptible to radiotherapy if within a treatment field. As many children are receiving 'combination therapy' they may already have significant alopecia from their chemotherapy, but for those receiving cranial irradiation alone there may be only sporadic hair loss within the field that is being treated (Strohl, 1990). This may actually cause more problems than the widespread alopecia that accompanies chemotherapy as it is more straightforward to wear a wig or present a fashionable bald look. Hair loss due to chemotherapy is most often a temporary state and it will grow back several weeks after completion of treatment, but the proportion of those who sustain permanent hair loss is higher in children who have undergone radiotherapy. Some children experience permanent thinning, whereas others may have areas where there is no new growth at all.

This is usually dependent on the dose of radiotherapy given. Temporary hair loss occurs if the child receives up to 30 Gy, however, the loss is permanent at doses above 55 Gy (McDonald, 1992). Hair regrowth normally begins about two to three months post-treatment and continues for up to a year post-irradiation. When regrowth occurs the hair may be a slightly different colour and texture (Dunne-Daly, 1994).

Care of the scalp is as for any other skin area and therefore the guidelines described earlier (Campbell & Lane, 1996) can be used. The scalp may be far too sensitive to wear a wig during and immediately after radiotherapy. Soft cotton scarves or baseball caps are therefore recommended. The prophylactic use of moisturising creams on the scalp is essential to prevent significant skin trauma. The effect on body image of this hair loss depends on the individual and the permanence of the loss. It is most important that the child is prepared for this adverse effect and, although accuracy of predictions of permanent loss are not very high, this issue will need to be introduced with older children.

Fatigue

This symptom, so often described by patients after undergoing any form of radiotherapy, is often attributed to myelosuppression, somnolence in cases of brain irradiation, or the adverse effects of pain and poor nutrition. Indeed, Tiesinga et al. (1996) suggest that fatigue is a complex, multidimensional and non-specific subjective phenomenon, for which no definition is widely accepted. Their extensive literature review unfortunately only discusses adult literature from the 1980s and confirms general feelings of malaise that are poorly attributed in cause. There is a considerable amount of literature concerning the experience of fatigue whist receiving treatment for cancer (Piper, 1988; Winningham et al., 1994), but little to describe the effect of radiotherapy alone (Haylock & Hart, 1979; King, 1985). There appears to be no paediatric literature on the subject except in discussion of nutrition or myelosuppression in radiotherapy. Tiesinga et al. (1996) do acknowledge that continued fatigue can be psychologically compromising. Winningham et al. (1994) recommend that patients and their families require preparation for fatigue and continued support throughout treatment.

Although it is often a recommended strategy to encourage frequent rest periods between daily activities, or to reduce levels of activity, this advice may actually contribute to further debilitation in the older child, especially if this is for prolonged periods (Winningham, 1992). Young children will often take naps as and when they feel the need, but for older children it may be more useful to promote strategies such as gentle exercise or a change of activity to one that interests and distracts the individual (Graydon et al., 1995). Physical activity helps to maintain energy levels, whereas enforced immobility or resting may lead to a cycle of increased fatigue, i.e. the less the individual does the more fatigued they feel and the less they feel able to do. Winningham (1992) proposes that this may be enhanced by the structural and biochemical changes that take place when skeletal muscle is inactive for prolonged periods. Gentle exercise, frequent changes of activity and interesting distractions may all increase feelings of well-being and also increase activity tolerance (Bloom et al., 1990).

Brain

Acute toxicity is possible in children after whole or partial brain irradiation. The mechanisms of the acute reactions are inflammation, oedema and increased intracranial pressure (Berger, 1992). This acute damage results in symptoms of headache, nausea and vomiting (Moore, 1995). Iwamoto (1992) highlights the fact that symptoms may also progress to visual disturbances, seizures, motor function difficulties, slurred speech and altered states of consciousness. Medical management is based on steroidal therapy and the role of the nurse is to provide education and support to the family to help cope with these distressing symptoms. Pain control, as per unit protocol, is required for severe and possibly debilitating headaches. The prompt instigation of antiemetic support is also required and ondansetron is the drug of choice (Sullivan et al., 1992; Zoubek et al., 1993).

Subacute damage to the brain can manifest itself several weeks after therapy due to damage to the oligodendroglial cells which results in inhibition of myelin formation and a transient demyelinisation of brain tissue (Berger, 1992). In children, the main presenting reaction is somnolence syndrome. This may manifest as extreme drowsiness (William & Karcon, 1978) or, in some severe cases, dysphasia, fever and ataxia (Bleyer, 1981).

Research studies have concentrated mainly on children who have reported experiencing this condition when receiving prophylactic cranial radiation for lymphoblastic leukaemia (Littman et al., 1984;

Mandell et al., 1989). There is no literature describing its prevalence in children receiving TBI or with brain tumours, but what has been described and not documented is generalised fatigue rather than the more debilitating symptoms of somnolence. Studies which have aimed to estimate the cause and effect of this condition have shown a wide variety of results. There have also been a number of criteria used to diagnose it (Faithful, 1991). Although some studies have used EEG readings to try to determine criteria for diagnosis. Littman et al. (1984) argued that they had established clinical criteria based on the subjective interpretations of the observing researcher. The internal and external validity of such studies could be called into question.

Faithful (1991) therefore undertook a qualitative study whereby adult patients kept a radiotherapy diary. Although the subjects were adults and the study utilised a distinctly different methodology, the results were remarkably similar to previous studies. Descriptions of feeling exhausted, that any effort would be a struggle, in addition to sensory changes, impaired hearing and limb weakness, were all documented by patients. In common with many other research samples the patients complained that the experience had left them afraid that something was 'dreadfully wrong' and that they had relapsed. This study concluded, in keeping with previous literature, that more education and preparation should be undertaken with patients and their families prior to anticipated somnolence. Symptoms of somnolence have been consistently described as being less severe in those children who received cranial radiation as a prophylactic leukaemic measure than in those who were treated for a brain tumour (Faithful, 1991). In addition, there has been some work to suggest that the incidence of somnolence in children receiving prophylactic cranial radiation can be reduced by giving concurrent doses of steroids (Mandell et al., 1989).

Many texts argue that somnolence is only a minor side effect, which will pass quickly (Moore, 1995). However, experience has taught health professionals not to be complacent about it. It is extremely important to ensure that the parents and the child are aware of the potential effects of somnolence. Teenagers may find it devastating to their social interactions which are so vital for their well-being. It is true, however, that some children will experience very little in the way of symptoms, so much so that they may not realise they have even had any degree of somnolence. However, it can be the cause of a great deal of concern and distress for the family. The child may sometimes sleep around the clock and carers often become concerned about the lack of fluid and dietary intake they are able to manage. Occasionally, the effects experienced can be very similar to those experienced at diagnosis and can place the family under a great deal of stress (Freeman et al., 1993).

Nursing care

Nutritional and hydration status of the child should be monitored at clinic visits and, indeed, through education of the parents to observe for signs of dehydration and nutritional deficit. The parents must be reassured by staff that this is a temporary effect of treatment and the child will become more and more alert. A dietetic referral may be required if there is a prolonged weight loss associated with decreased nutritional intake. Supplements to oral intake or to 'top up' naso-gastric feeds may be indicated in the younger child. However, most children are able to maintain their intake by small high-calorie meals and frequent fluids when awake.

Pneumonitis

Radiation pneumonitis is an acute side effect of irradiation of the chest and lungs (Strohl, 1992). This acute pneumonitis is charac-terised by oedema and sloughing of endothelial cells in the smaller vessels, which allows fluid to accumulate in the interstitial tissues. The cells lining the alveoli are also affected and the swelling and sloughing of these cells also causes excess exudate (Strohl, 1992). Fibrosis and vascular changes contribute to decreased lung compli-ance and volume. The pneumonitis begins to subside when the exudate is finally absorbed and regeneration of cells begins. Fibrosis may remain after cellular repair and forms the basis of the late-occurring effects.

The child suffers from dyspnoea, cough and fever, which gener-ally subsides after two to three months. With larger doses of radia-tion, symptoms can present within two to three weeks (Moss & Cox, 1989). Pneumonitis can occur with doses above 7.5 Gy, even as a cumulative fractionated dose (Van Dyk et al., 1981). The child requiring radiotherapy that includes the lung fields requires observa-tion for signs of respiratory distress and compromise. Admission for respiratory monitoring, support and anti-inflammatory medication may be necessary, although this is a rare complication in paediatric oncology as care is taken when irradiating the chest, keeping the dose to a minimum. The child and the family must be adequately informed of this potential side effect and must be prepared for its occurrence. They need to know what symptoms to look for and when they should contact the unit if they are at all concerned. Paediatric oncology outreach nurse specialists and community children's nurses will be able to offer ongoing advice and support in the community.

Cystitis

In aggressive radiation therapy to the pelvic area in children, often to treat rhabdomyosarcoma, the bladder receives significant doses of radiation. General symptoms of acute inflammation or cystitis are common, such as dysuria, decreased bladder capacity, frequency, urgency and nocturia (Iwamoto, 1992). Assessment and monitoring of symptoms are a primary nursing objective. An increased fluid intake should be encouraged and analgesic and antispasmodic medications may be required to relieve dysuria (McCarthy, 1992). In combination with myelosuppression from chemotherapy, the infection risk is high and symptoms should always be assessed with this in mind; urinary tract infections require prompt antibiotic treatment. Preparation of the child and the parents is a primary objective in nursing care. Advice on maintaining fluid intake, despite frequency and nocturia, is essential, as is the use of highly acidic fluids, such as cranberry juice, which can decrease bacterial growth within the bladder. In older children, items such as coffee, tea, alcohol and tobacco should be discouraged as they further irritate the lining of the bladder. Loose cotton underclothing and trousers are also thought to have some positive effect also. Acute effects on the bladder subside within two to eight weeks.

The immediate effects of treatment can be distressing, painful and perhaps life-threatening and nurses play a pivotal role in the prompt identification of symptoms. Good preparation of the child and the family before therapy helps to alleviate some of the anxiety and trauma engendered by such symptoms. It is essential that nurses caring for children undergoing radiotherapy are aware of and understand the basis of the radiation injury and the most appropriate evidence-based care. It is clear that the literature on research-based care in this area is scant and much more is needed. In the meantime, care must be based on a sound theoretical rationale using reflective experiential learning.

Chapter 24
The role of radiotherapy in palliation

Monica Hopkins and Jane Pownall

Radiotherapy in Oncological Emergencies

Spinal cord compression

Spinal cord compression may be caused by either an extradural or intradural lesion, or perhaps even a combination of both. It may be due to an extension of a primary lesion, such as an ependymoma or an astrocytoma (Knight-Morse, 1992a), or metastases from a non-CNS tumour that has developed extradurally to the cord, such as neuroblastoma, primitive neuroectodermal tumour, rhabdomyosarcoma, Ewing's sarcoma or a non-Hodgkin's lymphoma. After extensive investigation which should include MRI and the commencement of corticosteroids (Neal & Hoskin, 1994) palliative radiotherapy can be extremely effective in radiosensitive tumours (Goldman, 1992).

The literature is extremely positive about the use of radiotherapy to relieve this difficult situation (Baldwin, 1983; Kanner, 1987; Wilson, 1989; Schafer, 1994) and it is argued that it can be as effective as surgery and radiotherapy together (Baldwin, 1983; Byrne, 1992; Ingham et al., 1993). Yet there is still a school of thought that recommends the use of surgery if the compression is progressing rapidly; if it is a radio-resistant tumour; the child has already received maximal tolerated doses of radiotherapy; or if neurological deterioration continues throughout therapy (Schafer, 1994).

Fractionated radiotherapy is recommended to prevent compromising oedema that may result from a larger single dose (Kornblith & Cassidy, 1985). However, the exact dose and number of fractions varies considerably in the literature, Dietz and Flaherty (1990) recommend 27–30 Gy over a two-week period as an adult dose but no reference is made to children. What is suggested is a single posterior field that extends the length of the compression plus two vertebral bodies above and below as margins. Should vital structures anterior to the cord need to be shielded, parallel opposing fields can be used instead.

Prognosis for neurological recovery depends on the speed of diagnosis and commencement of treatment. Children who are still mobile at the time of treatment are usually able to walk again following treatment (Neal & Hoskin, 1994).

Care of the child and family is principally concerned with support through such frightening symptoms and intensive investigation. This must be coupled with detailed and accurate neurological assessment throughout the experience, including movement, sensation, bowel and bladder control (Schafer, 1994). Care must be taken to ensure respiratory function is closely monitored and supported, depending on the position of the compression. In addition, pain control should be assessed as well as necessary prophylactic measures to avoid the complications of prolonged immobility (Schafer, 1994).

Superior vena cava obstruction

This is a serious though fortunately rare complication of a large tumour load, that constitutes a significant oncological emergency in the pre-terminal child. An upper mediastinal tumour of any histology can potentially lead to the compression of this vessel but T-cell non-Hodgkin's lymphoma is often the cause in children (Glover & Glick, 1991). It can also be caused by thoracic neuroblastoma, Hodgkin's lymphoma and Ewing's sarcoma (Pinkerton et al., 1994). This condition is often accompanied by other symptoms, such as dysphagia and stridor (Neal & Hoskin, 1994). Obstruction may signal the beginning of the child's distress, but thrombosis will inevitably follow and become life-threatening (Neal & Hoskin, 1994). Clinical signs and symptoms are described below:

- Signs:

  oedema of face, neck and upper thorax
  peri-orbital oedema, with or without protrusion of the eye
  subconjuctival haemorrhage
  plethora of the face

increased pressure of the jugular veins
dilation and prominence of the collateral vessels of the neck and
upper thorax
inspiratory wheeze
tachycardia

- Symptoms:

swelling of the face and upper limbs
breathlessness, dry cough, stridor (wheeze)
headache
visual disturbances and dizziness, bloodshot eyes
hoarseness, rare
chest pain, rare
swelling of the fingers/hands
(Schafer (1994) cited by Otto (1994)).

Following diagnosis using radiography and CT scanning, treatment is initiated as quickly as possible. Although chemotherapy is often the treatment modality of choice, especially if the causal lesion is a lymphoma (Neal & Hoskin, 1994, Pinkerton et al., 1994), radiotherapy is also very effective when the disease is acute and a rapid response is needed (Knight-Morse, 1992b). A combination of modalities may be used with the dose of radiotherapy being dependent upon:

- Tumour type
- Tumour size
- Condition of the child
- The response required
  (Schafer, 1994).

Acute observational skills are needed to recognise respiratory and cardiac compromise before, during and immediately after therapy. The child and the family require explanations and reassurance about the process of the condition and the rationale for treatment. The child should be helped to find a more comfortable position for ease of breathing whilst encouraging chest expansion and deep breathing at least two-hourly (Schafer, 1994). Oxygen may be prescribed and requires administration in a controlled and humidified form through either nasal cannulae or a mask, depending on the flow rate and the child's preference. Oxygen saturation monitoring should be undertaken as gaseous exchange may be compromised due to vena cava congestion.

The cardiovascular system must also be observed, as obstruction may be affecting venous return to the heart (and thus stroke volume) even in the period immediately after therapy whilst the mass is still present. This may lead to compromise of the peripheral vascular system and the child should be assessed for levels of perfusion and signs of peripheral shutdown. There is a potential for alteration in cerebral perfusion as evidenced by an altered state of consciousness, which should be assessed at each interaction and carefully documented (Schafer, 1994).

The child should be monitored closely for fluid and electrolyte destabilisation when there is a risk of tumour lysis syndrome. Large amounts of fluid may be infused to irrigate the kidneys and, as a result, blood biochemistry should be assessed frequently.

Following therapy, as the mass decreases, observation for respiratory and cardiovascular compromise can be less frequent. Kidney function and radiotherapy site skin integrity assessment must be maintained and carefully documented for alterations in status.

Radiotherapy in palliative care

It is asserted that approximately half of the courses of radiotherapy administered in the care of people with cancer are delivered with palliative intent (Richter & Coia, 1985). This fact does, of course, refer to adults who may require several courses. Radiotherapy has proved to be extremely useful in the treatment of many neoplasms in children, when the aim of care is to cure. It is, however, also an extremely useful tool in the palliation of distressing symptoms of advancing disease in the dying child.

Palliative radiotherapy can be used in many situations where radiation would not be considered a useful modality for cure, i.e. with apparently radio-resistant tumours. These neoplasms may be thought incurable by standard dose radiotherapy, but palliative radiotherapy may be able to reduce the tumour sufficiently to relieve the symptoms (Kirkbride, 1995). Radiation has been used with considerable success to arrest pain, obstruction, compression and bleeding caused by the disease.

Despite this testimony to its efficacy, the use of radiotherapy must be considered very carefully in caring for a child in the terminal and pre-terminal stages of disease, as this modality of treatment has its costs. The child and the parents must be active members of the treatment decision, and be in full possession of all the facts about its use, efficacy and adverse consequences in terms of comfort, freedom and the loss of precious time at home with loved ones (Spinetta & Deasy-Spinetta, 1989). They must be aware, as should all professionals involved, that this is not a last attempt at cure, but a palliative measure, that although it may convey symptom relief for a period of time it is not a permanent measure. The child and the family should not be offered this therapy in order to create hope in a desperate situation (Maher et al., 1993). The tumour may, indeed, respond in a significant manner to radiotherapy, but it will not put the child into a state of remission. It must be clear to all involved that the expenditure in time, travelling, effort and discomfort will be worth the possible benefits (Kirkbride, 1995). The possibility of failure must also be considered, as even a radiosensitive tumour may be so large that it may not shrink sufficiently to alleviate the symptoms. Also, tumour shrinkage is not always required to remove discomfort, for example, it is the cellular changes induced in bone tissue that decreases the excruciating pain (Kirkbride, 1995).

In many cases the use of palliative radiotherapy entails only short courses of therapy at relatively low doses, but the healthy surrounding tissue may still be damaged. In children, it is often the case that only single fractions are given, so as to reduce hospital intervention to a minimum where possible.

The areas that are considered to respond most effectively to radiotherapy will now be discussed in detail.

Control of bone pain

It is not truly understood why it is that metastases in the bone tissue cause such incredible pain, nor why the cellular changes induced by radiotherapy relieve it. The area around the lesion is typically tender on palpation, and in more severe cases, in which the response to radiotherapy is greatest, pain is unable to be controlled by NSAIDs in conjunction with opiates (Price et al., 1986). Pain relief, however, once attained is usually durable for long periods of time (Gilbert et al., 1977). Painful bone metastases are most common in solid tumours such as neuroblastoma.

Control of bone pain is probably the most common use of palliative radiotherapy and, indeed, is where the most significant amount of evaluatory research has been carried out (Price et al., 1986; Crellin et al., 1989; MRC, 1991). In the last 15 years, the literature repeatedly quotes the same response statistics, i.e. that 55–66% of patients will receive total relief from their pain with radiotherapy and 90% will experience some partial relief of symptoms (Kirkbride, 1995). The method of administration is where the most controversy lies. Many centres are adamant that single-fraction doses are just as effective as protracted schedules of a fractionated dose (Price et al., 1986; Crellin et al., 1989; MRC 1991) except perhaps where bone pain arises from the vertebral column as many practitioners are concerned about giving such high doses to the spinal cord. Goldman (1992) has argued that in the past paediatric radio-oncologists were unfortunately not using single fractions as often as appropriate in children and were preferring to extend the course with smaller fractions, despite the evidence. This does appear to be changing. The situation is also unclear internationally. Surveys of practice outside the UK (Duncan et al., 1993) have found that the controversy has caused an extreme variety of practices to spring up in different oncology centres, despite evidence to the contrary (MRC, 1991). Extensive fractionation is thought to be of use, however, in the prevention and treatment of pathological fractures in lytic lesions. This is most often used effectively in conjunction with orthopaedic surgery to fixate the fracture internally. Prevention of such a problem is far more successful than trying to seal the bone after a fracture. It must therefore be remembered that before irradiating a large destructive bone metastases it is strongly recommended that an orthopaedic consultation is sought.

Whatever the course of radiotherapy, the role of the nurse is in the accurate assessment of pain before, during and after therapy. The child and the family are likely to be distressed and will require information, honest reassurance and support throughout the experience of palliative radiotherapy. Returning to a department previously associated with curative treatment may be stressful for the family and confusing for the child, especially if attempts have already been made to prepare the family unit for the eventual death of the child.

Control of bleeding

Radiotherapy will control bleeding from widespread malignant ulceration, as in soft tissue sarcomas such as rhabdomyosarcoma. External beam radiotherapy will also control haemoptysis in most cases where conventional haemostatic agents have not proved effective. Unfortunately, most of the information available on the use of radiotherapy for this problem is anecdotal and research in this area is not immediately evident. Haematuria has also been treated effectively with radiation and single fractions are used in such situations. The child who is not yet in the terminal stages of disease may also be treated to prevent haemorrhage due to tumour erosion, e.g epithelial haemangioma (Kirkbride, 1995), when conventional wound care is insufficient.

Bleeding is one of the most frightening and distressing symptoms, however small the actual blood loss. Here, the role of the nurse is speed of recognition of symptoms and reassurance to the family.

Troublesome metastases

Radiotherapy has a significant role to play in alleviating troublesome brain metastases that are causing unacceptable cerebral signs in a pre-terminal child. These lesions can cause disabling symptoms, such as headache, nausea, seizures and neurological impairment. Cranial radiation is most often the answer as the source of these problems is predominantly cerebral oedema. Use of a short course of radiation to reduce the lesion causing the cerebral oedema may mean it is possible to reduce a dose of steroids.

Lung metastases from any primary tumour, but especially from bone tumours, can lead to bronchial obstruction which can cause premature and extremely distressing respiratory impairment. Sometimes it may be appropriate to use single-dose therapy to relieve such a symptom.

Other distressing symptoms of advancing disease that can be treated by the use of radiotherapy are liver metastases causing pain from a stretched liver capsule, thoracic or pleuritic pain from mediastinal masses and metastatic lung deposits (Hilderley, 1992b).

Palliative therapy should aim for simplicity in procedure, for the quick relief of symptoms, in order to prevent complications that can lead to discomfort pain or distress.

Dosages and fractionation schedules are usually determined by the oncologist in response to the child's condition and the needs of the family. The concurrent use of steriods with single radiation doses to reduce associated oedema is also a clinical decision to be made by the oncologist, depending on the child's status. It is beyond the remit of this chapter to cover all the psychosocial aspects of good palliative care. Radiotherapy is merely a tool to be used to relieve physical discomfort so that the child can resume living a dignified life. Many of the symptoms described previously are disabling and visible to the child, and the issue of body image should be remembered, especially at this difficult time. Accepting a personal identity is part of making sense of existence and this can be a necessary step in working positively towards death.

Preparation and nursing care for the child undergoing palliative radiotherapy should be similar to the standards set in curative regimes but time may be short. Consequently, flexibility is required in caring for these children and their families. It may be beneficial to have the primary palliative care nurse accompany the child and the family to the unit so that continuity of care is maintained whilst the child is within the radiotherapy suite. The parents will then have a supportive professional present who can also be an advocate with intimate knowledge of the child's status and the family's wishes.

Chapter 25
Late effects of radiotherapy

Linda Scott, Jane Pownall and Monica Hopkins

Introduction

The primary goal in paediatric radiation oncology is to eradicate tumour cells without severely damaging the child's quality of life in the long term (Constine, 1991). Knowledge and awareness of the late effects, from considerable research in this area over the years, has resulted in the planning of treatment to minimise them. According to Jenney and Kissen (1996) some late effects can be predicted, for example, infertility from gonadal radiation, whilst others are less well-defined. Late tissue reaction depends on the interaction between the therapy utilised, the individual patient and the nature of the tumour. Therapy factors that influence the extent of tissue damage in the long term are total and fractionated dose, dose rate, treatment time, energy of the source and the volume of tissue treated (Constine & Rubin, 1988). Generally, as the intensity of radiotherapy increases, additional long term complications will be seen (Jenney & Kissen, 1996). The child's developmental status, individual genetic make up and inherent capacity for tissue repair and adaptation to abnormalities will also influence the extent of late tissue effects. Finally, the extent of the disease and its effects on organs, irrespective of therapy, will also influence the body's available response (Jones & Larkkarman, 1987).

Children's bodies are made up of a variety of tissues, each developing and maturing at different rates. These tissues are most at risk from significant damage during their individual periods of rapid growth. This window in development differs with each tissue (Rubin et al., 1982). Kroll et al. (1994) propose that many children suffer from late occurring adverse effects after radiotherapy. These authors estimate that 40% of children have some form of bone deformity, 21% have an endocrine problem, 30% atrophic skin changes, and 7% develop secondary malignancies. These statistics have not been confirmed by any other literature, but allude to the significance of this area of practice. There exists, therefore, a vast array of significant adverse effects. Intervention may be needed in some cases, such as growth hormone replacement, but for many children it is ongoing assessment, monitoring and psychosocial support that are the most useful professional interventions.

Central Nervous System

The greatest part of the brain's development is concentrated into the first three years of life, with very little taking place after the sixth year (Packer et al., 1987). There is no increase in the number of neurones during these periods of development, only in their size. It is growth in connective tissue and accessory cells which increases the size of the organ. Most areas are myelinised by the end of the second year, although this process continues until puberty. The main radiation damage that can occur to the CNS is demyelinisation (i.e. damage to the oligodendrocytes) and, consequently, white matter necrosis, either in localised lesions or diffusely across the whole system. For these reasons radiotherapy to the CNS is contraindicated in the very young child. Glial cells can also be damaged, as can the vascular endothelium in the brain. When a significant volume of vascular endothelium fails, vasogenic oedema is seen as there is a loss of support tissue to the neurones and cerebral cortical atrophy results (Constine, 1991).

Radiation necrosis occurs in a very small number of cases, and only after 50–60 Gy of radiation fractionated over a period of six weeks (Constine, 1991), although the risk increases with doses above this point. This is not a situation that arises routinely in the irradiation of children in this country. The signs and symptoms include headache, symptoms of raised intracranial pressure and focal deficits. On scanning it is seen as a mass surrounded by oedema. The condition is progressive and often fatal, and so if possible, surgical debulking of the mass is recommended although steroids will give temporary relief (Marks & Wong, 1985).

Cerebral necrosis was highlighted in an Australian study on adults who had received irradiation for brain tumours. Seizures, stroke-like episodes, dementia and somnolence were found in a minority of patients, indicating that necrosis is a rare but poorly recognised complication of radiation (Morris et al., 1994).

Leukoencephalopathy, when present, is identified as multiple necrotic foci in the white matter and is manifested by lethargy, seizures, spasticity, paresis and ataxia (Bleyer & Griffin, 1980). It is difficult to elucidate the exact cause when the child has received intrathecal or intravenous methotrexate with cranial radiation, as all three elements can contribute to the problem. However, radiotherapy and either form of methotrexate work synergistically to increase the risk in a child. Most of the children who were identified with this problem had received more than 20 Gy whole brain radiation for CNS leukaemia prophylaxis (Constine, 1991).

The CNS also includes the spinal cord, and the damage caused in irradiating it ranges from the transient to the irreversible. Chronic radiation myelitis is rare and can only be confirmed on autopsy. The clinical picture, however, is one of increasing paraesthesia and sensory changes, beginning about a year after treatment. Children are reported to be more vulnerable to this condition following smaller doses and a shorter post-treatment period. In addition, the administration of dactinomycin has been suggested to decrease the threshold for this problem. The larger the individual fraction sizes, shorter overall treatment time, larger cord length treated and higher total dose, the greater the risk of myelopathy (Goldwein, 1987).

Chronic brain tissue damage is due to both the inactivity of fully committed parenchymal cells and the impairment of their replacement over time. In addition to this there is damage to the underlying vasculature which continues to cause progressive injury (Rubin, 1984). This arteriolar damage is very prevalent in the late irreparable form of tissue damage and accentuates the cellular damage seen not only in the brain but also in the heart and kidneys. The time taken for this damage to be expressed decreases with higher doses of radiation. Mitchell et al. (1991) reported that cerebrovascular disease in large and medium vessels can be a common sequelae for children who have received radiotherapy for a brain tumour.

Radiation injury to the brain is not just confined to this organ's structure but also to its function. Christie et al. (1994) studied a sample of children who had all previously relapsed on leukaemia treatment regimes and then received a bone marrow transplant. They found that although all the children demonstrated problems with coordination, none had major motor difficulties. Unfortunately, all the children had cataracts and growth hormone deficiency. Verbal IQ scores and attention deficits were present in all the children. Girls exhibited significantly greater morbidity than the boys studied, and total dosage of radiation, age at relapse and time between cranial irradiation and bone marrow transplant were all prognostic influences.

It is also evident from the literature that radiotherapy that includes the brain within its field can cause significant harm to cognitive function and neuro-endocrine release.

Cognitive function

This particular late effect of radiation to the brain has probably been the adverse effect most concentrated upon in recent years. It certainly has profound implications for quality of life and may have a significant influence on the decision to treat children with radiotherapy.

Cognitive and educational abilities have been found to be the most severely affected in childhood cancer survivors who have received cranial radiotherapy. Verbal IQ and attention deficits appear to be the most significant areas of concern (Anderson et al., 1994). It has been argued that 18 Gy of cranial irradiation results in the same decrease in neuropsychological functioning as intravenous methotrexate in areas such as IQ tests, arithmetic and verbal reasoning (Ochs et al., 1991).

Christie et al. (1995) studied children who had received both cranial irradiation and intrathecal methotrexate. They found that children irradiated at age fours years or younger all had impairment in certain aspects of cognition, non-verbal ability, short term memory and attention. Verbal and non-verbal reasoning tests highlighted that the greatest impairment was found in children irradiated at a young age, especially the girls in the sample (Waber et al., 1992). This large and intensive study confirms previous research in this area.

Cognitive deficits are also prevalent in long term survivors of medulloblastoma and other non-cortical brain tumours, and once again children treated with whole brain radiotherapy at a younger age have significantly more cognitive impairment than older children (Radcliffe et al., 1994). It is hard to ascertain if these children eventually reach a plateau of impairment or continue to decline, as it is difficult to distinguish between evidence of continuing cognitive impairment and the failure to acquire new cognitive skills at the same rate as peers. Thus, it may be argued that the children's underlying defect does not progress but the limits it places on their ability to learn ensures the gap between them and their peers continues to widen. This theory is supported by the knowledge that concentration has also been found to be affected by cranial irradiation (Goff et al., 1980).

Neuro-endocrines

It has been argued that radiation has an effect on endocrine function by causing tissue injury to both the hypothalamus and pituitary gland. This may lead to dysfunction in the control of thyroxine, growth and gonadotrophic hormones.

Thyroid hormone

The production of thyroxine is a three-stage process which begins in brain tissue. The hypothalamus produces a neurotransmitter, called thyrotropin releasing hormone (TRH), which stimulates the anterior pituitary to release thyroid stimulating hormone (TSH). Finally, the TSH acts on the thyroid gland to produce thyroid hormone (TH). The whole process is a negative feedback loop to control thyroid hormone levels (Fergusson et al., 1986). TSH levels will be raised in the presence of decreased and normal thyroxine levels, depending on whether the gland is responding to the stimulation.

The thyroid gland can begin to dysfunction as a late response to radiation tissue damage to either itself or the hypothalamic/pituitary axis (Constine, 1991). Patients treated with head and neck radiotherapy or craniospinal irradiation may develop hypothyroidism (Constine et al., 1984; Constine et al., 1989). Thyroid dysfunction can also arise from direct sources of radiation damage in addition to cranial irradiation. The thyroid gland itself is extremely sensitive to the effects of radiotherapy and even low-dose scatter from adjacent radiation fields can lead to significant dysfunction (Jenney & Kissen, 1996). Radiotherapy to the neck, spinal, mantle and mediastinal fields, in addition to TBI and the intravenous administration of [131]ImIBG (Hobbie & Schwartz, 1989) may all result in radiation injury to this gland. This injury may lead to abnormalities in secretion or in structure, such as the development of benign or malignant tumours. These children require lifelong monitoring.

The frequency of hypothyroidism in spinal radiotherapy is unknown, although it has been studied extensively in children treated with mantle field irradiation for Hodgkin's disease (Kaplan et al., 1983). In these studies, increasing frequency was associated with increasing dose. Some patients do recover spontaneously (about 27%) and the rest require supplementation. Children who receive TBI as part of their conditioning regime for bone marrow transplant are also at risk from this problem, especially if it is given as a single dose (Sklar et al., 1982; Locatelli et al., 1993).

Implications for long term follow-up

For those children that have received radiotherapy treatment to the thyroid gland and low-dose cranial radiation, monitoring should be by palpation of the gland itself and by checking blood levels of T_4 and TSH. Should palpation reveal any abnormality, an ultrasound scan and endocrine referral is recommended. In addition, if the TSH is raised (although T_4 levels are normal), thyroxine should be introduced as the TSH is having to overwork to produce a normal T_4. Should the T_4 level remain low, even in the presence of a raised TSH, then not only should thyroxine be given but an endocrine referral will also be necessary (Kissen & Wallace, 1993).

Children who have received higher doses of radiation to the craniospinal fields require more detailed endocrine investigation of the injury to the hypothalamic–pituitary axis and its effects on thyroid function. Referral to a paediatric endocrinologist is essential.

Growth hormone

Growth hormone (GH), like many other pituitary hormones, does not exert its influence directly. It is not in direct control of bone growth. GH stimulates the production of somatomedin-C by the liver, which does affect linear growth (Fergusson et al., 1986). This hormone influences growth just before and during puberty. Radiation along the hypothalamic–pituitary axis, therefore, can have significant effects on its hormonal production and controlling influences.

Growth impairment in survivors of childhood leukaemia has been recognised since the 1960s, and radiotherapy has been seen as the main cause of this problem for some considerable time (Jenney & Kissen, 1996). Littley et al. (1990) identified that radiotherapy to the brain, spine and gonads contributes to bone and endocrine dysfunction. Both the hypothalamus and the pituitary can be affected by radiation. The hypothalamus, however, has been found to be affected even by doses of 24 Gy or less. These low doses disturb the frequency and rhythmic pulse secretion of the gland very slightly, and a quantitative decrease in GH may only be detected at puberty (Crowne et al., 1992).

A burning question for researchers has been to gain an understanding into where exactly in the brain the injury occurs. Ogilvy-Stuart et al. (1994) argue that patients with GH deficiency usually remain responsive to exogenous growth hormone releasing hormone (GHRH), implying that it is due to radiotherapy damage to the hypothalamus rather than to the pituitary.

The collective research data on spontaneous growth compared to final height have been conflicting in childhood leukaemia survivors. Therefore, Cicognani et al. (1994) undertook a longitudinal study of the growth of children who had received 18 or 24 Gy of cranial irradiation, with no spinal or testicular therapy. They found that the mean final height in girls was significantly lower at both dose levels compared to non-irradiated girls, and yet this situation was only evident in the boys at 24 Gy. It was also found that girls who were irradiated at less than four years of age showed greater height problems than those irradiated after this point (Leiper et al., 1987). These results were supportive of the work completed by Sklar et al. (1993). These researchers had also found that those children who had received 24 Gy or more radiation to the brain suffered the greatest loss of final height attainment. They concluded that radiotherapy at a young age and female gender are the greatest influencing factors in a reduced height attainment, although the effect of pubertal timing may also be a significant influence in these children.

Low-dose cranial radiation (18–24 Gy) used for CNS prophylaxis and treatment in children with ALL may also cause early or precocious puberty, especially in girls (Jenney & Kissen, 1996). Their lack of GH results in a lack of growth prior to this point. With the early onset of puberty there is much less opportunity to use GH supplementation before puberty begins and the epiphyses seal (Ogilvy-Stuart et al., 1994). It may be necessary, therefore, to arrest or decelerate puberty by hormonal manipulation to allow further growth to take place before the onset of menstruation. This is accomplished by using an analogue of a gonadotrophin-releasing hormone (GRH) (Wallace & Shalet, 1992).

There can also be a significant decrease in growth velocity in those children who receive TBI as part of their conditioning regime for transplant, especially in those children who have received previous prophylactic cranial irradiation (Locatelli et al., 1993).

In summary, it can be stated that radiation doses of less than 24 Gy to the hypothalamic–pituitary axis place children at risk of early puberty and an attenuated pubertal growth spurt. Doses over 24 Gy to the same axis put them at risk of GH deficiency, early puberty and multiple pituitary hormone deficiencies. These problems are obviously now anticipated and treatment with GH is standard management. However, there is still a modest risk of reduced final height attainment (Sklar et al., 1993).

Gonadotrophic hormones

The role of the pituitary gland in puberty, and so growth and fertility, is pivotal, and radiation injury to this gland has significant consequences for the child treated for cancer. Before highlighting the literature on the nature of these adverse consequences, the physiology of puberty and pubertal growth will be reviewed briefly.

The pituitary gland controls sexual development through the production of gonadotrophic hormones. In females puberty begins at approximately ten years of age when the pituitary begins to secrete luteinising hormone (LH) and follicle stimulating hormone (FSH). These two hormones stimulate the maturation of the ovaries and this will eventually lead to ovulation (Fergusson et al., 1986). It is at this point that oestrogen secretion, which has only been in very small amounts, now increases approximately 20-fold. This rise in oestrogen secretion then stimulates the sequence of events that leads to menstruation. Oestrogen also stimulates breast development (the first sign of impending puberty), pubic and axillary hair, and supports bone growth. Oestrogen has a greater effect on accelerating bone maturity than linear growth, in which it plays a supportive role. It is for this reason that women, on average, tend to be significantly shorter than men. Females reach their final adult height soon after the onset of menstruation when the epiphyses seal. The continued secretion of oestrogen is also required for continued bone maintenance, and consequently, should there be ovarian failure or inhibition of oestrogen from the pituitary gland then osteoporosis will appear.

In males the process is a little different. It begins somewhat later at approximately 11 years of age and lasts for five to six years. The first sign that puberty has begun is enlargement of the testicles in response to the gonadotrophins released by the pituitary. This is followed closely by an increase in the level of testosterone produced by the testes, the secondary sexual characteristic which this hormone produces, begin to appear. Enlargement of the penis, pubic and axillary hair growth, increase in linear growth, muscle development and, finally, facial hair all occur at this time. Testosterone, as already mentioned, is produced in the testes by the Leydig cells under the direct influence of LH. However, it is FSH that is required, along with testosterone, for the production of spermatozoa by the germinal epithelium.

Didcock et al. (1995) investigated pubertal growth in children who had received cranial irradiation at 18 and 24 Gy for CNS prophylaxis in ALL. These authors found that puberty occurred earlier in girls but not in boys, and that the velocity of growth was slowed in both sexes, although the duration of puberty was not altered. This may, therefore, have led to loss of height in both groups. Early puberty in girls after cranial irradiation has been demonstrated in many other studies (Leiper et al., 1987; Uruena et al., 1991).

Locatelli et al. (1993) describe the incidence of delayed puberty in males and females after TBI. Post-pubertal teenagers may develop amenorrhoea, azoospermia and gonadal failure after radiotherapy and may require hormonal substitute therapy if they are to enter puberty at all.

Implications for long term follow-up

Growth charting should be undertaken at least six-monthly until the child has been established on his normal pubertal growth spurt. Pubertal staging must also take place on a regular basis and must include monitoring testicular volume in boys. The child should be referred for endocrine assessment if height velocity pre-pubertally is less than 4 cm/year and so 'falls off' the centile chart. Also, if there is evidence of puberty beginning before the child is nine years of age and, finally, if there is a loss of synchronisation between growth and puberty (Kissen & Wallace, 1993).

Skin

Late stage reactions can be seen throughout the whole of the integumentary system: skin, hair, nails, sweat glands and sebaceous glands (Rodriguez & Ash, 1996). The latent injury may take months or even years to repair after completion of therapy, where radiotherapy has caused progressive structural changes throughout all the layers of skin, and the complementing tissues of the entire system. This acute stage of damage may go on to become a chronic health issue with implications for body image.

Sittom (1992) highlights the fact that more chronic tissue damage in the skin may actually decrease its elasticity and flexibility, and so its ability to maintain a protective layer around the body. Gallagher (1995) points out that the most commonly reported chronic skin changes are atrophy, telangiectasia, changes in pigmentation and fibrosis. This author also states that ulceration and necrosis may be seen in certain extreme cases where very high doses of radiation have been administered.

These reactions appear to be extreme and the literature unfortunately only reports on the experiences of adults. However, children are far more likely to encounter alopecia, dryness, and hyperplasia of vasculature, with some degree of damage to connective tissue (Marcus et al., 1994).

Nursing care for the child with chronic skin damage, like many late effects, focuses on education (Hagopian, 1991, 1996; Gomez, 1995). Firstly, an accurate history of previous skin problems should always be obtained, as well as an extensive physical examination of the area in question to identify the nature of the injury. These findings must be recorded graphically and accurately to form a baseline for longitudinal evaluation. Education programmes and informative literature should include advice on the avoidance of mechanical, thermal and chemical irritation of the area. This can be encouraged through the use of adequate clothing to protect the skin from extreme heat or cold; protective clothing should be worn when handling detergents, abrasive chemicals, paints and science materials (in school or at home), and direct avoidance of highly perfumed or exfoliating skin products (Sittom, 1992). Gentle cleansing of the skin, with scrupulous attention to moisturising, should be promoted in addition to the observation and identification of the signs of inflammation and infection so that prompt medical treatment can be sought. Further nursing research is urgently required in this area to guide practice in the care of children with altered skin integrity.

There is a gap in the radiotherapy literature when the focus turns to children and the nursing support required during and after therapy. Skin damage may lead to significant distress in the child on a physical and emotional level. Body integrity has been breached by the therapy and the testimony to it remains in the form of visible skin damage. Psychological support must be a priority when emotional distress has been identified. Nurses must seek to facilitate access to information to empower the child and the family to cope with these difficulties and to promote an open honest atmosphere where the concerns of the child regarding skin changes and methods of reducing their effect, can be discussed.

Bone

Bone growth is not uniform, rather, it falls into spurts or phases soon after birth and then again at puberty. Steady growth continues between five and ten years of age (Constine, 1991). Growth retardation therefore depends not only on the dose of radiation but also on the age of the child at therapy. Single doses of 2–20 Gy inhibit the proliferation of cartilage cells, causing disarray within the growth plates. However, there is little damage to bone growth with total fractionated doses of less than 10 Gy, there is partial growth arrest at 10–20 Gy, and complete arrest at more than 20 Gy (Constine, 1991). Severe stunting occurs when the epiphyseal plates are within the treatment field, consequently these are avoided wherever possible.

The long bones that contribute so much to final height are not the only casualties of radiotherapy. Larson et al. (1990) described the severe side effects that are noted in children treated with radiotherapy to the head and neck for soft tissue sarcomas and retinoblastoma. Adverse effects, such a hypoplasia of the jaw, orbit and facial bones, were not uncommon. The disfiguring effects of this bone growth retardation are further enhanced by atrophy of the soft tissue overlying them. This combination can happen elsewhere in the body and cause extreme body image difficulties for children and young teenagers alike. Osteoradionecrosis is also a possible effect seen primarily in the mandible, where hypoplasia of the bone leaves it vulnerable to infection or inflammation from dental decay or mucosal problems, eventually leading to complete breakdown of the tissue. Surgical removal and reconstruction of the bony area is often required (Iwamoto, 1994). For this reason, the child should be made aware of the risks of poor dental and oral hygiene after radiotherapy to the jaw. This should be the subject of continued health education for the child in long term follow-up.

A study by Rate et al. (1991) of children who had received radiotherapy for Wilms' tumour found that 10% of children developed late orthopaedic effects after abdominal radiotherapy. Larger fields and doses above 28.9 Gy were found to be characteristics of this subgroup of children. Abdominal radiotherapy for Wilms' tumour causes secondary changes in the skeleton, there are also growth disturbances and osteochondrosis of variable degree (Scheibel-Jost et al., 1991). Fortunately, modern techniques seek to avoid these problems by focusing treatment more accurately and using the minimum doses possible. Long term follow-up clinics, however, may still see children with such difficulties.

Scoliosis and kyphosis can also be seen as a result of unilateral flank irradiation; this is to be avoided wherever possible. If there has also been surgery in the area, asymmetrical growth can still be seen despite symmetrical irradiation of the skeleton, due to soft tissue vulnerability to damage after surgery (Probert et al., 1973). When evident, scoliosis progresses most rapidly at the pubertal growth spurt.

Probert et al. (1973) suggested that the greatest arrest of spinal growth took place when children were irradiated under six years of age and during puberty with more than 35 Gy.

Radiation fields that include the lower limbs may cause problems not only with bone growth but also structural damage, which may have severe consequences for bone integrity. Irradiation of the femoral head during pelvic radiotherapy can lead to slipped capital epiphyses as well as avascular necrosis (Taylor, 1996). The latter condition is particularly evident if the child is receiving steroids in addition to irradiation, and if the dose exceeds 30–40 Gy (Donaldson & Kaplan, 1982).

Discrepancies in leg length following abdominal, pelvic or lower extremity radiotherapy were described in 12 out of 67 children studied by Robertson et al. (1991). Leg length inequality was associated with increasing the total dose of pelvic radiotherapy, asymmetry of radio-therapy to the pelvic area and high-dose therapy to the lower limbs.

Short stature due to decreased bone growth can also occur with paratesticular radiotherapy. This treatment is extremely effective for malignant disease of the testicle, but the incidence of growth impair-ment when the radiation field includes the para-aortic nodes pre-puberty is a significant cause for concern (Hughes et al., 1994). This may be due to the radiation injury to bone plates within the field and also the concomitant reduction in testosterone production.

Additional growth problems after TBI

Growth after bone marrow transplant can be an extremely problem-atic area to deal with and this is largely due to the use of TBI as a conditioning regime (Ogilvy-Stuart et al., 1992). The reason for the difficulty in addressing this level of growth impairment is probably due to the combination of skeletal dysplasia, GH dysfunction, gonadal dysfunction and possibly the presence of chronic GVHD (Jenney & Kissen, 1996). The effects on growth velocity are more often seen in single-dose TBI but also in fractionated schedules. Supplementation with GH is not as effective in these children as its mechanism is impaired by the presence of skeletal dysplasia (Bozzola et al., 1993).

Implications for long term follow-up

Complaints of back pain or suspected fractures should be investi-gated seriously if craniospinal radiotherapy has been given. It may also be useful to consider measuring bone density to detect signs of hypoplasia, secondary malignancy or osteoporosis if there have been hormonal deficiencies.

The measurement and documentation of growth must be meticulously maintained and compared with the clinical picture of puberty and maturation to ensure there are no adverse problems in development.

Gonads

According to Sklar et al. (1990), damage to the gonads can be either as a result of direct radiation tissue damage, or indirectly from radiation effects on the hypothalamic–pituitary unit in cranial irradiation. The latter damage is well-documented in the literature, but far less is known about the nature of the effect of radiotherapy on the developing gonad (Table 25.1).

The gonads can be affected by radiotherapy directly, when radiation is administered to the spinal, abdominal or pelvic fields in girls, and to the pelvic fields or directly to the testes in boys. Both sexes can be affected by the use of TBI.

Testicular function is controlled by the release of FSH and LH from the pituitary gland. This, in turn, is controlled by the release of GRH from the hypothalamus. Leydig cells within the testes produce testosterone and the germinal epithelium produces sperm. The testosterone produced by the testes acts as a negative feedback control mechanism to the pituitary gland in its production of FSH and LH. Germinal cells are far more sensitive to radiation injury than Leydig cells.

Testicular failure is most commonly seen in the form of damage to the germinal epithelium, which can be induced by doses as low as 10 cGy (Clifton & Bremmer, 1983). Where there is some temporary reduction in the sperm count, 400–600 cGy can cause azoospermia that may be reversible in three to five years. At a dose of more than 600 cGy, it may be permanent (Ash, 1980). Leydig cell function is rarely impaired until after the administration of 2000 cGy, therefore the 2400 cGy received by boys with testicular relapse can cause significant injury to these cells (Blatt et al., 1985) and so to testosterone production.

Germ cell damage can be detected even when the testes have been exposed to scattered radiation from craniospinal fields (Sklar et al., 1990). Even shielding the testes during pelvic irradiation, for example in the treatment of Hodgkin's disease, may be insufficient to prevent tissue damage that would require several years of healing for sperm production to return (Pedrick & Hoppe, 1986).

Table 25.1: Male pubertal staging			
Genital size	Pubic hair	Concomitant changes	Prader orchidometer
Prepubertal	No pigmented hair	Long testis axis <2.5 cm	1, 2, 3
Early penile, testicular and scrotal growth	Minimal pigmented hair at base of penis	Early voice changes, testes length 2.5–3.3 cm	3, 4, 5, 6, 8
Increased penile length and width, scrotal and testes growth	Dark, coarse, curly hair extends to the mid-line above penis	Light hair on upper lip, acne, maximal growth, testes length 3.3–4.0 cm	10, 12, 15
Increased penile size (inc. width), pigmented scrotum	Considerable but less than an adult distribution	Early sideburns, testes length 4.0–4.5 cm	15, 20
Adult size and shape	Adult distribution that extends to medial thighs or beyond	Beard growth, testes 4.5 cm	25
Source: Tanner (1962) as cited by Lee (1993)			

From this information it can clearly be seen that focal radiotherapy to the testes, as a treatment for a leukaemic recurrence, may cause atrophy and testosterone insufficiency (Brauner et al., 1983). Indeed, those children who receive doses greater than 20 Gy directly to the testes are usually rendered sterile and often require androgen replacement therapy (Shalet et al., 1995). However, current technology in sperm banking means that there is some realistic hope for future procreation (Sweet et al., 1996).

Direct radiation exposure to the ovaries either from focal radiotherapy (Wallace et al., 1989) or TBI (Davies et al., 1989) causes tissue injury and ovarian failure. Ovarian dysfunction is evident when doses as low as 4–8 Gy are absorbed by the ovaries (Hobbie et al., 1993). If both ovaries are not destroyed there may certainly be a reduction in available ovarian follicles so menstruation may occur, but ova supplies soon empty and early menopause is seen. In some girls all ovarian tissue is injured and puberty will never commence without hormone replacement (Table 25.2). Ovarian failure and the resultant lack of oestrogen secretion has dramatic consequences for bone tissue. It results in a progressive loss of trabecular bone significantly increasing the risk of osteoporotic fractures (Hillard et al., 1991). Hormone replacement therapy (HRT) prevents such bone loss and therefore maintains a normal bone density in young women (Cust et al., 1990; Lindsey, 1993; Vermeulen, 1993). These hormones enable normal sexual function to be facilitated but they cannot reverse infertility if ova are destroyed. At this time ova banking is precluded due to the time required to prepare for this very invasive procedure. However, it may be possible in a small number of teenagers to surgically place an ovary out of the radiation field temporarily to preserve its function (Shalet, 1996), this procedure is called an *oöphoropexy*.

Table 25.2: Female pubertal development		
Breast development	Pubic hair	Concomitant changes
Prepubertal, papilla elevation	No pigmentation	–
Budding; larger areolae, palpable and visible elevated contour	Pigmented hair, mainly labial	Accelerated growth rate
Enlargement of the breasts and areola	Coarser spread of pigmented hair over mons	Peak growth rate, thicker vaginal mucosa, axillary hair
Secondary mound of areola and papilla	Adult type but smaller area	Menarche (stage 3 or 4), decelerated growth rate
Mature	Adult distribution	–
Source: Lee (1993)		

In cases where boys have received TBI, the germinal epithelium will undoubtedly have been damaged, if this actually results in ablation of the germinal epithelium then there is almost universal sterility and testosterone production may also cease (Jenney & Kissen, 1996). There may then also be a need for androgen therapy to compensate for the testes' hormonal role in puberty, and possibly after this point to maintain normal libido and sexual function. Lack of testicular growth as a result of these injuries may be cosmetically embarrassing and socially inhibitory. It is for this reason that Jenney and Kissen (1996) recommend that prosthetic implants be offered to these young men.

It is vitally important that nurses discuss these pertinent though often sensitive issues with teenagers and their families.

Nursing note:

Sperm banking is an extremely sensitive issue. It is, however, vital that it is addressed at the appropriate time if it is to have the best possible chance of success. With advances in technology it is now possible to obtain DNA under anaesthetic rather than the collection of sperm itself. Staff need to consider children of all ages rather than just teenagers who may be judged to be sexually aware. It has also been considered more often than not that if the young male has been able to produce sperm prior to therapy then he will be successful in having children in later life. It is important to prepare the teenager and the family for the possibility that sperm may not be viable. In the past, many health professionals have not been very enthusiastic about discussing the possibility of utilising these procedures, but they can have a major effect on the child's self-concept and body image in years to come.

Implications for long term follow-up

Growth charting, pubertal staging (including testicular volume), discussion of possible infertility, and semen analysis (when appropriate) must all be addressed by the multidisciplinary team at each clinic visit.

If there is no sign of puberty by 11 years of age, girls should be considered to be at risk of ovarian failure. In the case of boys, reduced testicular volume in relation to pubertal stage indicates dysfunction. Hormone levels should be monitored closely in all cases (Kissen & Wallace, 1993). Sex steroid therapy with oestrogen preparations for girls and testosterone for boys must be commenced promptly to ensure the development of secondary sexual characteristics; this is continued for life to allow for normal sexual activity. According to Lindsey (1993), dosages vary but blood levels should be kept in the mid-follicular range. There are reported risks of endometrial cancer with oestrogen therapy but this can be reduced if progesterone supplementation is added sequentially for 10–12 days during each cycle (Hillard et al., 1991). There is no further risk of ovarian or cervical cancer documented, and the literature on breast cancer is inconsistent (Davies et al., 1989).

Radiation injury to internal organ systems

Green (1993) draws the attention of health professionals to the greater need for awareness of the long term adverse consequences of radiotherapy in organs such as the heart, kidneys, lungs and bladder. These critical organs have a known level of tolerance of radiation before severe damage is incurred, and these doses should be limiting factors in any proposed therapy to each organ (Table 25.3).

Table 25.3: Normal tissue tolerance doses of radiation	
Tissue	Tolerance dose (Gy)
Whole lung	8
Kidney	15
Liver	20
Spinal cord	50–55

Heart

Shuey (1994) explains that radiotherapy directly to the heart and surrounding blood vessels causes heart disease in a variable number of patients; there is limited data on the long term effects. However, it has been linked with pericarditis, cardiomyopathy, valvular failure, pulmonary hypertension and coronary artery insufficiency (McCoy & Mierzejewski, 1993).

There are varying results found in studies of ECG traces in patients who have received radiotherapy to this area (Ilhan et al., 1995). Diastolic abnormalities have been found in some childhood cancer survivors, which have developed into systolic difficulties. There is also evidence to suggest that greater cardiac malfunction may be detected the longer the patient is past their treatment date. Indeed, generally, cardiac complications due to therapy are manifested approximately ten years after completion of treatment (Lipshultz & Sallan, 1993). Many treatment regimes and more recent dosaging schedules, therefore, may not reveal their true effects for some time to come. Recent studies have found much lower numbers of problems, probably due to the lower doses now used and the greater use of shielding (Kissen, 1996).

Pericarditis, valvular abnormalities, restrictive cardiomyopathy and coronary artery stenosis are all late cardiac complications occurring many years after mantle radiation for Hodgkin's disease (Morgan et al., 1985).

Mediastinal radiotherapy, although rare, can cause measurable heart injury if utilised. It appears to result in thinning of the walls of the left ventricle and to reduce the muscle mass performance (Leandro et al., 1994). Contractility measurement will appear normal but there is evidence of reduced contractile function. It may also produce a pericardial effusion up to five years after therapy (Potijola-Sintonen et al., 1987) in addition to early coronary artery atherosclerosis and atrioventricular valve damage (Hobbie et al., 1993). If the child has also received anthracycline therapy in a chemotherapy protocol then the radiation effects are potentiated.

Implications for long term follow-up

Annual assessment of exercise tolerance and blood pressure must be undertaken and investigated further only if there are clinical indications. Care must be taken to monitor further in pregnancy. All patients with abnormal examination results should be referred to a cardiologist. High risk patients:

- Have received mediastinal or whole lung radiation
- Are pregnant or going through puberty (where there are extra demands on the heart in foetal circulation or the teenage growth spurt)
- Are receiving sex steroid or GH replacement therapy
- Are undertaking strenuous exercise, such as weightlifting.

Lungs

Lung tissue injury is a potential risk in any child who has received radiotherapy to the thoracic, mediastinal, mantle, spinal or flank fields, for primary or metastatic disease. In addition, children who have received TBI may also cause concern.

There are two main problems associated with radiation injury to lung tissue in children: acute pneumonitis and chronic fibrosis. There is, however, also a chance of respiratory compromise when there is evidence of impaired growth of muscle, cartilage and bone of the thoracic cage due to the effects of radiation. Acute pneumonitis presents three to six months post-treatment as fever, congestion, 'hacking' productive cough, dyspnoea and pleuritic pain. Pulmonary investigations show a loss of lung volume and the child exhibits signs of decreased gaseous exchange (Jenney & Kissen, 1996). Chronic fibrosis, conversely, is not seen for months or even years after radiotherapy and although some patients may appear asymptomatic there are many who have chronic respiratory impairment. Steroid therapy is the primary mode of management in the acute phase to relieve symptoms, but their use must be monitored closely.

Flank radiotherapy in children treated for Wilms' tumour also impinges on the lower lung and can cause some degree of impairment of lung function. All children treated using this method may require pulmonary function tests as part of their long term follow-up (Shaw et al., 1991).

The greater the total dose of radiotherapy and the larger the dose per fraction, the greater the risk of significant lung damage. Bleomycin, dactinomycin and doxorubicin significantly increase the amount of damage to the lung. However, lowering radiation doses to 15–25 Gy essentially eliminates this complication (Constine, 1991).

Implications for long term follow-up

Although exercise tolerance should be investigated on each follow-up appointment, pulmonary function testing is only indicated if the child is symptomatic, i.e. has dyspnoea or a persistent cough. It is also necessary to advise strongly against smoking, as any further damage to lung tissue can be extremely hazardous (Hobbie et al., 1993). This is one of many topics that are central to the health education focus of the nurse's role in long term follow-up. As time passes and new issues and problems arise nurses must be able to inform the child or teenager on the most appropriate health behaviour to minimise the injury or its effect on their life and future health, for example flu vaccinations in the winter months. Education on diet, exercise, medications, vigilance in preventing infection and the dangers of smoking must be made available to these young people to ensure that they are given the opportunity to make informed health choices for the rest of their lives (Rose, 1989).

Liver

Upper abdominal and lower thoracic radiation fields that involve any portion of the liver and, of course, TBI, may result in liver toxicity.

If a large hepatic volume is irradiated with more than 30 Gy, signs of liver toxicity will begin to appear within three months. The clinical picture is one of increased abdominal girth, portal hypertension, ascites, jaundice and raised liver function tests (Constine, 1991). Children appear to be more susceptible to liver injury than adults. In addition, if the child has also been treated with dactinomycin, a drug potentially toxic to the liver, there can be sudden and severe thrombocytopenia. Veno-occlusive disease is a severe but rare complication of TBI in transplant patients. It can occur even in very low dose single-fraction radiotherapy (Woods et al., 1980).

Flentje et al. (1994) suggest that there is some evidence of liver toxicity in children receiving abdominal radiotherapy for Wilms' tumour. Symptoms of such toxicity may begin to present six weeks after the start of radiotherapy if the liver is within the main field, and the level of toxicity significantly increases if the majority of the liver receives over 20 Gy.

Implications for long term follow-up

The function of the liver should always be assessed at the end of treatment and then only revisited if there are clinical indications to do so. Any evidence of severe liver toxicity will require close follow-up and possible intervention from specialised medical personnel and dietetic consultants. Support and education may be required from nursing staff in the clinic on diet, fluids and protection from bleeding.

Kidneys

Renal function impairment is a late effect of radiotherapy that includes either kidney in the treatment field. Mild problems may be evidenced by hypertension but more severe damage may lead to acute renal failure (Taylor, 1996). The clinical signs of tissue damage may not be visible for two to three years after treatment.

The only early symptom of acute renal damage due to radiotherapy is likely to be a decreased glomerular filtration rate (GFR). As the condition becomes worse, symptoms such as headache, peripheral oedema, anaemia, hypertension, proteinurea and increasing levels of waste products in the blood will be observed, finally leading to renal failure and possible death from associated complications (Constine, 1991).

Abdominal radiation for Wilms' tumour, neuroblastoma and lymphoma have all been associated with renal damage (Cassady et al., 1981). The severity of impairment is dose-related, with the most severe problems occurring when the dose exceeds 25 Gy to both kidneys (Constine, 1991).

Implications for long term follow-up

A child who has received irradiation to the kidney must have their renal function monitored closely on follow-up if there are any signs of chronic nephritis or renal impairment. Prompt treatment of infection, as well as ensuring that the family is aware that they must alert medical staff to this fact if they are ever treated away from their oncology unit, is good prophylaxis.

Uterus

In girls receiving abdominal or pelvic radiation there is considerable risk of uterine injury even when ovarian function has been preserved (Shalet, 1996). Exposure to 20–30 Gy of radiation to the abdomen in childhood has been shown to result in severe difficulties in maintaining a successful pregnancy (Wallace et al., 1989). Prepubertal exposure may also have devastating structural effects on the vasculature and size of the developing uterus (Shalet, 1996). It appears that girls who receive significant doses of abdominal irradiation in their childhood are unlikely to carry a pregnancy to term. This has implications for consent to treatment, late effects, education and the importance of close monitoring and support of young women in this situation who become pregnant.

Bladder

Yeung et al. (1994) found that children who have received radiotherapy to the bladder, using external beam and brachytherapy, can be left with reduced functional capacity and an abnormal voiding pattern. This may result in the need for upper urinary tract dilatation or surgery for severe bilateral hydronephrosis. The researchers felt that this is an area that could benefit from accurate assessment to help pinpoint the problem, including charting the frequency and volume of voiding patterns. This may be a potentially distressing and serious complication for many children and requires effective education and ongoing nursing support for the child and the family.

There is also evidence of problems of chronic inflammation leading to fibrosis of the bladder and recurrent cystitis after pelvic radiotherapy (Green, 1989). Each symptom can be extremely painful, distressing and socially inhibitory. Faithful (1995) comments that urinary symptoms after pelvic radiotherapy can be debilitating, especially in males. She further proposes that health care professionals are not much further forward in dealing with it although it significantly reduces quality of life. Nurses must be sensitive to these distressing symptoms, assessing pain and discomfort, and planning appropriate care. Advice may be necessary on pain control, fluid intake and planning daily routines to allow for increased frequency of micturition. It may also be necessary to facilitate the expression of negative feelings by the child on having such a distressing and potentially embarrassing problem.

Eyes

There are several tissue groups within the eye and each varies considerably in its sensitivity to radiation. Acute reactions observed on irradiating the eye include iridocyclitis, keratitis and conjunctivitis. Late reactions (often six months or more after treatment) manifest as retinopathy, optic neuropathy, lachrymal gland atrophy or duct stenosis, glaucoma, cataract, corneal vascularisation and scarring, conjunctival telangiectasia and eyelid atrophy (Heyn et al., 1986). Servodidio and Abramson (1993) state that late effects of direct radiation to the eye can be even more severe and may include melting, cataract, corneal neovascularisation, retinopathy, retarded bone growth and secondary malignancies. All these symptoms can cause pain, visual disturbance and even visual loss.

Until 1985 it was common practice to irradiate the whole eye when radiotherapy was chosen above enucleation as the prime modality of treatment for retinoblastoma. Although this was effective in eradicating the tumour, it left behind significant morbidity: eyelid damage, impaired tear production and a high incidence of cataract formation (Hungerford et al., 1995). Since this time, however, it has become common practice in conservative treatment for this tumour to use a lens-sparing technique with little loss of efficacy in tumour control. The immediate side effect is mild erythema only, but more worrying is the long term effect of middle facial bone growth retardation (Hungerford et al., 1995). In some cases, there remains the risk of slight cataract formation and it appears there may be an increased risk of tumour arising in the unirradiated anterior chamber.

TBI may also have adverse effects on the eyes if they are not shielded, which may not be the case if insuring against leukaemic infiltrates. Low-dose radiation causes damage to the germinal layer of epithelium on the lens which leads to cataract formation (Constine, 1991). Calissendorff et al. (1991) documented the development of cataracts in children after bone marrow transplant by use of a single fraction of 10 Gy TBI as a conditioning regime.

They were, however, able to prove that doses of 8 Gy rather than 10 Gy administered with eye shields did not result in cataract formation.

Although single-fraction TBI is the known cause of cataracts and lachrymal gland dysfunction, Locatelli et al. (1993) found that these problems may occasionally also be found in children with fractionated regimes.

Implications for long term follow-up

Annual history-taking should include any visual problems and ophthalmoscopy should be performed to examine the lens. If cataracts are discovered an ophthalmic referral should be instigated. Many of the severe effects stated will have an extreme effect on the visual appearance of the child and therefore may cause problems with body image. It is imperative that these children have access to trained psychological support, to enable them to work through these issues.

Teeth

Severe abnormal ondontogenesis can be seen in children that have received radiotherapy to the area in addition to chemotherapy (Kaste et al., 1994). The damage caused to children's teeth by inclusion in a radiation field is likely to result in permanent functional and cosmetic problems which may have a profound psychological effect. Injury may only be apparent in some children when their teeth actually erupt in the buccal cavity. Treatment for head and neck tumours is the most likely cause of such irradiation damage. All health professionals, especially dentists, must anticipate this potential problem and monitor the situation closely.

In addition, approximately 40% of children who receive cranial radiation for CNS leukaemia prophylaxis, also exhibit some molar damage (Constine, 1991). TBI has also been associated with impaired root development, microdontia and enamel hypoplasia (Dalhllof et al., 1988).

Permanent injury may also be inflicted on the salivary glands when irradiating the head and neck at doses above 50 Gy (Fromm et al., 1986). Secretions may be permanently lost with significant long term consequences for infection control and mastication.

With such potential for problematic dentition, it is essential that regular dental assessment is performed and corrective orthodontics instigated promptly.

Bone Marrow

The bone marrow is extremely sensitive to radiation, hence the use of TBI as part of the conditioning regime for transplant. The immediate effects of radiation have already been outlined in some detail, as some degree of injury occurs with any fractionated dose. The increased sensitivity of children's bone marrow to radiotherapy may be linked to the differing extent of active bone marrow at different ages (Cristy, 1981). In the neonatal period, conversion to functional yellow fatty marrow progresses from the extremities to the axial skeleton and from the diaphysis to metaphysis in the long bones. Some researchers suggest that this young marrow has a greater regenerative capacity for, as yet, unknown reasons.

Radiation damage may cause permanent aplasia if localised regions receive doses of 20 Gy or more in a single fraction (Constine, 1991). This is not a normal occurrence in paediatric oncology but 40 Gy in fractionated doses can mean that bone marrow may take up to two years to recover, and in 45% of patients recovery may not be complete.

Secondary Malignancies

The precise mechanism of how secondary malignancy occurs in some childhood cancer survivors is not fully understood (Rodriguez & Ash, 1996). However, D'Angio and Green (1995) propose that there is malignant cell transformation in individuals due to their genetic predisposition. In addition, the radiotherapy acts not only as an immunosuppressor but also as a cell mutation initiator. They go on to suggest that promotion of tumour growth is enhanced by the combination of chemotherapy and radiotherapy. Hawkins (1990) states that there is confirmation that radiotherapy is associated with an increased risk of further malignancies. Over 9000 cases of childhood cancer, treated in the UK before 1980, were reviewed and it was found that these children were about five times more at risk of a second primary tumour than the general population. In those treated with radiotherapy alone, the risk increased to six times and in those treated with radiotherapy and chemotherapy the risk rose to nine times that expected in the general population.

Many papers have been written on the most potent influencing factors (Fraser & Tucker, 1988; Biti et al., 1994; Meadows & Fenton, 1994; Bokemeyer & Schmoll, 1995) and the most common recurring factors are:

- Larger total doses
- Larger number of fractions
- The use of orthovoltage rather than megavoltage (this form of radiation is no longer used in the treatment of children)
- The use of combinations of chemotherapy and radiotherapy
- The younger the child at exposure, whilst there is still active proliferation in body tissues.

This information has implications for long term follow-up and health education. Girls who have received radiotherapy to fields that have incorporated breast tissue should be taught regular self-examination and awareness to monitor for possible malignancies. Regular follow-up should include physical examination of the breast and discussion of the risk of failure to lactate after pregnancy.

Effects on Children of Long Term Adverse Effects of Radiotherapy

Physical changes have a profound effect on children's growth when they receive cancer therapy. They may experience severe difficulties in adjusting to physical changes, especially reduced growth and development, and there may be significant problems with body image (see Chapter 4). This may lead to distress and frustration and perhaps even to psychological morbidity. The social impact and psychological demands of such difficulties can be greater than the diagnosis of cancer (Gray et al., 1992; Hoffman, 1992; Ruccione 1994).

Residual physical and cognitive problems may result in limited job performance and decreased participation in activities of daily living, which will lead to poor daily functioning and dependency (Ruccione, 1994). Rodriguez and Ash (1996) suggest that nurses should consider the following in planning appropriate support for these children and their families:

- Education
- Physiological monitoring
- Promotion of existing coping abilities
- Taking all concerns seriously, especially about secondary malignancies
- Psychological support referrals.

Health promotion

Health promotion is an important role of the paediatric oncology nurse in the long term follow-up setting. As children grow up they start making health choices for themselves and this sometimes includes taking health risks as part of their normal adolescent development. Smoking cigarettes, drinking alcohol, experimenting with recreational drugs and unprotected sexual intercourse may be some of the options open to them in today's society. Children's nurses cannot ignore these issues simply because they are not recommended for continued health. After many months or even years of overprotection by family and professionals the desire to rebel may be significant. Young men and women who have been prepared that they may be infertile may see contraception, and more especially condoms, as unnecessary, thus leaving themselves vulnerable to infection (HIV, hepatitis, sexually transmitted diseases) and unwanted pregnancies. Consuming alcohol and smoking tobacco may seem attractive, yet they may aggravate underlying heart, liver and lung injury. Finally, recreational drugs are a common concern for many parents, and the acute side effects of tachycardia and severe dehydration are well-documented. To a child with underlying cardiac injury these problems may be extremely harmful. However, a dictatorial authoritarian approach to discouraging these pursuits is often unrewarding. Nurses must discuss these topics openly and calmly with information that is accurate and up-to-date for each child/teenager. Perhaps encouraging other more positive ways of expressing independent thought and action may be more useful. As risk-taking is a normal part of development, outdoor pursuits and sports may be less dangerous. However, there is a duty to educate these young people about the facts and allow them to make some decisions in full cognisance of the likely consequences of their actions.

Martinez-Clement et al. (1994) developed a scale for assessing quality of life in survivors of childhood brain tumours. It focused on three main concerns: physical, psycho-intellectual and endocrine/growth. These authors found when using this tool that children treated with radiotherapy before four years of age demonstrated lower scores. The same applied to children who had received treatment for posterior fossa tumours where incomplete resection required significant use of radiotherapy. Their results were comparable to the literature so far in these areas that has indicated multiple problems in such children. Indeed, Syndikus et al. (1994), in a study of children treated successfully for brain tumours, discovered that morbidity was disabling in 58% of children treated at or below three years of age.

It is therefore essential for those involved in the care of children receiving radiotherapy treatment to develop a more thorough knowledge base and utilise up-to-date research in the provision of care. This is a most important issue in relation to informed consent, when ensuring that the child and the family are able to make an informed decision about treatment.

Once treatment has taken place and the child is no longer in immediate danger of dying from disease the long term follow-up team must begin their work in earnest.

Livesey et al. (1990) observed that diligent endocrine follow-up is required for children treated for brain tumours, and that anticipation of hormone deficiencies, leading to early diagnosis and treatment, can improve the quality of life for survivors. Quigley et al. (1989) also stress the importance of regular and accurate monitoring, including good baseline data prior to treatment, which incorporates an assessment of standing height, sitting height, weight, bone-age, pubertal assessment and testicular volume, measured by means of an orchidometer. Larson et al. (1990) reiterate the fact that although treatment for childhood cancer now results in a greater than 60% cure rate, whether used alone or in combination with chemotherapy, the treatment also carries the potential of multiorgan system morbidity which may last a lifetime. Although it is not within the nurse's power to prevent many of these problems, knowledge of them can assist in preparing families and responding swiftly and accurately to acute and chronic needs, physical or emotional.

The recommendations for all oncological follow-up in regional late effects clinics are as documented in the UKCCSG guidelines for long term follow-up (Kissen & Wallace, 1993).

Nursing Care Issues in Long Term Follow-up

Nurses have an important part to play in the development of these recommendations, and are able to assist in dealing with issues such as sexuality, body image, family relationships and adaptation. As previously stated, nurses must have a sound knowledge base about the late effects of radiotherapy. Almost all of the late effects of radiotherapy directly or indirectly affect either function, self-image or growth potential (physically or cognitively), and in all likelihood a combination of all three (Commeau Lew, 1992).

In addition to the medical support that can be offered by additional specialist members of the interdisciplinary team to deal with some of the more severe physical injuries, psychosocial support for the child and the family is the main focus for nursing care in long term follow-up.

The success of psychosocial support for childhood cancer survivors depends upon early assessment, prevention and intervention (Lansky et al., 1993). It is recommended that in view of the increasing timespan between clinic appointments, a small group of professionals, representing all aspects of the multidisciplinary team, takes responsibility for this area of care in order to build on relationships and to facilitate continuity of care (Kissen, 1996).

Successful coping with physical and psychosocial developments, as a result of treatment or disease, demands adaptation to many new concepts, experiences and realities once therapy for cancer is completed. The legacy of diagnosis, treatment and the concept of survivorship is left for the child and the family to comprehend, adapt to and work with for the rest of their lives. The literature on psychosocial morbidity is still exploratory and at times confusing. In addition, much of it was carried out on children who were actually treated many years ago, however, psychologists of today still find aspects of their conclusions valid. Many eminent authors (Koocher et al., 1980; Koocher & O'Malley, 1981; Lansky et al., 1993; Mulhern et al., 1989) discuss the significant prevalence of psychosocial morbidity in children when treatment is complete, whereas there is literature to argue that this is not always the case and, indeed, there have been some more positive developments (Teta et al., 1986; Tebbi & Mallon, 1987; Fritz & Williams, 1988; Spirito et al., 1990). This apparent dichotomy in the literature may be explained by a hypothesis of Lansky et al. (1993), who propose that these children are not at greater risk of psychosocial morbidity but rather that they are more vulnerable to intermittent adjustment problems (Barbarin, 1987). That is, as each new stage of child or family development becomes evident, there may be some difficulty in the childhood cancer survivor responding effectively immediately.

Research evidence to support appropriate intermittent intervention to meet these adjustment problems is scarce (Kazak, 1994), except strategies for dealing with acute anxiety and the problems of returning to school. The promotion of recognised coping strategies, therefore, must be utilised to guide nursing practice in this area.

Adjustment, adaptation and coping are the goals of nursing care for the child and the family in a partnership framework of care. Nursing care can facilitate these achievements by building on the work of Spinetta (1977) and Koocher and O'Malley (1981) who adapted recognised frameworks for coping to the needs of the childhood cancer survivor. They proposed that the child must learn to manage periods of distress and anxiety, maintain self-value and esteem, maintain rewarding interpersonal relationships with family and friends and, finally, access and use available resources for support and guidance. This can be facilitated by health professionals using interventions that concur with positive coping strategies (Hurwitz et al., 1962). The child and the family must understand the implications of disease, treatment, and long term survival, as well as being able to express and manage complex emotions (Kupst, 1994). These issues can be translated into nursing interventions for long term care and support of childhood cancer survivors and their families.

Nurses must develop teaching programmes to facilitate education of the parents and the child on the possible symptoms of radiation injury that may occur, based on their dose of radiotherapy and the field treated (Mullen, 1984; Hobbie et al., 1993; Kissen, 1996). Symptoms will therefore be interpreted by the family as treatment-related and not recurrence, which may cause extreme distress and anxiety. Understanding what may happen to the body and why promotes a sense of control in the child. In addition, it allows them to plan for differing situations and so facilitate more effective coping. Health education is an essential component of these programmes.

Effective listening, communication and interviewing skills are essential in all team members to assess many factors influencing the coping abilities of the child and the family:

- The situation at home
- Issues concerning body image
- Coping with functional problems
- Re-integration and rehabilitation into normal daily routine and responsibilities
- The evolving roles and functions of family, school and peer relationships
  (Barbarin, 1987; Hymovich & Roehnart, 1989).

In addition, use of such skills may encourage the expression of negative emotions by family members and children themselves regarding misconceptions or perceived lack of knowledge related to the long term consequences of therapy. It is not uncommon for the family to feel that they were left with extremely difficult choices between potentially hazardous therapy and overwhelming disease at diagnosis.

Extensive health assessments should be carried out at clinic reviews to ensure early detection of late effects or treatment consequences (Hobbie et al., 1993; Kissen, 1996). In this way early intervention or further referral can be expedited. Paediatric oncology nurses should have the necessary knowledge and skill to play a significant role in ascertaining this information from the child and the family.

The medical care and intervention for the treatment of any late effects will vary slightly from centre to centre, however, in each case the child and the family require information and support to ensure their informed consent to treatment and knowledge of possible outcomes (Everhart, 1991). It is essential that they are prepared for all further investigations to monitor the extent of radiation injury and are involved fully in the discussion of investigative results and proposed treatment plans.

Positive self-image is widely cited within the literature as a possible area of difficulty for the child after treatment, especially in view of the many potential problems associated with growth and development after irradiation. Helping the child and the family to focus and work with positive aspects of their life and society has been found to be an effective coping strategy (Chesler & Barbarin, 1987).

Counselling may be a further role to be undertaken by appropriately trained nursing staff to faciliatate the child and/or family members in their growing understanding of their developing needs, and in planning strategies to cope with them (Mullen, 1984). The many realities and concepts facing these children and their families include:

- Becoming more independent of the close observation of the hospital (Edbaugh, 1988)
- Coping with the threat of recurrence (Koocher & O'Malley, 1981)
- Coping with impaired physical functioning (Meadows & Silber, 1985) and perhaps learning disabilities (Mulhern et al., 1992)
- Developing and promoting a positive body image within the child (Fritz & Williams, 1988; Kazak, 1994)
- The promotion of exploration of the child's own sexuality in view of possible infertility (Byrne et al., 1987)
- Coping with delayed or early puberty (Wasserman et al., 1987)
- Changing peer relationships (Kazak, 1994).

Referral to a psychologist or psychiatrist must be considered when there is concern about increasing difficulties in adaptation to life after cancer and treatment (Hobbie et al., 1993; Kazak, 1994). There may be difficulties in working through what has and is happening within the family, in addition to understanding and building coping strategies and adaptations. It is essential that paediatric oncology nurses recognise their own limitations in dealing with such complex needs and utilise the resources within the team to ensure the most appropriate support for the whole family.

Communication between members of the family is necessary for each member to support one another through the adaptation process which may be life long. Facilitation of this process can create an environment in which family members, including the child who has been treated for cancer, can express feelings, concerns and needs, in addition to listening to one another (Koocher & O'Malley, 1981; Chesler & Barbarin, 1987; Fritz et al., 1988).

It is imperative that the family becomes increasingly independent of intensive services in order to carry on with its own life. Ultimate self-care skills will be the ability to support, seek support (Chesler & Barbarin, 1987; Kupst & Schulman, 1988) and facilitate coping in one another but this can only become possible if communication pathways are open and functional within a family group.

Also needed are ongoing support and guidance from the multi-disciplinary team to facilitate the family's access to further supportive networks, such as voluntary agencies and support groups (Hobbie et al., 1993). Continuing health education is also required, including school liaison to assist the child and the family to continue to develop their coping mechanisms and to deal with each new situation or difficulty in an informed and controlled manner (Rose, 1989).

Future Trends in Radiotherapy

It is well-known that cranial or spinal radiotherapy should not be considered in children under two years of age in normal circumstances, due to their neural state of incomplete myelinisation making them at extremely high risk for long term neurological side effects. However, it is worth noting that the highest incidence of childhood malignancy is in the 0–4-year-olds (Doyle, 1984). Stereotactically implanted sealed sources to deliver brachytherapy in brain tumours may be one way to avoid full brain toxicity in young children. Radioactive silver (Ag^{98}) and iridium (Ir^{192}) are used as they can achieve fast-falling dose gradients at the periphery of the tumour and protect healthy brain tissue from damage (Thompson et al., 1989).

In addition, use of the stereotactical multiple arcing rotational technique may be a revolution in more efficiently targeting radiotherapy (Plowman, 1992). A linear accelerator is mounted so that it can move rapidly to create arcs whereby the lesion is constantly in the path of the beam. Healthy tissue is excluded from the arc and so is spared irradiation. So far, this has only been used on small spherical tumours, such as a low grade astrocytoma. Targeted radiotherapy can also be delivered using monoclonal antibodies (Pizer & Kemshead, 1994) and may increase in efficacy in coming years.

Athough radiotherapy has and will continue to play a significant role in the effective treatment of childhood malignancies, the consequences of its use must be addressed in both research, practice and professional issues such as consent. It is a complex and potentially harmful therapy, but it can be exceptionally effective for a number of highly malignant neoplasms.

Nurses have an important role in the preparation and education of children and their families to make an informed decision about treatment and to facilitate their coping with the possible adverse effects on the child physically and psychosocially, both before and after treatment. Caring for the child who has received radiotherapy is challenging both in the short term with acute effects, but perhaps more especially in the long term follow-up clinics. Evening clinics with appointment times, crèche facilities and a dedicated interdisciplinary team of personnel committed to late effects care are developing around the country.

The literature on the experience of children after treatment is extensive and overwhelmingly it indicates that although treatment may be increasingly effective in curing cancer it is crucial to ensure that children are able to survive and live rather than exist afterwards. The critical influence determining the difference between effective non-traumatic therapy and patient distress are the team members that care for these children and their families throughout the treatment experience. All team members have a responsibility to ensure that there is disease irradication with the least possible harm to children and their families.

The future: what does it hold?

A practical approach focusing on the detailed nursing management of care, underpinned by theory and research, has been the realised aim of this textbook. The book is grounded in a philosophy of family-centred care and negotiation, with an emphasis on a multi-disciplinary approach. The ultimate aim is to inform practice so that the quality of care is improved by increasing the body of knowledge; knowledge that is embedded in the practice itself (Benner, 1983; Benner et al., 1996), recognising that 'a wealth of untapped knowledge is embedded in the practices and the "know how" of expert clinicians' (Benner, 1984, p. 11). This 'know how' is acquired through experience (Benner, 1983), experience being a requisite for expertise (Benner, 1984) and for the development of knowledge (Urden, 1989). It is this knowledge that is difficult to capture in a nursing textbook and within nursing theory. However, central to the advancement of nursing practice and the development of a nursing knowledge base, is the recognition and understanding of clinical knowledge (Benner & Wrubel, 1982). It is this clinical knowledge that is well described within this book, providing the focus for the explication of nursing practice. To this end the content has begun to map the domain of nursing practice in paediatric oncology, 'a domain that has both theoretical and practical boundaries' (Meleis, 1997, p. 102).

This book has enabled expert practitioners to 'unlock the knowledge they hold in their heads' (Pearson, 1992, p. 213), and to reveal the 'know how' of practising nurses. Many nursing practices are inherently difficult to describe and convey to others, and yet often they are the very things that make a difference to care. Participants in a study by Macleod (1994) make reference to 'the little things that count' (p. 365), not to be thought of as insignificant, especially as Benner (1984) argues that it is these 'little things' of patient care that are the hallmarks of nursing expertise. The 'Nursing notes' within

503

the text are examples of those little things, where expert paediatric nurses attempt to articulate those everyday, taken-for-granted practices that are imbued with nursing knowledge and skill. These practices often reflect their ability to successfully transfer theoretical knowledge into practice, and are central to skilled clinical judgement (Facione & Facione, 1996).

The theoretical basis of this book is well established and provides a common ground for communication for nurses. The book is evidence that theory and theoretical thinking are not limited to the theoreticians within our profession; theoretical thinking is integral to all the roles played by nurses (Meleis, 1997). Meleis (1997) defines nursing theory as 'a conceptualization of some aspect of nursing reality communicated for the purpose of describing phenomena, explaining relationships between the phenomena, predicting consequences, or prescribing nursing care' (p. 12). This definition is not unlike the description of theoretical knowledge by Benner (1984), identified as 'knowing that' and includes formal statements about the interactional and causal relationships between events (p. 298). Elements of this are well articulated within each section of this text.

The two areas of knowledge clearly distinguishable within this book are what Benner (1983), citing Polanyi (1958) and Kuhn (1962), refers to as 'know how' and 'know that'. These are terms seeking to distinguish between practical and theoretical knowledge, 'where often the "know how" knowledge has been acquired through practice and experience and often cannot be theoretically accounted for by "know that" knowledge' (Manley, 1991, p. 2). The practitioners examining paediatric oncology practice are clearly involved in both practical and theoretical achievements, where one is used for the benefit of the other. Their description and use of practical knowledge thus charts the existence of 'know how' developed through clinical experience and 'is essential to the development and extension of nursing theory' (Benner, 1984, p. 11). The importance of this practice-based knowledge is well recognised by Benner (1983, 1984) and Schön (1983) with the 'know how' and 'know that' domains of knowledge being apportioned equal importance and therefore equal value, a view endorsed throughout this book.

Knowledge can be gained from a number of different sources, each of which has something to offer in our total understanding or 'knowing' (Vaughan, 1992). The contribution of knowledge gained from other disciplines is in evidence within this book. The benefits of such knowledge cannot go unrecognised, however; it must also be recognised how expert practitioners have applied that knowledge to create something different. It is this that makes the knowledge unique to nursing. A nursing perspective on these different sources of knowledge is apparent throughout, and has been shaped by what Meleis (1997, p. 93) refers to as 'defining characteristics' of nursing: the nature of nursing science as a human science; practice aspects of nursing; caring relationships that nurses and patients develop; and a health and wellness perspective. These perspectives reflect shared views that define the way that nurses assess their patients and their situations in order to identify an individual plan of care. Visintainer (1986) suggests that it is nurses who 'assemble the package, using different perspectives, or different maps ... from many different disciplines' (p. 35). Multidisciplinary teamwork, affirmed within this book, ensures that sources of knowledge from all disciplines are used, with all roles complementing one another. The particular knowledge and theories of the various disciplines used will depend on the demands of the care situation (Visintainer, 1986) in addition to the knowledge of individuals and their environments.

Knowing the patient is now considered to be a key component of excellent nursing practice (Jenny & Logan, 1992). It has been considered a 'central theme in nurses' everyday discourse about their practice' (Tanner et al., 1993, p. 273) and is essential for success when making clinical decisions (Jenks, 1993). Throughout this book, expert practitioners reveal the knowledge of children that facilitates their decision-making, resulting in their ability to personalise the nursing care being prescribed. It is this process of knowing the patient that shapes caring activities and is inextricably linked to patient outcomes (Macleod, 1994). The skill of caring is a core activity in nursing practice (Benner & Wrubel, 1989), with the child and the family benefiting from theoretical and practical knowledge that is enhanced by 'knowing the patient'. The nature of knowing in nursing has yet to be fully articulated, however, it will emerge if the world can be viewed through the eyes of practising nurses and their patients (Schultz & Meleis, 1988). This book has provided one such opportunity for a group of expert practitioners within the field of paediatric oncology.

Expert nurses bring to a caring situation 'knowing that', 'knowing how' and 'knowing self'; a connected knowing where 'knowing self' is part of understanding what is known (Schultz & Meleis, 1988). 'Knowledge is the product of knowing' (Manley, 1991, p. 1) and experience is the essential component for the development of that knowledge (Urden, 1989). The work of Carper (1978) (referred to within this book) offers a taxonomy of nursing knowledge in which all parts are inter-related and interdependent. She suggests that there are four 'fundamental patterns of knowing in nursing giving attention to what it means to know and what kinds of knowledge are held to be of most value in the discipline of nursing' (p. 13). The four areas referred to are: empirics, the science of nursing; aesthetics, the art of nursing; personal knowledge; and ethics, moral knowledge in nursing. Notions of these can be seen in this book, providing an understanding of clinical experience (Vaughan, 1992), as expert practitioners attempt to articulate what they know of nursing. In addition, Carper's (1978) work provides a useful framework when reflecting on the content. 'Knowing nursing' may, therefore, incorporate all four patterns of knowledge (Pearson, 1992), not all of which have been easy to articulate and document.

Practitioners within this book have attempted to unlock the knowledge that they hold in their heads and to begin to describe the notions of 'know how' and 'know that' resulting from clinical experience gained within their speciality. Their ability to do so can only benefit other paediatric oncology nurses, as well as the profession, ultimately improving care for children and their families. As nursing advances (Autar, 1996; Manley, 1997; Goodman, 1998; UKCC, 1998), evidenced by the emergence of advanced nurse practitioner roles (Hockenberry-Eaton & Jordan, 1992; Read, 1995; Fergusson & Diserens, 1996; Barnes & Shaw, 1998), our knowledge base, theoretical and practical, must also advance: education and clinical experience together preparing paediatric oncology nurses for practice (Gibson & Langton, 1998).

We must take every opportunity to examine nursing expertise and experience in order to reveal the new complexities within nursing practice. The expert practitioners here have demonstrated successfully how it is possible to describe and document practice. Only then 'will the knowledge embedded in these skilled practices be recognised, enhanced, and communicated' (Benner & Wrubel, 1982, p. 17), revealing the link between theoretical knowledge and practice (Macleod, 1994).

Faith Gibson and Margaret Evans

References

Autar R (1996) The scope of professional practice in specialist practice. British Journal of Nursing 5(16): 984–989.

Barnes K, Shaw D (1998) Advanced practice in the US: part one the paediatric nurse practitioner. Paediatric Nursing 10(9): 30–34.

Benner P (1983) Uncovering the knowledge embedded in clinical practice. Image: Journal of Nursing Scholarship 15(2): 36–41.

Benner P (1984) From Novice to Expert: Excellence and Power in Clinical Nursing Practise. Menlo Park, CA: Addison-Wesley.

Benner P, Wrubel J (1982) Skilled clinical knowledge: the value of perceptual awareness. Nurse Educator 7: 11–17.

Benner P, Wrubel J (1989) The Primacy of Caring: Stress and Coping in Health and Illness. Menlo Park, CA: Addison-Wesley.

Benner P, Tanner CA, Chesla CA (1996) Expertise in Nursing Practice: Caring, Clinical Judgement and Ethics. New York: Springer.

Carper BA (1978) Fundamental patterns of knowing in nursing. Advances in Nursing Science 1(1): 13–23.

Facione NC, Facione PA (1996) Externalizing the critical thinking knowledge development and clinical judgement. Nursing Outlook 44(3): 129–136.

Fergusson JH, Diserens D (1996) A comparison of the educational needs of advanced practice nurses in pediatric oncology: 1987 and 1995. Journal of Pediatric Oncology 13(4): 204–211.

Gibson F, Langton H (1998) Paediatric oncology nurse education: past, current and future pathways for specialist preparation. European Journal of Oncology Nursing 2(3): 178–181.

Goodman I (1998) Evaluation and evolution: the contribution of the advanced practitioner to cancer care. In Rolfe G, Fulbrook P (eds), Advanced Nursing Practice. Oxford: Butterworth Heinemann.

Hockenberry-Eaton M, Jordan C (1992) The pediatric nurse practitioner and the physician assistant: how are we different? Journal of Pediatric Health Care 6(6): 383–384.

Jenks JM (1993) The pattern of personal knowing in nurse clinical decision making. Journal of Nursing Education 32(9): 399–405.

Jenny J, Logan J (1992) Knowing the patient: one aspect of clinical knowledge. Image: Journal of Nursing Scholarship 24(4): 254–258.

Macleod M (1994) 'It's the little things that count': the hidden complexity of every-day clinical nursing practice. Journal of Clinical Nursing 3(6): 361–368.

Macleod MLP (1996) Practicing Nursing — Becoming Experienced. New York: Churchill Livingstone.

Manley K (1991) Knowledge for nursing practice. In Perry A, Jolley M (eds), A Knowledge Base for Practice. London: Edward Arnold.

Manley K (1997) A conceptual framework for advanced practice: an action research project operationalizing an advanced practitioner/consultant nursing role. Journal of Clinical Nursing 6(3): 179–190.

Meleis AL (1997) Theoretical Nursing: Development and Progess (third edition). Philadelphia: Lippincott.

Pearson A (1992) Knowing nursing: emerging paradigms in nursing. In Robinson K, Vaughan B (eds), Knowledge for Nursing Practice. Oxford: Butterworth Heinemann, pp. 213–226.

Read S (1995) Catching the tide: new voyages in nursing? SCHARR, Occasional Paper No. 1.

Schön DA (1983) The Reflective Practitioner: How Professionals Think and Act. New York: Basic Books.

Schultz PR, Meleis AI (1988) Nursing epistemology: traditions, insights, questions. Image: Journal of Nursing Scholarship 20(4): 217–221.

Tanner CA, Benner P, Chesla C, Gordon DR (1993) The phenomenology of knowing the patient. Image: Journal of Nursing Scholarship 25(4): 273–280.

United Kingdom Central Council for Nursing, Midwifery and Health Visiting (1998) Higher level of practice — specialist practice project phase II. London: UKCC.

Urden LD (1989) Knowledge development in clinical practice. Journal of Continuing Education in Nursing 20(1): 18–22.

Vaughan B (1992) Exploring the knowledge of nursing practice. Journal of Clinical Nursing 1(3): 161–166.

Visintainer MA (1986) The nature of knowledge and theory in nursing. Image: Journal of Nursing Scholarship 18(2): 32–38.

References
Section One

Abu-Saad H (1993) Pediatric Pain Management: An Intervention Study. Paper presented at Royal Collge of Nursing 1st International Conference in Paediatrics, Cambridge, UK.

Adams L (1993) Managing chemotherapy-induced nausea and vomiting. Professional Nurse 9(2): 91–94.

Adwani SS, Whitehead BF, Rees PH, Whitmore P, Elliot MJ, De Leval MR (1995) Heart transplantation for dilated cardiomyopathy. Archives of Disease in Childhood 73(5): 447–452.

Aistars J (1987) Fatigue in the cancer patient: a conceptual approach to a clinical problem. Oncology Nurses Forum 14(6): 25–29.

Aitken TJ (1992) Gastrointestinal manifestations in the child with cancer. Journal of Pediatric Oncology Nursing 9(3): 99–109.

Akers JA, Bell SK (1994) Should children be used as research subjects? Nursing Forum 29(3): 28–33.

Albano EA, Pizzo PA (1988) Infectious complications in childhood acute leukemias. Pediatric Clinics of North America 35(4): 873–901.

Alderson P, Montgomery J (1996) Participation and Consent. Health Care Choices: Making Decisions with Children series. London: Institute for Public Policy Research.

Allegretta GJ, Weisman SJ, Altman AJ (1985) Oncologic emergencies 1. Pediatric Clinics of North America 32(3): 601–611.

Allison K, Kellick M, Meyers P (1996) Administration of high-dose methotrexate (12 g/m²) and management of toxicity in the outpatient setting. (Abstract) Medical and Pediatric Oncology 27(4): 274.

Andrejak M, Lafon B, Decoq G, Chetaille E, Dupas JL, Ducroix JP, Capron JP (1996) Antibiotic associated pseudomembranous colitis: retrospective study of 48 cases diagnosed by colonoscopy. Therapie 51(1): 81–86.

Andrews PLR, Davis CJ (1993) The mechanism of emesis induced by anti-cancer therapies. In Andrews PLR, Sanger G (eds), Emesis in Anti-cancer Therapy: Mechanism and Treatment. London: Chapman & Hall.

Andrews PLR, Rapeport WG, Sanger GJ (1988) Neuropharmacology of emesis induced by anti-cancer therapy. Trends in Pharmacology Science 9: 334–341.

Atra A, Richards S, Chessels JM (1993) Remission death in acute lymphoblastic leukaemia: a changing pattern. Archives of Disease in Childhood 69(5): 550–554.

BACUP (1996) Understanding Clinical Trials. London: BACUP.

Baehner RL (1986) The value of nutritional support in children with cancer. Cancer (Suppl.) 58(8): 1904–1910.

Balis FM, Hockenberry JS, Poplack DG (1993) General principles of chemotherapy. In Pizzo PA, Poplack DG (eds), Principles and Practice of Pediatric Oncology (second edition). Philadelphia: JB Lippincott, pp. 197–245.

Balis FM, Poplack DG, Horowitz ME (1996) Randomized trial of the cardioprotective agent ICRF-187 in pediatric sarcoma patients treated with doxorubicin. Journal of Clinical Oncology 14(2): 362–372.

Balsom WR, Bleyer WA, Robinson LL, Heyn RM, Meadows AT, Sitarz A, Blatt J, Sather HN, Hammond DG (1991) Intellectual function in long term survivors of childhood acute lymphoblastic leukaemia: protective effect of pre-irradiation methotrexate? A children's cancer study group study. Medical and Paediatric Oncology 19(6): 486–492.

Barkvoll P, Attramadal A, Odont D (1989) Effect of nystatin and chlorhexidine digluconate on Candida albicans. Oral Surgery, Oral Medicine and Oral Pathology 67(3): 279–281.

Barton Burke M, Wilkes GM, Berg D, Bean CK, Ingwerson KI (1991) Cancer Chemotherapy: A Nursing Process Approach. Boston, MA: Jones & Bartlett.

Bassan R, Rambaldi A, Amaru RM, Otta T, Barbui T (1994) Unexpected remission of acute myeloid leukaemia after GM-CSG. British Journal of Haematology 87(4): 835–838.

Beck SL (1992) Prevention and management of oral complications in the cancer patient. Current Issues in Cancer Nursing Practice Updates 1(6): 1–12.

Beck WT, Grogan TM, Willman CL, Cordon-Cardo C, Parham DM, Kuttesch JF, Andreef M, Bates SE, Berard CW, Boyett JM, Brophy NA, Broxterman HJ, Chan HSL, Dalton WS, Dietel M, Fojo AT, Gascoyne RD, Head D, Houghtan PJ, Srivastava DK, Lehnert M, Leith CP, Paietta E, Pavelic ZP, Rimsza L, Roninson IB, Sikic BI, Twentyman PR, Warnke R, Weinstein R (1996) Methods to detect p-glycoprotein-associated multidrug resistance in patients' tumors: consensus recommendations. Cancer Research 56(13): 3010–3020.

Behrend SW (1994) Documentation in the ambulatory setting. Seminars in Oncology Nursing 10(4): 264–280.

Benjamin E, Leskowitz S (1991) Immunology: A Short Course (second edition). USA: Wiley–Liss.

Benson P, Burkey ED, Martin Mitchell B, Clark JC (1993) Home and hospice care for the child or adolescent with cancer. In Foley GV, Fochtman D, Hardin Mooney K (eds), Nursing Care of the Child with Cancer (second edition). Philadelphia: WB Saunders.

Bernstein IL (1978) Learned taste aversions in children receiving chemotherapy. Science 200(16): 1302–1303.

Bertelli G et al. (1994) Hyaluronidase as an antidote to extravasation of vinca alkaloids: clinical results. Journal of Cancer Research and Clinical Oncology 120(8): 505–506.

Bertino JR, O'Keefe P (1992) Barriers and strategies for effective chemotherapy. Seminars in Oncology Nursing 8(2): 77–82.

Beyer WA (1990) The impact of childhood cancer on the United States and the world. Cancer Journal for Clinicians 40(6): 355–367.

Bignold S, Ball S, Cribb A (1994) Nursing Families with Children with Cancer: The Work of the Paediatric Oncology Nurse Specialist. London: Department of Health.

Billet EA, Sallan SE (1993) Management of nausea and vomiting. In Pizzo PA, Poplack DG (eds), Principles and Practice of Pediatric Oncology (second edition). Philadelphia: JB Lippincott, pp. 1051–1057.

Bingham CA (1978) The cell cycle and cancer chemotherapy. American Journal of Nursing (July): 1201–1205.

Bird C (1990) A prescription for self-help. Nursing Times 86(43): 52–55.

Bird C, Hassal J (1993) Self-administration of Drugs. London: Scutari Press.

Blackledge G, Lawton F (1992) The ethics and practical problems of Phase I and II studies. In Williams CJ (ed.), Introducing New Treatments for Cancer: Practical, Ethical and Legal Problems. Chichester: John Wiley.

Blackmore C (1988) Body image: the oncological perspective. In Salter M (ed.), Altered Body Image — The Nurse's Role. London: John Wiley.

Bleiberg H (1992) Antiemetic agents. Current Opinion in Oncology 4(4): 597–604.

BNF (1996) British National Formulary 31. London: BMA and Royal Pharmaceutical Society of Great Britain.

Bozzetti F (1995) Nutrition support in patients with cancer. In Payne-Jones J, Grimble G, Silk D (eds), Artificial Nutrition Support in Clinical Practice. London: Edward Arnold, pp. 511–534.

Bray GL (1993) Inherited and acquired disorders of hemostasis. In Holbrook PR (ed.), Textbook of Critical Care. Mexico: WB Saunders, pp. 783–801.

British Paediatric Association (1992) Guidelines for the Ethical Conduct of Medical Research Involving Children. London: British Paediatric Association.

Brodeur GM, Castleberry RP (1993) Neuroblastoma. In Pizzo PA, Poplack DG (eds), Principles and Practice of Pediatric Oncology (second edition). Philadelphia: JB Lippincott.

Bronchud M (1992) The Importance of Dose in Cancer Chemotherapy. Consultant series no. 8. Macclesfield: Gardiner-Caldwell Communications.

Bru G (1989) Using and documenting nursing diagnosis in an ambulatory setting. Journal of the Association of Pediatric Oncology Nurses 6(2): 7–10.

Bru GA, Viamontes M, Nirenberg A, Poremba FA, Houlihan NG (1985) Short form for short stay. American Journal of Nursing 85(4): 401–403.

Buchanan GR (1993) Hematologic supportive care of the pediatric cancer patient. In Pizzo PA, Poplack DG (eds), Principles and Practice of Pediatric Oncology (second edition). Philadelphia: JB Lippincott, pp. 973–986.

Buckley MM, Benfield P (1993) Eutetic lidocaine/prilocaine cream; a review of the topical anaesthetic/analgesic efficacy of a eutetic mixture of local anaesthetics. Drugs 46(1): 126–151.

Bu'Lock FA, Gabriel HM, Oakhill A, Mott MG, Martin RP (1993) Cardioprotection by ICRF 187 against anthracycline toxicity in children with malignant disease. British Heart Journal 70(2): 187–188.

Bu'Lock FA, Mott M, Oakhill A (1996) Early identification of anthracycline cardiomyopathy: possibilities and implications. Archives of Disease in Childhood 75(5): 416–422.

Burish TG, Tope DM (1992) Psychological techniques for controlling the adverse side effects of cancer chemotherapy: findings from a decade of research. Journal of Pain and Symptom Management 7(5): 287–301.

Burt K (1995) The effects of cancer on body image and sexuality. Nursing Times 91(7): 36–37.

Bushkin E (1993) Signposts of survivorship. Oncology Nursing Forum 20(6): 870–887.

Calman K (1982) Malignancy cancer cachexia. British Journal of Hospital Medicine 27(1): 28–34.

Campbell SJ (1987) Mouthcare in cancer patients. Nursing Times 83(29): 59–60.

Campbell ST, Evans MA, MacTavish F (1995) Guidelines for Mouthcare. London: The Paediatric Oncology Nursing Forum, Royal College of Nursing.

Capizzi RL, Poole M, Cooper MR, Richards F, Stuart JJ, Jackson DV, White DR, Spott CL, Hopkins JO, Muss HB, Rudnick SA, Wells R, Gabriel D, Ross D (1984) Treatment of poor risk acute leukaemia with sequential high-dose ARA-C and asparaginase. Blood 63(3): 694–698.

Casey A (1995a) Nursing assessment and communication. In Campbell S, Glasper EA (eds), Whaley and Wong's Children's Nursing. London: CV Mosby.

Casey A (1995b) Partnership nursing: influences on involvement of informal carers. Journal of Advanced Nursing 22(6): 1058–1062.

Casper ES, Gaynor JJ, Hajdu SI, Magill GB, Tan C, Friedrich C, Brennan MF (1991) A prospective randomised trial of adjuvant chemotherapy with bolus versus continuous infusion of doxorubicin in patients with high-grade extremity soft tissue sarcoma and an analysis of prognostic factors. Cancer 68(6): 1221–1229.

Cass Y, Musgrave CF (1992) Guidelines for the safe handling of excreta contaminated by cytotoxic agents. American Journal of Hospital Pharmacy 49(8): 1957–1958.

Cass Y, Ferguson L, Wright P (1997) Health and safety aspects of cytotoxic services. In Allwood M, Stanley A, Wright P (eds), The Cytotoxics Handbook (third edition). Oxford: Radcliffe Medical Press, 35–53.

Castaigne S, Chomienne C, Daniel MT, Ballerini P, Berger R, Fenaux P, Degos L (1990) All-trans retinoic acid as a differentiating therapy for acute promyelocytic leukaemia. Blood 76(9): 1704–1709.

Caudell KA (1988) Quantification of urinary mutagens in nurses during antineoplastic exposure. Cancer Nursing 11(1): 41–50.

Chambas K (1991) Sexual concerns of adolescents with cancer. Journal of Pediatric Oncology Nursing 8(4): 165–172.

Chandraseka PH, Gatny CM (1994) Effect of fluconazole on fever and use of amphotericin in neutropenic patients. Chemotherapy 40(2): 136–143.

Chessells JM (1995) Maintenance treatment and shared care in lymphoblastic leukaemia. Archives of Disease in Childhood 73(4): 368–373.

Chessells JM, Cox TCS, Kendall B, Cavanagh NPC, Jannou NL, Richards S (1990) Neurotoxicity in lymphoblastic leukaemia: comparison of oral and intramuscular methotrexate and two doses of radiation. Archives of Disease in Childhood 65(4): 416–422.

Chiron (1995) Cardioxane (Dexrazoxane). Product monograph.

Clark JW (1996) Targeted therapy. In Chabner BA, Longo DL (eds), Cancer Chemotherapy and Biotherapy (second edition). Philadelphia: JB Lippincott–Raven.

Clarke G (1993) Mouth care and the hospitalized patient. British Journal of Nursing 2(4): 225–227.

Clayton PE, Shalet SM, Price DA, Campbell RHA (1988) Testicular damage after chemotherapy for childhood brain tumours. Journal of Paediatrics 112(6): 922–926.

Cloak MM, Connor TH, Stevens KR, Theiss JC, Alt JM, Matney TS, Anderson RW (1985) Occupational exposure of nursing personnel to antineoplastic agents. Oncology Nursing Forum 12(5): 33–39.

Close P, Burkey E, Kazak A, Danz P, Lange B (1995) A prospective, controlled evaluation of home chemotherapy for children with cancer. Pediatrics 95(6): 896–900.

Cogliano-Shutta NA (1986) Pediatric Phase I Clinical Trials: Ethical issues and nursing considerations. Oncology Nursing Forum 13(2): 29–32.

Cohen IJ, Zehavi N, Buchwald I, Yaniv Y, Goshen Y, Kaplinsky C, Zaizov R (1995) Oral ondansetron: an effective ambulatory complement to intravenous ondansetron in the control of chemotherapy-induced nausea and vomiting in children. Pediatric Hematology and Oncology 12(1): 67–72.

Cohen LF, Barlow JE, Macgrath IT, Poplack DG, Zieger JL (1980) Acute tumour lysis syndrome: a review of 37 patients with Burkitt's lymphoma. American Journal of Medicine 68(4): 486–491.

Cohen LF, Barlow JE, Macgrath IT, Poplack DG, Collins JM (1996) Pharmacokinetics and clinical monitoring. In Chabner BA, Longo DL (eds), Cancer Chemotherapy and Biotherapy (second edition). Philadelphia: Lippincott–Raven.

Cohen PA, Hwu P, Rosenberg SA (1996) Adoptive cellular immunotherapy and gene therapy. In Chabner BA, Longo DL (eds), Cancer Chemotherapy and Biotherapy (second edition). Philadelphia: Lippincott–Raven.

Coleman S (1995) An overview of the oral complications of adult patients with malignant haematological conditions who have undergone radiotherapy or chemotherapy. Journal of Advanced Nursing 22(6): 1085–1091.

Collins JM (1996) Pharmacokinetics of clinical monitoring. In Chabner BA, Longo DL (eds), Cancer Chemotherapy and Biotherapy (second edition). Philadelphia: Lippincott–Raven.

Cotanch PH (1983) Relaxation training for control of nausea and vomiting in patients receiving chemotherapy. Cancer Nursing 6(4): 277–283.

Cotanch PH (1984) Measuring nausea and vomiting in clinical nursing research. Oncology Nursing Forum 11(3): 92–94.

Cotanch P, Hockenberry-Eaton M, Herman S (1985) Self-hypnosis as antiemetic therapy in children receiving chemotherapy. Oncology Nurses Forum 12(4): 41–46.

Cowie F, Meller ST, Cushing P, Pinkerton R (1994) Chemoprophylaxis for pulmonary aspergillosis during intensive chemotherapy. Archives of Disease in Childhood 70(2): 136–138.

Crounse Van Scott (1960). Cited in Price B (ed.) (1990), Body Image: Nursing Concepts and Care. London: Prentice Hall.

Cuttner J, Holland JF, Norton L et al. (1983) Therapeutic leukopheresis for hyper-leukocytosis in acute myelocytic leukemia. Medical Pediatric Oncology 11(2): 76–78.

Daeffler R (1980) Oral hygiene measures for patients with cancer. Cancer Nursing 3(5): 347–353.

D'Angio GJ (1992) An overview and historical perspective of late effects of treatment for childhood cancer. In Green DM, D'Angio DJ (eds), Late Effects of Treatment for Childhood Cancer. New York: Wiley–Liss.

Daniels L (1995) The physical and psychosocial implications of central venous devices in cancer patients — a review of the literature. Journal of Cancer Care 4(4): 141–145.

Daniels LE (1995) Developing a home chemotherapy service. International Journal of Palliative Nursing 1(2): 81–85.

Darbyshire P (1986) Body image: when the face doesn't fit. Nursing Times 82(36): 28–29.

Darbyshire P (1990) Handle with care. Nursing Times 86(1): 37–38.

Darovic GO (1984) Septic shock. In Carolan JM (ed.), Shock: A Nursing Guide. Bristol: Wright, Medical Economics Books, pp. 85–102.

David J, Speechley V (1987) Scalp cooling to prevent alopecia. Nursing Times 83(32): 36–37.

Davies HA, Lennard L, Lilleyman JS (1993) Variable mercaptopurine metabolism in children with leukaemia: a problem of non-compliance? British Medical Journal 306(6887): 1239–1240.

Davis C (1990) Chemotherapy and patient information. Nursing Standard 4(26): 25–27.

Dean JC, Salmon SE, Griffith KS (1979) Prevention of doxorubicin-induced hair loss with scalp hypothermia. New England Journal of Medicine 301(26): 1427–1429.

Degregorio MW, Lee WMS, Ries CA (1982) Candida infections in patients with acute leukaemia: ineffectiveness of nystatin prophylaxis and relationships between oropharyngeal and systemic candidasis. Cancer 50(2): 2780–2784.

DeLaat CA, Lampkin BC (1992) Long-term survivors of childhood cancer: evaluation and identification of sequelae of treatment. Cancer Journal for Clinicians 42(5): 263–282.

Department of Health (1989) Reprt of the advisory group on nurse prescribing (Crown Report). London: DoH.

Department of Health (1998) Review of prescribing, supply and administration of Medicines. A report on the supply and administration of medicines under group protocols. London: DoH.

Devita VT (1989) Principles of chemotherapy. In Devita VT, Hellman S, Rosenberg S (eds), Principles and Practice of Oncology. Philadelphia: JB Lippincott.

Dietz KA, Flaherty AM (1993) Oncologic emergencies. In Groenwald SL, Frogge HM, Goodman M, Yarbo CH (eds), Cancer Nursing Principles and Practice (third edition). Boston, MA: Jones & Bartlett, pp. 801–839.

Dimond B (1990) Parental acts and omissions. Paediatric Nursing 2(1): 23–24.

Dolgin MJ, Katz ER, McGinty K, Siegal SE (1985) Anticipatory nausea and vomiting in pediatric cancer patients. Pediatrics 75(3): 547–552.

Dolgin MJ, Katz ER, Doctors SA, Siegal SE (1986) Caregivers' perceptions of medical compliance in adolescents with cancer. Journal of Adolescent Health Care 7(1): 22–27.

Donovan M (1980) Relaxation with guided imagery: a useful technique. Cancer Nursing 3(1): 1880–1896.

Dorr RT (1990) Antidotes to vesicant chemotherapy extravasation. Blood Review 4(1): 41–60.

Eagan AP, Taggart JR, Bender CM (1992) Management of chemotherapy-related nausea and vomiting using a serotonin antagonist. Oncology Nurses Forum 19(5): 791–795.

Eden OB (1994) Children deserve better. Pediatric Hematology and Oncology 11(3): 241–242.

Eilers J, Berger AM, Peterson MC (1988) Development, testing and application of the oral assessment guide. Oncology Nurses Forum 15(3): 325–330.

Eiser C (1996) The impact of treatment: adolescents' views. In Selby P, Bailey C (eds), Cancer and The Adolescent. London: BMJ Publishing.

Eiser C, Havermans T (1994) Long term adjustment after treatment for childhood cancer. Archives of Disease in Childhood 70(1): 66–70.

Erikson E (1965) Childhood and Society. London: Penguin.

Evans M (1990) The child receiving chemotherapy. In Thompson J (ed.), The Child with Cancer — Nursing Care. London: Scutari Press.

Evans M (1993) Paediatric oncology. In Glasper EA, Tucker A (eds), Advances in Child Health Nursing. London: Scutari Press.

Evans M (1996) Interacting with teenagers with cancer. In Selby P, Bailey C (eds), Cancer and The Adolescent. London: BMJ Publishing Group.

Evans M, Kelly P (1995) Bringing support home for families of children with cancer. British Journal of Nursing 4(7): 395–398.

Evans S, Radford M (1995) Current lifestyle of young adults treated for cancer in childhood. Archives of Disease in Childhood 72(5): 423–426.

Falck K, Grohn P, Sorsa M (1979) Mutagenicity in urine of nurses handling cytostatic drugs. Lancet 1(8): 1250–1251.

Fanurik D, Zeltzer LK, Roberts MC, Blount RL (1993) The relationship between children's coping styles and psychological interventions for cold pressor pain. Pain 53(2): 213–222.

Faulkner A, Peace G, O'Keefe G (1995) When a Child has Cancer. London: Chapman & Hall.

Favrot MC, Michon J, Floret D, Cochat C, Negrier S, Mathiot C, Coze C, Zucker JM, Franks CR, Bouffet E, Philip T (1990) Interleukin-2 immunotherapy in children with neuroblastoma after high-dose chemotherapy and autologous bone marrow transplantation. Pediatric Hematology and Oncology 7(3): 275–284.

Fawcett H (1995) Nutritional support for hospital patients. Nursing Standard 9(48): 25–28.

Fay L, Evans M (1997) Direct line to home. Nursing Times 93(37): 29–30.

Feit F, Slater W, Blum R, Muggia F (1988) Protective effect of the bispiperaznedione ICRF-187 against doxorubicin-induced cardiac toxicity in women with advanced breast cancer. New England Journal of Medicine 319(12): 745–752.

Ferguson JH (1981) Cognitive late effects of treatment of acute lymphocytic leukaemia in childhood. Topics in Clinical Nursing 2(4): 21–29.

Fischer DS, Tish Knobf M, Durivage HJ (1993) The Cancer Chemotherapy Handbook (fourth edition). USA: CV Mosby–Year Book Inc.

Flavell D, Boehm DA, Emery L, Noss A, Ramsay A, Flavell SU (1995) Therapy of human B-cell lymphoma-bearing SCID mice is more effective with anti-CD19 and anti-CD23-saporin immunotoxins used in combination than with either immunotoxin used alone. International Journal of Cancer 62: 337–342.

Foley GV, Hochtrian D, Hardin Mooney K (1993) Nursing Care of the Child with Cancer. Philadelphia: WB Saunders.

Foot ABM, Hayes C (1994) Audit of guidelines for effective control of chemotherapy and radiotherapy induced emesis. Archives of Disease in Childhood 71(5): 475–480.

Fradd E (1990) Sharing accountability. Paediatric Nursing 2(3): 6–8.

Frazer MC, Tucker MA (1988) Late effects of cancer therapy: chemotherapy related malignancies. Oncology Nursing Forum 15(1): 67–77.

Furman WL, Crist WM (1992) Biology and clinical applications of hemopoeitins in pediatric practice. Pediatrics 90(5): 716–728.

Gajraj NM (1994) Eutectic mixture of local anaesthetics (EMLA) cream. Anaesthesia and Analgesia 78(3): 574–583.

Galassi A (1996) Chemotherapy administration: practical guidelines. In Chabner BA, Longo DA (eds), Cancer Chemotherapy and Biotherapy (second edition). Philadelphia: Lippincott–Raven.

Galbraith I, Bailey D, Kelly L, Rehn K, Spear S, Steinle G, Vaughn G, Wehage S (1991) Treatment for alteration in oral mucosa related to chemotherapy. Paediatric Nursing 17(3): 233–237.

Galvin H (1994) The late effects of treatment of childhood cancer survivors. Journal of Cancer Care 3(2): 128–133.

Gandi V, Estey E, Keating MJ, Plunkett W (1993) Fludarabine potentiates metabolism of cytarabine in patients with acute myelogenous leukemia during therapy. Journal of Clinical Oncology 11(1): 116–124.

Gault DT (1993) Extravasation injuries. British Journal of Plastic Surgery 46(2): 91–96.

Ghadile Harris M, Bean CA (1991) Changing the role of the nurse in the haematology–oncology outpatient setting. Oncology Nursing Forum 18(1): 43–46.

Gibson CH (1991) A concept analysis of empowerment. Journal of Advanced Nursing 16(3): 354–361.

Gibson F (1994) The Phenomena of Chemotherapy-associated Nausea and Vomiting Examined in Relation to the Ability of Children to Use a Self-report Instrument. Unpublished MSc Dissertation. University of Surrey.

Gibson F, Horsford J, Nelson W (1997) Oral care; ritualistic practice reconsidered within a framework of action research. Journal of Cancer Nursing 1(4): 183–190.

Glaus A, Crow R, Hammond S (1996) A qualitative study to explore the concept of fatigue/tiredness in cancer patients and in health individuals. European Journal of Cancer Care 5(2) (Suppl.): 8–23.

Glen S (1988) Altered body image in children. In Salter M (ed.) Altered Body Image: The Nurse's Role. Chichester: John Wiley.

Goede IA, Betcher DL (1994) EMLA. Journal of Pediatric Oncology Nursing 11(1): 38–41.

Goldberg M, Ginsburgh D, Mayer R, Stone R, Maguire M, Rosenthal D, Autin J (1987) Is heparin administration necessary during induction chemotherapy for patients with acute promyelocytic leukaemia. Blood 69(1): 187–191.

Goldie JH, Coldman AJ (1984). The genetic origin of drug resistance in neoplasms: implications for systemic therapy. Cancer Research 44(9): 3643–3653.

Goldie JH, Coldman AJ (1986) Theoretical considerations regarding the early use of adjuvant chemotherapy. Recent Results in Cancer Research 103: 30–35.

Goldman A, Beardsmore S, Hunt J (1990) Palliative care for children with cancer —home, hospital or hospice? Archives of Disease in Childhood 65(6): 641–643.

Goldstein L, Galaski A, Fojo M (1989) Expressions of multidrug resistance gene in human cancers. Journal of the National Cancer Institute 81(2): 116–124.

Goodinson SM (1987) Biochemical assessment of nutritional status. The Professional Nurse 2(12): 8–12.

Goodman M (1987) Management of nausea and vomiting induced by outpatient cisplatin therapy. Seminars in Oncology Nursing 3(1): 23–35.

Gould D (1995) Hand decontamination: nurses' opinions and practices. Nursing Times 91(17): 42–45.

Graham-Pole J, Weare J, Engel S, Gardner R, Mehta P, Gross S (1986) Antiemetics in children receiving cancer chemotherapy: a double blind prospective randomized study comparing metoclopramide with chlorpromazine. Journal of Clinical Oncology 4(7): 1110–1113.

Grahame-Smith DG, Aronson JK (1992) Oxford Textbook of Clinical Pharmacology and Drug Therapy (second edition). Oxford: Oxford University Press.

Grant MM, Rivera LM (1995) Anorexia, cachexia and dysphagia: the symptom experience. Seminars in Oncology Nursing 11(4): 266–271.

Graubert TA, Ley TJ (1996) How do lymphocytes kill tumour cells? Clinical Cancer Research 2(5): 785–789.

Green DM, D'Angio GJ (1992) Late Effects of Treatment for Childhood Cancer. New York: Wiley–Liss.

Groenwald SL, Frogge MH, Goodman M, Yarbo CH (1993) Cancer Nursing Principles and Practice (third edition). Boston, MA: Jones & Bartlett.

Gross R (1991) Psychology: The Science of Mind and Behaviour. London: Hodder & Stoughton.

Gullo SM (1988) Safe handling of antineoplastic drugs: translating the recommendations into practice. Oncology Nursing Forum 15(5): 595–601.

Gullo SM (1995) Safe handling of antineoplastic drugs: translating the recommendations into practice. Oncology Nursing Forum 22(3): 517–525.

Gussack GS, Brantley BA, Farmer JC (1984) Biology of tumours and head and neck cancer chemotherapy. Laryngoscope 94(9): 1181–1187.

Hammond E (1988) Anaphylactic reactions to chemotherapeutic agents. JAPON 5(3): 16–19.

Hammond GD (1992) Late adverse effects of treatment among patients cured of cancer during childhood. Cancer Journal for Clinicians 42(5): 261–262.

Hanada T, Ono I, Hiranon C, Kurosaki Y (1990) Successful treatment of neutropenic enterocolitis with recombinant granulocyte colony stimulating factor in a child with acute lymphoblastic leukaemia. European Journal of Paediatrics 149(11): 811–812.

Hanigan MJ, Walter GA (1992) Nutritional support of the child with cancer. Journal of Pediatric Oncology Nursing 9(3): 110–118.

Hardy JR, Pinkerton CR (1992) Cancer chemotherapy and mechanisms of resistance. In Plowman PN, Pinkerton CR (eds), Paediatric Oncology: Clinical Practice and Controversies. London: Chapman & Hall.

Harris CV, Bradlyn AS, Ritchey K, Olsen BR, Pisaruk AK (1994) Individual differences in pediatric cancer patients' reactions to invasive medical procedures: a repeated measure analysis. Pediatric Hematology and Oncology 11(3): 293–299.

Hawkins MM, Draper GJ, Kingston JE (1987) Incidence of secondary primary tumours among childhood cancer survivors. British Journal of Cancer 56(3): 339–347.

Hawkins MM, Kinnier Wilson LM, Stovall MA, Marsden HB, Potok MHN, Kingston J, Chessells JM (1992) Epipodophyllotoxins, alkylating agents, and radiation and risk of secondary leukaemia after childhood cancer. British Medical Journal 304(6832): 951–958.

Hawkins MM, Stevens MCG (1996) The long term survivors in cancer in children. British Medical Bulletin 32(4): 898–923.

Hawthorn J (1991) The management of nausea and vomiting induced by chemotherapy and radiotherapy: a comprehensive guide for nurses. European Journal of Cancer 1(1): 23–26.

Hawthorn J (1995) Understanding and Management of Nausea and Vomiting. Oxford: Blackwell Science.

Health and Safety Executive (1988a) The Control of Substances Hazardous to Health (COSHH) Regulations. London: HMSO.

Health and Safety Executive (1988b) Guidance Note: Precautions for the Safe Handling of Cytotoxic Drugs. London: HMSO.

Hemminki K (1985) Spontaneous abortions and malformations in the offspring of nurses exposed to anaesthetic gases, cytostatic agents and other potential hazards in hospitals, based on registered information of outcome. Journal of Epidemiology and Community Health 39(2): 141–147.

Hendrick J (1997) Legal Aspects of Child Health Care. London: Chapman & Hall, p. 238.

Hill BT (1978) Cancer chemotherapy: the relevance of certain concepts of cell cycle kinetics. Biochimica et Biophysica Acta 516: 389–417.

Hill BT (1986) Neuroblastoma — an overview of laboratory studies aimed at inducing tumour regression by initiation of differentiation or administration of antitumour drugs. Pediatric Hematology and Oncology 3(1): 73–88.

Hinchliffe RF (1992) Reference values. In Lilleyman JS, Hann IM (eds), Paediatric Haematology. Singapore: Churchill Livingstone, pp. 1–28.

Hirst M, Tse S, Mills DG (1984) Occupational exposure to cyclophosphamide. Lancet 1(8370): 186–188.

Ho CS (1994) The future direction of clinical trials. Cancer 74(9) (Suppl.): 2739–2744.

Hobbie W, Ruccione K, Moore IK, Truesdell S (1993) Late effects in long term survivors. In Foley GV, Fochtman D, Mooney KH (eds), Nursing Care of the Child with Cancer (second edition). Philadelphia: WB Saunders.

Hockenberry-Eaton M, Benner A (1990) Patterns of nausea and vomiting in children: nursing assessment and intervention. Oncology Nurses Forum 17(14): 575–584.

Hockenberry-Eaton M, Herman SB, Katz SL (1986) Management of infections. In Hockenberry MJ, Coody DK (eds), Pediatric Oncology and Hematology: Perspectives on Care. St Louis, MO: CV Mosby, pp. 380–393.

Hogan CM (1990) Advances in the management of nausea and vomiting. Nursing Clinics of North America 25(2): 475–497.

Holmes S (1990) Cancer Chemotherapy. London: Austen Cornish.

Holmes S (1991a) The oral complications of specific anticancer therapy. International Journal of Nursing Studies 28(4): 343–360.

Holmes S (1991b) Support can boost the body's defences: nutrition in cancer care. Professional Nurse 7(2): 83–89.

Holmes S, Mountain E (1993) Assessment of oral status: evaluation of three oral assessment guides. Journal of Clinical Nursing 2(1): 35–40.

Hooker L (1996) An evaluation of parent-administered home intravenous drug therapy. (Abstract) Medical and Pediatric Oncology 27(4): 274.

Hooker L, Williams J (1996) Parent-held shared care records: bridging the communication gaps. British Journal of Nursing 5(12): 738–741.

Hoppe JE, Klingebiel T, Niethammer D (1994) Selection of *Candida glabrata* in pediatric bone marrow transplant recipients receiving fluconozole. Pediatric Hematology and Oncology 11(2): 207–210.

Howarth H (1977) Mouthcare procedures for the very ill. Nursing Times 73(10): 354–355.

Hubbard SM (1981) Chemotherapy and the nurse. In Marino LB, Cancer Nursing. St Louis, MI: CV Mosby.

Hughes W, Armstrong D, Bodey G, Feld R, Mandell G, Meyers J, Pizzo P, Schimpff S, Shenep J, Wade J, Young L, Yow M (1990) Guidelines for the use of antimicrobial agents in neutropenic patients with unexplained fever. Journal of Infectious Diseases 161(3): 381–396.

Hully M, Hyne J (1993) Using parent-held records in an oncology unit. Paediatric Nursing 5(8): 14–16.

Human Fertilisation Embryology Authority (1992) Sperm and Egg Donors and the Law. London: HFEA.

Human Fertilisation Embryology Authority (1995) Treatment Clinic: Questions to Ask. London: HFEA.

Hunt JA (1995) The paediatric oncology community nurse specialist: the influence of employment location and funders on models of practice. Journal of Advanced Nursing 22(1): 126–133.

Hymes JA, Spraker MK (1986) Racial differences in the effectiveness of a topically applied mixture of local anesthetics. Register of Anaesthetics 11(1): 11–13.

Irwin MM (1986) Enteral and parenteral nutrition support. Seminars in Oncology Nursing 21(1): 44–54.

James JA, Harris DJ, Mott MG, Oakhill A (1988) Paediatric oncology information pack for general practitioners. British Medical Journal 296 (9 Jan): 97–98.

Jayabose S, Escobedo V, Tugal O, Nahaczewski A, Donohue P, Fuentes V, Devereau, Sunkara S (1991) Home chemotherapy for children with cancer. Cancer 69(2): 574–579.

Jenns K (1994) Importance of nausea. Cancer Nursing 17(6): 488–493.

Junghans RP, Sgouros G, Scheinberg DA (1996) Antibody-based immunotherapies for cancer. In Chaber BA, Longo DL (eds), Cancer Chemotherapy and Biotherapy (second edition). Philadelphia: Lippincott–Raven.

Juranek DD (1995) Cryptosporidiosis: sources of infection and guidelines for prevention. Clinical Infectious Diseases 21(Suppl. 1): 57–61.

Jürgens H, McQuade B (1992) Ondansetron as prophylaxis for chemotherapy and radiotherapy-induced emesis in children. Oncology 49(4): 279–285.

Kamp AA (1988) Neoplastic diseases in a paediatric population; a survey of the incidence of oral complications. Paediatric Dentistry 10(1): 25–29.

Kantarjian H, Keating M, Walters RS, Estey EH, McCreedie KB, Smith TL, Dalton WT, Cork A, Trujillo JM, Freireich EJ (1986) Acute promyelocytic leukaemia: MD Anderson experience. American Journal of Medicine 80(5): 789–797.

Kartner N, Ling V (1989) Multidrug resistance in cancer. Scientific America 260(3): 44–51.

Kaszyk LK (1986) Cardiac toxicity associated with cancer therapy. Oncology Nursing Forum 13(4): 81–87.

Kaufman C, Chabner BA (1996) Clinical strategies for cancer treatment: the role of drugs. In Chabner BA, Longo DL (eds), Cancer Chemotherapy and Biotherapy (second edition). Philadelphia: Lippincott–Raven.

Keller VE (1995) Management of nausea and vomiting in children. Journal of Pediatric Nursing 10(5): 280–286.

Kelly KM, Womer RB, Barr FG (1996) Minimal disease detection in patients with alveolar rhabdomyosarcoma using reverse transcriptase–polymerase chain reaction. Cancer 78(6): 1320–1327.

Kerr DJ (1994) Phase I clinical trials: adapting methodology to face new challenges. Annals of Oncology 5(Suppl. 4): S67–S70.

Kinrade LC (1988) Typhlitis: a complication of neutropenia. Pediatric Nursing 14(4): 291–295.

Kissen GDN, Wallace WHB (1995) United Kingdom Children's Cancer Study Group. Late Effects Group: Long Term Follow-up Therapy-based Guidelines. Leicester: UKCCSG.

Knopf MKT, Fischer DS, Welch-McCaffrey D (1984) Cancer Chemotherapy: Treatment and Care (second edition). Boston, MA: GK Hall Medical.

Kohler JA, Radford M (1985) Terminal care for children dying of cancer: quantity and quality of life. British Medical Journal 291(6488): 574–579.

Krishnasamy M (1995) The nurse's role in oral care. European Journal of Palliative Care (Suppl. 1): 8–9.

Kulkarni V, Webster N (1996) Management of sepsis. Care of the Critically Ill 12(4): 122–127.

Kurtz A (1993) Disseminated intravascular coagulation with leukaemia patients. Cancer Nursing 16(6): 456–463.

Lange B, D'Angio G, Ross AJ, O'Neill JA, Packer RJ (1993) Oncologic emergencies. In Pizzo PA, Poplack DG (eds), Principles and Practice of Pediatric Oncology (second edition). Philadelphia: JB Lippincott, pp. 951–972.

Lansdown R, Goldman A (1988) The psychological care of children with malignant disease. Journal of Child Psychology and Psychiatry 29(5): 555–567.

Lansky SB, Smith SB, Cairns NU, Cairns GF (1983) Psychological correlates of compliance. American Journal of Pediatric Hematology/Oncology 5(1): 87–92

Lanzkowsky P (1995) Manual of Pediatric Hematology and Oncology (second edition). London: Churchill Livingstone.

Larcombe IJ, Walker J, Charleton A, Meller S, Morris Jones P, Mott MG (1990) Impact of childhood cancer on return to normal schooling. British Medical Journal 301: 169–171.

Lau R, King S, Richardson S (1994) Early discharge of pediatric febrile neutropenic cancer patients by substitution of oral for intravenous antibiotics. Pediatric Hematology and Oncology 11(4): 417–421.

Lawrence J (1994) Critical care issues in the patient with haematologic malignancy. Seminars in Oncology Nursing 10(3): 198–207.

Leadbetter M (1991) Increasing knowledge. Nursing Times 87(3): 32–35.

LeBaron S, Zeltzer LK, LeBaron C, Scott SE, Zeltzer PM (1988) Chemotherapy side effects in pediatric oncology patients: drugs, age and sex as risk factors. Medical and Pediatric Oncology 16(4): 262–268.

Lee L (1992) Ethical issues related to research involving children. Journal of Pediatric Oncology Nursing 8(1): 24–29.

Lehne RA (1990) Pharmacology for Nursing Care. Philadelphia: WB Saunders.

Lendrum S, Syme G (1992) Gift of Tears. London: Routledge.

Lennard L, Lilleyman JS, Van Loon J, Weinshilboum RM (1990) Genetic variation in response to mercaptopurine in childhood lymphoblastic leukaemia. Lancet 336(8709): 225–229.

Lever SA, Dupuis LL, Chan HS (1987) Comparative evaluation of benzydamine oral rinse in children with antineoplastic-induced stomatitis. Drug Intelligence and Clinical Pharmacy 21(4): 359–361.

Ley P (1988) Communicating with Patients. London: Croom Helm.

Lie SO (1990) 13-Cis Retinoic acid as continuation therapy in children with advanced neuroblastoma in complete or good partial remission. Medical and Pediatric Oncology 18(5): 384–388.

Lieschke GJ, Maher D, O'Connor M, Green M, Sheridan W, Rallings M, Bonnem E, Burgess AW et al. (1990) Phase I study of intravenously administered GM-CSF and comparison with subcutaneous administration. Cancer Research 50(30): 606–614.

Lilleyman JS, Hann IM (eds) (1992) Paediatric Haematology. Singapore: Churchill Livingstone.

Lindsey AM (1986) Cancer cachexia; effects of the disease and its treatment. Seminars in Oncology Nursing 2(1): 19–29.

Ling J, Penn K (1995) The challenges of conducting clinical trials in palliative care. International Journal of Palliative Nursing 1(1): 31–34.

Lupulescu AP (1996) Hormones, vitamins, and growth factors in cancer treatment and prevention. Cancer 78(11): 2264–2280.

Lydon J (1986) Nephrotoxicity of cancer treatment. Oncology Nursing Forum 13(2): 68–77.

Lynam MJ (1987) The parent network in pediatric oncology: supportive or not? Cancer Nursing 10(4): 207–216.

McCalla JL (1985) A multidisciplinary approach of identification and remedial intervention for adverse late effects of cancer therapy. Nursing Clinics of North America 20(1): 117–129.

McCalla JL, Santacroce SJ, Woolery-Antill M (1993) Nursing support of the child with cancer. In Pizzo PA, Poplack DG (eds), Principles and Practice of Pediatric Oncology (second edition). Philadelphia: JB Lippincott, pp. 1059–1077.

McClelland B (1996) Handbook of Transfusion Medicine (second edition). London: The Stationery Office.

McClure RJ, Prasad VK, Brocklebank JT (1994) Treatment of hyperkalaemia using intravenous and nebulised salbutamol. Archives of Disease in Childhood 70(2): 126–128.

McDonald AD, McDonald JC, Armstrong B (1988) Congenital defects and work in pregnancy. British Journal of Industrial Medicine 45(4): 141–147.

McEvoy M, Duchon D, Schaefer DS (1985) Therapeutic play for patients and siblings in a pediatric oncology ambulatory care unit. Topics in Clinical

Nursing 7(1): 10–18.

McEvoy MD, Cannon I, MacDermott ML (1991) The professional role of nurses in clinical trials. Seminars in Oncology Nursing 7(4): 268–274.

McEwing G (1996) Children's understanding of their internal body parts. British Journal of Nursing 5(7): 423–429.

McGhee MF, Jeffree P (1993) A Guide to Laboratory Investigations (second edition). Oxford: Radcliffe Medical Press.

MacGinley KJ (1993) Nursing care of the patient with altered body image. British Journal of Nursing 2(22): 1098–1102.

McHaffie HE (1992) Coping: an essential element of nursing. Journal of Advanced Nursing 17(8): 933–940.

McHaney V, Kovnar E, Meyer W, Furmai W, Schell M, Kun L (1992) Effects of radiation therapy and chemotherapy on hearing. In Green DM, D'Angio G (eds), Late Effects of Treatment for Childhood Cancer. New York: Wiley–Liss.

Macleod A (1994) Parenteral nutrition. In Shaw V, Lawson M (eds), Clinical Paediatric Dietetics. Oxford: Blackwell Scientific.

Marcus R, Goldman J (1986) Management of infection in the neutropenic patient. British Medical Journal 293(6543): 406–408.

Martinson IM, Armstrong GD, Geis DP, Anglim MA, Gronseth EC, MacInnes H, Kersey JH, Nesbit ME (1978) Home care for children dying of cancer. Pediatrics 62(1): 106–113.

Martinson IM, Gilliss C, Colaizzo DC et al. (1990) Impact of childhood cancer on healthy siblings. Cancer Nursing 13(3): 183–190.

Maurer HS, Steinherz PG, Gaynon PS (1988) Management of hyperleukocytosis in childhood with acute lymphoblastic leukaemia. Journal of Clinical Oncology 6(10): 1425.

Meadows AT, Evans AE, Pritchard J (eds) (1990) Practical Paediatric Oncology. London: Edward Arnold, pp. 95–102.

Meeske K, Ruccione KS (1987) Cancer chemotherapy in children: nursing issues and approaches. Seminars in Oncology Nursing 3(2): 118–127.

Mertens F, Heim S (1994) Cytogenetic analysis in the examination of solid tumors in children. Pediatric Hematology and Oncology 11(4): 361–377.

Michie B (1988) Total parenteral nutrition. Nursing Times 84(20): 46–47.

Millam D (1988) Managing the complications of IV therapy. Nursing 88 18(3): 34–43.

Morris-Jones PH, Craft AW (1990) Childhood cancer: cure at what cost? Archives of Disease in Childhood 65(6): 638–640.

Morrow GR (1985) The effect of a susceptibility to motion sickness on the side effects of cancer chemotherapy. Cancer 55(12); 2766–2770.

Morrow GR, Morrell C (1982) Behavioural treatment for the anticipatory nausea and vomiting induced by cancer chemotherapy. New England Journal of Medicine 307(24): 1476–1480.

Mulhern RK, Wasserman AL, Fairclough D, Ochs JJ (1988) Memory function in disease free survivors of childhood acute lymphoblastic leukaemia given CNS prophylaxis with or without 1800 cGy cranial radiation. Journal of Clinical Oncology 6(2): 315–320.

Mulvihill JJ, Byrne J (1992) Genetic counseling for the cancer survivor. Possible germ cell effects of cancer therapy. In Green DM, D'Angio GJ (eds), Late Effects of Treatment for Childhood Cancer. New York: Wiley–Liss.

Murata A, Matsuzaki M, Mityashita H, Kodama F, Taguchi J, Tomita N, Sakai R, Fujisawa S, Okubo T, Amano K (1995) Successful pregnancy after allogenic bone marrow transplantation following conditioning with total body irradiation. Bone Marrow Transplantation 15(4): 637–638.

Muzzin LM, Anderson NJ, Figueredo AT, Gudelis SO (1994) The experience of cancer. Social Science and Medicine 38(9): 1201–1208.

Nace C, Nace G (1993) Acute tumour lysis syndrome. Critical Care Nurse 5(3): 26–34.

Nail LM, Winningham ML (1995) Fatigue and weakness in cancer patients: the symptom experience. Seminars in Oncology Nursing 11(4): 272–278.

Nail LM, Greene D, Jones LS, Flannery M (1986) Nursing care by telephone: describing practice in an ambulatory oncology center. Oncology Nursing Forum 16(3): 387–395.

Neff JA (1990) Body knowledge and concerns. Nursing Times 86(20): 67–71.

Newell DR (1992) Recent advances and future trends in cancer chemotherapy. In Plowman PN, Pinkerton CR (eds), Paediatric Oncology: Clinical Practice and Controversies. London: Chapman & Hall.

Nexstar Pharmaceuticals (1995) Daunoxome (liposomal daunorubicin). Product information.

Nicholson RH (1986) Medical Research with Children: Ethics, Law and Practice. Oxford: Oxford University Press.

Ninane K (1992) Neuroblastoma. In Plowman PN, Pinkerton CR (eds), Paediatric Oncology: Clinical Practice and Controversies. London: Chapman & Hall.

Nordin C, Rosenquist M, Hollstedt C (1988) Sniffing of ethyl chloride — an uncommon form of abuse with serious mental and neurological symptoms. International Journal of Addictions 23: 623–627.

Norman AD, Brandeis L (1992) Addressing the needs of survivors: an action research approach. Journal of Psychosocial Oncology 10(1): 3–17.

Norville R (1995) Role opportunities in nursing research. Journal of Pediatric Oncology Nursing 12(1): 42–45.

Norville R, Hinds P, Wilmas J, Fairclough D, Fischl S, Kunkel K (1994) Platelet count, morphology, and corrected count increment in children with cancer: *in vitro* and *in vivo* studies. Oncology Nursing Forum 21(10): 1669–1673.

Noyes NF (1986) Chemotherapy. In Hockenberry MJ, Coody DK (eds), Pediatric Oncology and Hematology: Perspectives on Care. St Louis, MO: CV Mosby, pp. 309–337.

Nygaard R, Clausen N, Simems A, Marky I, Skjeldestad FE, Kristinsson JR, Vuoristo A, Wegelius R, Moe JP (1991) Reproduction following treatment for childhood leukaemia: a population-based prospective cohort study of fertility and offspring. Medical and Paediatric Oncology 19(6): 459–466.

O'Berle K, Davies B (1992) Support and caring: exploring the concepts. Oncology Nursing Forum 19(5): 764–767.

Ochs J, Mulhern RK (1992) Prospective evaluation of neuropsychological function following cranial radiation or intermediate dose methotrexate. In Green DM, D'Angio GJ (eds), Late Effects of Treatment for Childhood Cancer. New York: Wiley–Liss.

Ochs JJ, Parvey LS, Whitacker JN (1983) Serial cranial computed-tomography scans in children with leukaemia given two different forms of central nervous system prophylaxis with or without 1800 cGy cranial nervous system therapy. Journal of Clinical Oncology 1(12): 793–798.

Oncology Nursing Society (1992) Cancer Chemotherapy Guidelines — Module V: Recommendations for the Management of Extravasation, Hypersensitivity and Anaphylaxis. Pittsburgh: ONS.

Panzarella C, Duncan J (1993) Nursing management of physical care needs. In Foley GV, Fochtman D, Mooney KH (eds), Nursing Care of the Child with Cancer (second edition). Philadelphia: WB Saunders.

Paradise RL, Kendall VM (1985) Ambulatory care: primary nursing brings continuity. Nursing Management 16(12): 27–30.

Parkinson DR, Pluka JM, Cazenave L, Ho P, Sorensen JM, Sznol M, Christian MC (1996) Investigational cancer agents. In Chabner BA, Longo DL (eds), Cancer Chemotherapy and Biotherapy (second edition). Philadelphia: Lippincott–Raven.

Parrillo JE (1993) Pathogenetic mechanisms of septic shock. New England Journal of Medicine 328(20): 1471–1477.

Patient Education Group (1994) Clinical Trials: Your Questions Answered (second edition). London: Royal Marsden Hospital NHS Trust.

Patterson KL, Klopovich P (1987) Metabolic emergencies in pediatric oncology: the acute tumor lysis syndrome. JAPON 4(3/4): 19–24.

Pearson LS (1996) A comparison of the ability of foam swabs and toothbrushes to remove dental plaque. Implications for nursing practice. Journal of Advanced Nursing 23(1): 62–69.

Peate I (1993) Nurse-administered oral hygiene in the hospitalised patient. British Journal of Nursing 2(9): 459–462.

Philpott-Howard JN, Wade JJ, Mufti GJ, Brammer KW, Ehninger G (1993) Randomised comparison of oral fluconazole versus oral polyenes for the prevention of fungal infection in patients at risk of neutropenia. Journal of Antimicrobial Chemotherapy 31(6): 973–984.

Pickard-Holley S (1991) Fatigue in cancer patients. Cancer Nursing 14(1): 13–19.

Pickett RR (1992) Outpatient oncology chemotherapy documentation tool. Oncology Nursing Forum 19(3): 515–517.

Pike S, Gibson F (1991) A programme to support your extended role: chemotherapy training for paediatric nurses. Professional Nurse April: 362–364.

Pinkerton CR (1992) Avoiding chemotherapy related late effects in children with curable tumours. Archives of Disease in Childhood 67(9): 1116–1119.

Pinkerton CR, Phillip T (1991) Treatment Strategies in Paediatric Cancer: The Role of Haematopoietic Growth Factors. (Consultant series, no 7). Macclesfield: Gardiner-Caldwell Communications.

Pinkerton CR, Williams D, Wooten C, Meller ST, McElwain TJ (1990) 5-HT3 antagonist ondansetron — an effective outpatient antiemetic in cancer treatment. Archives of Disease in Childhood 65(8): 822–825.

Pinkerton CR, Cushing P, Sepion B (1994) Childhood Cancer Management: A Practical Handbook. London: Chapman & Hall.

Piper BF, Lindsey AM, Dodd MJ (1987) Fatigue mechanisms in cancer patients: developing nursing theory. Oncology Nurses Forum 14(6): 17–23.

Pizzo PA, Young RC (1989) Infections in the cancer patient. In Devita VT, Hellman S, Rosenberg SA (eds), Cancer: Principles and Practice of Oncology. Volume 3. Philadelphia: JB Lippincott.

Price B (1990) Body Image: Nursing Concepts and Care. London: Prentice Hall, p. 644.

Price B (1992) Living with altered body image: the cancer experience. British Journal of Nursing 1(13): 641–645.

Price B (1993) Diseases and altered body image in children. Paediatric Nursing 5(6): 18–21.

Price B (1996) Illness careers: the chronic illness experience. Journal of Advanced Nursing 24(2): 275–279.

Priestman TJ (1989) Cancer Chemotherapy: An Introduction (third edition). Berlin: Springer-Verlag.

Pritchard P, David J (1988) The Royal Marsden Hospital Manual of Clinical Nursing Procedures. London: Harper & Row.

Reams CA (1990) Inpatients and outpatients on one unit. Journal of Paediatric Oncology Nursing (conference proceedings) 7(2): 77–78.

Rechner M (1990) Adolescents with cancer: getting on with life. Journal of Paediatric Nursing 7(4): 139–144.

Redd WH, Andresen CV, Minagwa RY (1982) Hypnotic control of anticipatory emesis in patients receiving cancer chemotherapy. Journal of Consulting and Clinical Psychology 50(1): 14–19.

Renick-Ettinger A (1993) Chemotherapy. In Foley GV, Fochtman D, Mooney KH (eds), Nursing Care of the Child with Cancer (second edition). Philadelphia: WB Saunders.

Reville B, Almadrones L (1989) Continuous infusion chemotherapy in the ambulatory setting: the nurse's role in patient selection and education. Oncology Nursing Forum 16(4): 529–535.

Reynolds JEF (1996) Martindale: The Extra Pharmacopoeia (31st edition). London: Royal Pharmaceutical Society.

Rhodes VA (1990) Nausea, vomiting and retching. Nursing Clinics of North America 24(4): 885–900.

Richardson A (1987) A process standard for oral care. Nursing Times 83(32): 38–40.

Rickard KA, Coates TD, Grosfeld JL, Weetman RM, Baehner RL (1986) The value of nutritional support in children with cancer. Cancer 58(8): 1904–1910.

Rikonen P, Jalanko H, Hovi L, Saarinen U (1993) Fever and neutropenia in children with cancer: diagnostic parameters at presentation. Acta Paediatrica 82(3): 271–275.

Robinson S, Collier J (1997) Holding children still for procedures. Paediatric Nursing 9(4): 12–14.

Robison LL, Mertens A (1993) Second tumours after treatment of childhood malignancies. Hematology/Oncology Clinics of North America 7(2): 401–415.

Rogers TR (1995) Infectious complications of treatment. Ballière's Clinical Paediatrics 3(4): 683–698.

Roitt I (1991) Essential Immunology (seventh edition). Oxford: Blackwell.

Rosenthal D, Autin J (1987) Is heparin administration necessary during induction chemotherapy for patients with acute promyeolytic leukaemia. Blood 69(1): 187–191.

Ross AJ, O'Neill JA (1992) Surgical emergencies. In D'Angio GJ, Sinniah D, Meadows AT, Evans AE, Pritchard J (eds), Practical Paediatric Oncology. London: Edward Arnold, pp. 57–67.

Roth PT, Creason NS (1986) Nurse-administered oral hygiene; is there a scientific basis? Journal of Advanced Nursing 11(3): 323–331.

Rowe PM (1994) Monoclonal antibodies in cancer therapy. Lancet 344(8932): 1288.

Rowinsky EK, Donehower RC (1996) Antimicrotubule agents. In Chabner BA, Longo DA (eds), Cancer Chemotherapy and Biotherapy (second edition). Philadelphia: Lippincott–Raven.

Royal College of Nursing: Oncology Nursing Society (1989) Safe Practice with Cytotoxics. London: Scutari Press.

Royal College of Nursing (1994) Disposal of Health Care Waste in the Community. London: RCN.

Royal College of Nursing: Paediatric Community Nurses Forum (1994) Administering Intravenous Therapy to Children in the Community (second edition). London: RCN.

Royal College of Nursing: Paediatric Oncology Nurses Forum (1994) Guidelines for Paediatric Oncology Training in the Giving of Intravenous Drugs, including Cytotoxics (second edition). London: RCN.

Salisbury DM, Begg NJ (1996) Immunisation Against Infectious Diseases. London: The Stationery Office.

Saunders J and the Seattle Marrow Transplant Team (1992) Effects of bone marrow transplantation in reproductive function. In Green DM, D'Angio GJ (eds), Late Effects of Treatment for Childhood Cancer. New York: Wiley–Liss.

Schaison G (1993) Cytogenetic abnormalities in childhood acute lymphoblastic leukaemia. Pediatric Hematology and Oncology 10(1): 1–2.

Schering-Plough International (1994) Amifostine Product Monograph.

Scott DB (1986) Topical anaesthesia of the skin. British Journal of Parenteral Therapy Nov/Dec: 574–583.

Selevan SG, Lindbohm ML, Hornung RW (1985) A study of occupational exposure to antineoplastic drugs and fetal loss in nurses. New England Journal of Medicine 313(19): 1173–1178.

Senturia YD, Peckham CS (1990) Children fathered by men treated with chemotherapy for testicular cancer. European Journal of Cancer 26(4): 429–432.

Shalet SM (1989) Endocrine consequences of treatment of malignant disease. Archives of Disease in Childhood 64(11): 1635–1641.

Shalet SM, Wallace WHB (1992) Reproductive physiology. In Green DM, D'Angio GJ (eds), Late Effects of Treatment for Childhood Cancer. New York: Wiley–Liss.

Siddall S (1988) Chemotherapy problems and precautions. In Oakhill A (ed.), The Supportive Care of the Child with Cancer. London: Wright.

Sieve R, Betcher D (1994) Pentamidine. Journal of Paediatric Oncology Nursing 11(2): 85–87.

Sinniah D, Belasco JB (1992) Immunization in the immunocompromised patient. In D'Angio GJ, Smith D, Meadows AT, Evans AE, Pritchard J (eds), Practical Paediatric Oncology. London: Edward Arnold, pp. 97–102, 128–138.

Skinner R, Sharkey IM, Pearson ADJ, Craft AW (1993) Ifosphomide, mesna and nephrotoxicity in children. Journal of Clinical Oncology 11(1): 173–190.

Skov SD, Maarup B, Olsen J, Rorth M, Winthereik H, Lynge E (1992) Leukaemia and reproductive outcome among nurses handling antineoplastic drugs. British Journal of Industrial Medicine 49(2): 855–861.

Smith DE, Handy DJ, Holden CE, Stevens MCG, Booth IW (1992) An investigation of supplementary naso-gastric feeding in malnourished children undergoing treatment for malignancy; results of a pilot study. Journal of Human Nutrition and Dietetics 5: 85–91.

Smith LH, Van Gulick AJ (1992) Management of neutropenic enterocolitis in the patient with cancer. Oncology Nurses Forum 19(9): 1337–1344.

Smith RN (1989) Safety of ondansetron. European Journal of Cancer and Clinical Oncology 25 (Suppl. 1): 47–50.

Smith SD, Rosen D, Trueworthy RC, Lowman JT (1979) A reliable method for evaluating drug compliance in children with cancer. Cancer 43(8): 169–173.

Smith SD, Cairns NU, Sturgeon JK, Lanksy SB (1981) Poor drug compliance in an adolescent with leukemia. American Journal of Pediatric Hematology/ Oncology 3(3): 279–300.

Sonis A, Sonis S (1979) Oral complications of cancer chemotherapy in pediatric patients. Journal of Pedodontics 3(2): 122–128.

Spears N (1994) In vitro growth of oocytes. Human Reproduction 9(6): 169–176.

Speyer JL, Green MD, Kramer E, Rey M, Sanger J, Ward C, Dubin N, Ferrans V, Stecy P, Zelemich-Jacquotte A, Wernz C, Feit F, Slater W, Blum R, Muggia F (1988) Protective effect of the bispiperaznedione ICRF-187 against doxorubicin-induced cardiac toxicity in women with advanced breast cancer. New England Journal of Medicine 319(12): 745–752.

Stanley A (1993) Extravasation: Diagnosis, Treatment and Prevention. Oxford: Radcliffe Medical Press.

Stannard D (1989) Pressure relieves nausea. Nursing Times 85(4): 33–34.

Steger Osterhaus JK (1995) Telephone protocols in pediatric ambulatory care. Pediatric Nursing 21(4): 351–355.

Stehbens AA, Maclean WE, Kaleita TA, Noll RB, Schwartz E, Cantor NL, Woodard A, Whitt JK, Wasterwitz MJ, Ruymann FB, Hammond GH (1994) Effects of CNS prophylaxis on the neuropsychological performance of children with acute lymphoblastic leukaemia: nine months post-diagnosis. Children's Health Care 23(4): 231–250.

Steinherz LJ, Steinherz PG, Sklar C, Wollner N, Tan C (1994) Cardiac status of 42 patients over 15 years post-anthracycline treatment. (Abstract). Medical and Pediatric Oncology 23(3): 176.

Stevens RF (1991) The role of ondansetron in paediatric patients: a review of three studies. European Journal of Cancer 27(Suppl. 1): 20–22.

Stillwell TJ, Benson RC (1988) Cyclophosphamide-induced hemorrhagic cystitis: a review of 100 patients. Cancer 61(3): 451–457.

Stone M (1993) Lending an ear to the unheard; the role of support groups for siblings with cancer. Child Health 1(2): 54–58.

Stucky LA (1993) Acute tumour lysis syndrome; assessment and nursing implications. Oncology Nursing Forum 20(1): 49–57.

Sutton A (1988) Cancer cachexia. Nursing Times 84(3): 65–66.

Syntex Pharmaceuticals (1994) Product information: ethyl chloride BP.

Tebbi CK, Cummings KM, Zevon MA, Smith L, Richards M, Mallon J (1985) Compliance of pediatric and adolescent cancer patients. Cancer 58(5): 1179–1184.

Teich CJ, Raia K (1984) Teaching strategies for an ambulatory chemotherapy program. Oncology Nursing Forum 11(5): 24–28.

Terrin BN, McWilliams NB, Maurer HM (1984) Side effects of metaclopramide as an antiemetic in childhood cancer chemotherapy. Journal of Pediatrics 104(1): 138–140.

Theologides A (1979) Cancer cachexia. Cancer 43(3): 2004–2012.

Thornes R (1993) Bridging the Gaps. London: Action for Sick Children.

Thorpe G (1992) Experiments on the dying. In Williams CJ (ed.), Introducing New Treatments for Cancer — Practical, Ethical and Legal Problems. Chichester: Wiley.

Thurgood G (1994) Nurse maintenance of oral hygiene. British Journal of Nursing 3(7): 332–353.

Tierney AJ (1987) Preventing chemotherapy-induced alopecia in cancer patients: is scalp cooling worthwhile? Journal of Advanced Nursing 12(13): 300–310.

Tighe MG, Fisher SG, Hastings C, Heller B (1985) A study of the oncology nurse role in ambulatory care. Oncology Nursing Forum 12(6): 23–27.

Torrance C (1990) Oral hygiene. Surgical Nurse 3(4): 16–20.

United Kingdom Central Council for Nursing, Midwifery and Health Visiting (1993) Standards for Records and Record Keeping. London: UKCC.

United Kingdom Children's Cancer Study Group: Late Effects Group (1995) Long Term Follow-up Therapy-based Guidelines. Leicester: UKCCSG.

United Kingdom Children's Cancer Study Group (1996) Scientific Report. Leicester: Cancer Research Campaign.

United Kingdom Children's Cancer Study Group (1998) Extravasation Guidelines. Leicester: UKCCSG

Valanis B, Shortridge L (1987) Self-protective practices of nurses handling antineo-plastic drugs. Oncology Nursing Forum 14(3): 23–27.

Valente S (1991) Using hypnosis with children for pain management. Oncology Nurses Forum 18(4): 699–704.

Van Eys J (1979) Malnutrition in children with cancer. Cancer 43(5): 2030–2035.

Vennitt S, Criften-Sleigh C, Hunt J et al. (1984) Monitoring exposure of nursing and pharmacy personnel to cytotoxic drugs: urinary mutation assays and urinary platinum as markers of absorption. Lancet 1(8368): 74–77.

Vessey JA, Mahon MM (1990) Therapeutic play and the hospitalised child. Journal of Pediatric Nursing 5(5): 328–333.

Vitetta ES, Stone M, Amlot P, Fay J, May R, Newman J, Clark P, Collins R, Cunningham D, Ghetie V, Uhr J, Thorpe PE (1991) Phase I immunotoxin trial in patients with B-cell lymphoma. Cancer Research 51(15): 4052–4058.

Vlasveld LT, Ten-Bok K, Hunink WW, Rodenhuis S (1990) Neutropenic entero-colitis in a patient with ovarian cancer after treatment with high dose carbo-platin and granulocyte macrophage colony stimulating factor (GM-CSF). Netherlands Journal of Medicine 37(3/4): 156–161.

Walker G (1993) Data Sheet Compendium. UK: Datapharm Publications.

Wall DT, Gabriel LA (1983) Alterations of taste in children with leukaemia. Cancer Nursing 6(6): 447-542.

Ward P (1988) Antiemesis. In Oakhill A (ed.), The Supportive Care of the Child with Cancer. London: Wright.

Waterworth S (1992) Long-term effects of cancer on children and their families. British Journal of Nursing 1(8): 373–377.

Wawrzynczak EJ (1991) Systemic immunotoxin therapy of cancer: advances and prospects. British Journal of Cancer 64(4): 624–630.

Wenisch C, Parschalk B, Hasenhundl M, Hirschl AM, Graninger W (1996) Comparison of vancomycin, teicoplanin, metronidazole and fuscidic acid for treatment of *Clostridium difficile*-associated diarrhoea. Clinical Infectious Diseases 22(5): 813–818.

Wesdrop RI, Krause R, Van-Meyenfeldt M (1983) Cancer cachexia and its nutritional implications. British Journal of Surgery 70(6): 352–355.

Wesley JR, Coran AG (1986) Infants and children. In Barnett J, Nyhus L (eds), Treatment of Shock: Principles and Practice (second edition) Philadelphia, PA: Lea & Febiger, pp. 211–223.

Wetzel RC, Tobin JR (1992) Shock. In Rogers MC (ed.), Textbook of Pediatric Intensive Care (second edition). Baltimore, MD: Williams & Wilkins, pp. 563–613.

Wexler LH, Andrich MP, Venzon D, Berg SL, Weaver-McClure L, Chen CC, Dilsizian V, Avila N, Jarosinski P, Balis FM, Poplack DG, Horowitz ME (1996) Randomized trial of the cardioprotective agent ICRF-187 in pediatric sarcoma patients treated with doxorubicin. Journal of Clinical Oncology 14(2): 362–372.

Whaley LF, Wong DL (1987) Nursing Care of Infants and Children (third edition). St Louis, MO: CV Mosby.

Wheeler VS (1995) Gene therapy: current strategies and future applications. Oncology Nursing Forum 22(2) (Suppl.): 20–26.

While AE (1991) An evaluation of a paediatric home care scheme. Journal of Advanced Nursing 16(12): 1413–1421.

Wiernikowski J, Rothney M, Dawson S, Andrew M (1991) Evaluation of a home intravenous antibiotic program in pediatric oncology. American Journal of Pediatric Hematology/Oncology 13(2): 144–147.

Williams CJ (1985) Handling cytotoxics. British Medical Journal 291(6506): 1299–1300.

Williss J (1991) A Preliminary Study to Evaluate the Effectiveness of Acupressure 'Seabands' in Reducing Nausea and Vomiting in Children Receiving Chemotherapy. Unpublished BSc dissertation. King's College London.

Wingard JR, Merz WG, Rinaldi MG, Johnson TR, Karp JE, Salal R (1991) Increase in *Candida krusei* infection among patients with bone marrow transplantation and neutropenia treated prophylactically with fluconazole. New England Journal of Medicine 325(18): 1274–1277.

Witt PL, Lindner DJ, D'Cunha J, Borden EC (1996) Pharmacology of interferons: induced proteins, cell activation and antitumour therapy. In Chabner BA, Longo DL (eds), Cancer Chemotherapy and Biotherapy (second edition). Philadelphia: Lippincott–Raven.

Wittes RE (1986) Adjuvant chemotherapy — clinical trials and laboratory models. Cancer Treatment Reports 70: 87–103.

Wong D (1995) Whaley and Wong's Nursing Care of Infants and Children. St Louis, MO: CV Mosby.

Wong D, Baker C (1988) Pain in children: comparison of assessment scales. Pediatric Nursing 14(1): 9–17.

Woodhouse S (1990) Why have medicine rounds? Paediatric Nursing 2(10): 9–12.

Wujcik D (1993a) An odyssey into biologic therapy. Oncology Nursing Forum 29(6): 879–887.

Wujcik D (1993b) Infection control in oncology patients. Nursing Clinics of North America 28(3): 639–650.

Yasko JM (1985) Holistic management of nausea and vomiting caused by chemotherapy. Topics in Clinical Nursing 7(1): 26–38.

Yaster M, Tobin JR, Fisher QA, Maxwell LG (1994) Local anesthetics in the management of acute pain in children. Journal of Pediatrics 124(2): 165–176.

Zeltzer LK, LeBaron S (1983) Behavioural intervention for children and adolescents with cancer. Behavioural Medicine Update 5(2/3): 17–22.

Zeltzer LK, Le Baron S, Zeltzer PM (1984) A prospective assessment of chemotherapy-related nausea and vomiting in children with cancer. American Journal of Pediatric Hematology/Oncology 6(1): 5–16.

Zeltzer LK, LeBaron S, Richie M, Reed D, Schoolfield J, Prihoda TJ (1988) Can children understand and use a rating scale to quantify somatic symptoms? Assessment of nausea and vomiting as a model. Journal of Consulting and Clinical Psychology 56(4): 567–572.

Zeltzer LK, Dolgin MJ, LeBaron S, LeBaron C (1991) A randomized, controlled study of behavioral intervention for chemotherapy distress in children with cancer. Pediatrics 88(1): 34–42.

Ziegar JL (1980) Acute tumor lysis syndrome: a review of 37 patients with Burkitt's lymphoma. American Journal of Medicine 68(4): 486–491.

References
Section Two

Abramovitz L, Senner A (1995) Pediatric bone marrow transplantation update. Oncology Nursing Forum 22(1): 107–115.

Ainamo J, Asikainen S, Paloheimo L (1982) Gingival bleeding after chlorhexidine mouthrinses. Journal of Clinical Peridontology 9(4): 337–345.

Andrykowski M, Brady M, Greiner C, Altmaier E, Burish T, Antin J, Gingrich R, McGarighe C, Henslee Downley P (1995) 'Returning to normal' following bone marrow transplantation: outcomes, expectations and informed consent. Bone Marrow Transplantation 15(4): 573–581.

Anthony Nolan Bone Marrow Trust (1996) A guide for potential bone marrow donors. Information sheet for potential donors.

Apperley JF (1994) Umbilical cord blood progenitor cell transplantation. Bone Marrow Transplantation 14(2): 187–196.

Atkinson (1991) Chronic graft versus host disease — review. Bone Marrow Transplantation 5: 69–82.

Baglin T (1994) Veno-occlusive disease of the liver complicating bone marrow transplantation. (Review). Bone Marrow Transplantation 13(1): 1–4.

Baglin T, Harper P, Marcus R (1990) Veno-occlusive disease of the liver complicating ABMT successfully treated with recombinant tissue plasminogen activator (rt-PA). Bone Marrow Transplantation 5(3): 439–441.

Barnes DW, Loutit JF, Micklem HS (1962) Secondary disease of radiation chimeras; a syndrome due to lymphoid aplasia. Annals of the New York Academy of Science 99: 374–385.

Barnes R (1992a) Infections following bone marrow transplantation. In Treleaven J, Barrett J (eds), Bone Marrow Transplantation in Practice. London: Churchill Livingstone, pp. 281–287.

Barnes R (1992b) Treatment of bacterial, fungal and viral infections in hospital. In Treleaven J, Barrett J (eds), Bone Marrow Transplantation in Practice. London: Churchill Livingstone, pp. 299–306.

Barrett J (1993) Graft versus host disease. In Treleaven J, Barrett J (eds), Bone Marrow Transplantation in Practice. London: Churchill Livingstone, pp. 257–272.

Barrett J, Horowitz MM, Pollock BH (1994) Bone marrow transplants from HLA-identical siblings as compared with chemotherapy for children with acute lymphoblastic leukaemia in a second remission. New England Journal of Medicine 331(19): 1253–1258.

Bearman S (1995) The syndrome of hepatic veno-occlusive disease after marrow transplantation. (Review article 'Blood'). Journal of the American Society of Hematology 85(11): 3005–3020.

Beck S (1979) Impact of systematic oral care protocol on stomatitis after chemotherapy. Cancer Nursing 2(10): 185–199.

Beck S (1992) Prevention and management of oral complications in the cancer patient. In Hubbard S, Greene P, Knobf M (eds), Current Issues in Cancer Nursing Practice Updates. Pennsylvania: JB Lippincott.

Benner P (1983) Uncovering the knowledge embedded in clinical practice. Journal of Nursing Scholarship 15(2): 36–41.

Benner P (1984) Novice to Expert: Excellence and Power in Clinical Nursing and Practice. Menlo Park: Addison-Wesley.

Benner P, Wrubel J (1989) A phenomenological view of stress and coping. In Benner P, Wrubel J (eds), The Primacy of Caring; Stress and Coping in Health and Illness. California: Addison-Wesley, pp. 57–103.

Blotcky AD, Cohen DG, Conatser C (1985) Psychosocial characterisation of patients who refuse cancer treatment. Journal of Consulting Clinical Psychology 53(5): 729–731.

Borgna-Pignatti C (1992) Bone marrow transplantation for the haemoglobinopathies. In Treleaven J, Barrett J (eds), Bone Marrow Transplantation in Practice. London: Churchill Livingstone, pp. 151–159.

Brack G, LaClave L, Blix S (1988) The psychological aspects of bone marrow transplant. Cancer Nursing 11(4): 221–229.

Brykczynska G (1990) The gift of an organ. Paediatric Nursing, Oct 12, p.12.

Buckner CD, Clift RA, Saunders JE (1984) Marrow harvesting from normal donors. Blood 64(3): 630–634.

Butterworth T, Faugier J (1992) Clinical Supervision and Mentorship in Nursing. London: Chapman & Hall.

Carney B (1981) Bone marrow transplantation: nurses' and physicians' perceptions of informed consent. Cancer Nursing 10(5): 252–259.

Carper B (1978) Fundamental ways of knowing in nursing. Advances in Nursing Science 1(1): 13–23.

Casey A (1988) A partnership with child and family. Senior Nurse 8(4): 8–9.

Casey A, Mobbs S (1988) Partnership in practice. Nursing Times 84(44): 67–68.

Caudell K, Adams J (1990) Cyclosporin administration practices on bone marrow transplant units: a national survey. Oncology Nurses Forum 17(4): 563–568.

Chessells JM, Bailey CC, Wheeler K, Richards SM (1992) Bone marrow transplantation for high-risk childhood lymphoblastic leukaemia in first remission: experience in MRC UKALL X. The Lancet 340(8819): 565–568.

Clarke M (1986) Action and reflection: practice and theory. Journal of Advanced Nursing 11(1): 3–11.

Cleary J (1992) Caring for Children in Hospital. Parents and Nurses in Partnership. London: Scutari Press.

Cleaver S (1993) The Anthony Nolan Bone Marrow Research Centre and other matching registries. In Treleaven J, Barrett J (eds), Bone Marrow Transplantation in Practice. London: Churchill Livingstone, pp. 361–366.

Coody D (1985) High expectations: nurses who work with children who might die. Nursing Clinics of North America 20(1): 131–141.

Darbyshire P (1994) Living in Hospital with a Sick Child. The Experience of Parents and Children. London: Chapman & Hall.

Deeg HJ, Flourney N, Sullivan K, Sheehan K, Buckner CD, Sanders J, Storb Witherspoon R, Thomas ED (1984) Cataracts after total body irradiation: a sparing effect of dose fractionation. International Journal of Radiation Oncology Biology Physics 10(7): 957–964.

De Koning J, Van Bekkum D, Dicke K, Dooren L, Radl J, Van-Rood K (1969) Transplantation of bone marrow cells and foetal thymus in an infant with lymphopenic immunological deficiency. The Lancet 1(608): 1223–1227.

Delaney L (1996) Protecting children from forced altruism: the legal approach. British Medical Journal 312(7025): 240.

Department of Health (1989) The Children Act. London: HMSO.

Department of Health and Social Services (1995) The Children (Northern Ireland) Order. Belfast: HMSO.

Downs S (1994) Clinical issues in bone marrow transplantation. Seminars in Oncology Nursing 10(1): 58–63.

Dunleavy R (1996) Isolation in BMT: a protection or a privation? British Journal of Nursing 5(11): 663–668.

Dunn K (1988) Sibling influence on childhood development. Journal of Child Psychology and Psychiatry 29(2): 119–123.

Eilers J, Berger A, Peterson M (1988) Development, testing and application of the oral assessment guide. Oncology Nurses Forum 15(3): 325–330.

Eiser C (1989) Psychological effects of chronic disease. Journal of Child Psychology 31(1): 85–98.

Eiser C (1993) Growing Up with a Chronic Disease. London: Jessica Kingsley.

Eland J (1988) Pain in children. Nursing Clinics of North America 25(4): 871–884.

Ellis P (1992) A child's right to die: who should decide? British Journal of Nursing 1(8): 406–408.

Emery J (1993) Perceived sources of stress among pediatric oncology nurses. Journal of Pediatric Oncology Nursing 10(3): 87–92.

Evans M (1994) An investigation into the feasibility of parental participation in the nursing care of their children. Journal of Advanced Nursing 20(3): 477–482.

Ezzone S, Jolly D, Repogle K, Kapoor N, Tutschka P (1993) Survey of oral hygiene regimes among bone marrow transplant centres. Oncology Nurses Forum 20(9): 1375–1381.

Fenelon L (1995) Protective isolation: who needs it? Journal of Hospital Infection (Suppl.) 30: 18–22.

Ferrell B, Grant M, Schmidt G, Rheiner M, Whitehead C, Fonbuenu R, Foreman S (1992a) The meaning of quality of life for bone marrow transplant survivors. Part 1: The impact of bone marrow transplant on quality of life. Cancer Nursing 15(3): 153–160.

Ferrell B, Grant M, Schmidt G, Rheiner M, Whitehead C, Fonbuenu P, Foreman S (1992b) The meaning of quality of life for bone marrow transplant survivors. Part 2: Improving quality of life for bone marrow transplant survivors. Cancer Nursing 15(4): 247–253.

Ferretti G, Ash R, Brown A, Largent B, Kaplan A, Lillich T (1987) Chlorhexadine for prophylaxis against oral infections and associated complications in patients receiving bone marrow transplantation. Journal of the American Dental Association 114(4): 461–467.

Fischer A, Landais P, Friedrich W, Morgan G, Gerritsen B, Fasth A, Porta F, Griscelli C, Goldman S, Levinksy R, Vossen J (1990) European experience of bone marrow transplantations for severe combined immunodeficiency. The Lancet 2(8515): 850–854.

Fliedner RM, Steinbach KH (1988) Repopulating potential of hematopoietic precursor cells. Blood Cells 14(2–3): 393–410

Fox R, Swanley J (1974) The Courage to Fail: A Social View of Organ Transplants and Dialysis. Chicago: University of Chicago Press.

Frederick B, Hanigan MJ (1993) Bone marrow transplantation. In Foley GV, Fochtman D, Mooney KH (eds), Nursing Care of a Child with Cancer. Philadelphia: WB Saunders, pp. 130–178.

Freireich EJ, Judson G, Levin RH (1965) Separation and collection of leukocytes. Cancer Research 25(9): 1516–1520.

Freund B, Siegel K (1986) Problems in transition following bone marrow transplantation: psychosocial aspects. American Journal of Orthopsychiatry 56(2): 244–252.

Futerman AD, Wellisch DK (1990) Psychodynamic themes of bone marrow transplant — when I becomes thou. Hematology/Oncology Clinics of North America 4(3): 699–709.

Gauvreau J, Lenssen P, Cheney C, Aker S, Hutchinson M, Barale K (1981) Nutritional management of patients with graft-versus-host disease. Journal of the American Dietetic Association 79(6): 673–675.

Gibbs N (1990) The gift of love — or else. Time, September 10.

Gibson F (1989) Parental involvement in bone marrow transplant. Paediatric Nursing 1(7): 21–22.

Gluckman E (1995) Allogeneic sibling umbilical cord blood transplantation in children with malignant and non-malignant disease. The Lancet 346(8969): 214–219.

Gluckman E, Broxmeyer H, Auerbach AD (1989) Hematological reconstitution in a patient with Fanconi's anemia by means of umbilical cord blood from a HLA identical sibling. New England Journal of Medicine 321(17): 1174–1187.

Goldman JM, Ciale RP, Horowitz MM, Biggs SC, Chapman E, Gluckman E (1988) Bone marrow transplant in CML chronic phase: increased risk for relapse associated with T-cell depletion. Annals of Internal Medicine 108(6): 806–814.

Goodman JW, Hodgson GS (1962) Evidence for stem cells in peripheral blood of mice. Blood 19(6): 702–713.

Gordon H (1983) Fissure sealants. In Murray JJ (ed.), The Prevention of Renal Disease. Oxford: Oxford University Press, pp. 175–187.

Gordon-Box M, Senior Donor Welfare Officer, The Anthony Nolan Bone Marrow Trust (1996) personal communication.

Gould D (1991) Nurses' hands as vectors of hospital-acquired infection: a review. Journal of Advanced Nursing 16(10): 1216–1225.

Graham K, Pecoraro D, Ventura M, Meyer C (1993) Reducing the incidence of stomatitis using a quality assessment and improvement approach. Cancer Nursing 16(2): 117–122.

Grandt N (1989) Hepatic veno-occlusive diseases following bone marrow transplantation. Oncology Nurses Forum 16(6): 813–817.

Gratwohl A, Hermans J, Baldomero H (1996) Hematopoietic precursor cell transplants in Europe: activity in 1994. Report from the European Group for Blood and Marrow Transplantation (EBMT). Bone Marrow Transplantation 17(2): 137–148.

Gray T, Shea T (1994) Current status of peripheral blood progenitor cell transplantation. Seminars in Oncology 21(5) (Suppl. 12): 93–101.

Groenwald SL, Hansen Frogge M, Goodman M, Henke Yarbo C (1992) Treatment modalities. Boston: Jones and Bartlett.

Gureno M, Reisinger C (1991) Patient controlled analgesia for the young pediatric patient. Pediatric Nursing 17(3): 251–254.

Haberman M (1988) Psychosocial aspects of bone marrow transplantation. Seminars in Oncology Nursing 4(10): 251–254.

Hanigan M, Walter G (1992) Nutritional support for the child with cancer. Journal of Pediatric Oncology Nursing 9(3): 110–118.

Harding R (1996) Children with cancer: the needs of siblings. Professional Nurse 11(9): 588–590.

Hare J, Skinner D, Kliewer D (1989) Family systems approach to paediatric bone marrow transplantation. Children's Health Care 18(1): 30–36.

Heiney S (1989) Adolescents with cancer: sexual and reproductive issues. Cancer Nursing 12(2): 95–101.

Heiney S, Neuberg R, Myers D, Bergman L (1994) The aftermath of bone marrow transplantation for parents of pediatric patients: a post-traumatic stress disorder. Oncology Nurses Forum 21(5): 843–847.

Hinds PS, Quargnetti AG, Hickey SS (1994) A comparison of the stress response sequence in new and experienced pediatric oncology nurses. Cancer Nursing 17(1): 61–71.

Hogbin B (1989) Getting it taped: the bad news consultation with cancer patients. British Journal of Hospital Medicine 41(4): 330–333.

Hooper PJ, Santas EJ (1993) Peripheral blood stem cell transplantation. Oncology Nurses Forum 20(8): 1215–1221.

Hopkins M (1991) Sperm banking. Nursing Times 87(47): 38–40.

Jacobson L, O'Simmons EL, Marks EK, Marks E, Robson M, Bethard W, Gaston E (1950) The role of the spleen in radiation injury and recovery. Journal of Laboratory and Clinical Medicine 35(5): 746–751.

Jecker NS (1990) Conceiving a child to save a child: reproductive and filial ethics. Journal of Clinical Ethics 1(2): 99–102.

Jenkins J, Wheeler V, Albright L (1994) Gene therapy for cancer. Cancer Nursing 17(6): 447–456.

Kaempfer S, Hoffman D, Willey F (1983) Sperm banking: a reproductive option in cancer therapy. Cancer Nursing 6(1): 31–38.

Kanfer E (1993) The diagnosis and management of early complications. In Trealeven J, Barrett J (eds), Bone Marrow Transplantation in Practice. London: Churchill Livingstone, pp. 247–256.

Kennedy P, Grey N (1997) High pressure areas. Nursing Times 93(29): 26–28.

Kessinger A, Armitage JO, Landmark JD, Weisenburger DD (1986) Reconstitution of human hematopoietic function with autologous cryopreserved circulating stem cells. Experimental Hematology 14(3): 192–196.

Kinrade LC (1987) Preparation of a donor for bone marrow transplant harvest procedure. Cancer Nursing 10(2): 77–81.

Kolb HJ, Schattenburg A, Goldman J, Hertenstein B, Jacobsen N, Arcese W, Ljungman P, Ferrant A, Verdouk L, Niederweiser D, Rhee F, Mittermueller J, de Whitte T, Holler E, Ansari H (1995) Graft versus leukaemia effect of donor lymphocyte transfusions in marrow engrafted patients. Blood 86(5): 2041–2050.

Korbling M (1993) Some principles of blood stem cell transplantation. Transfusion Science 14(1): 61–64.

Korbling M, Fleidner TM (1996) The evolution of clinical peripheral blood stem cell transplantation. Bone Marrow Transplantation 17(2): S4–S11.

Kramer R, Moore I (1983) Childhood cancer: meeting the special needs of healthy siblings. Cancer Nursing 6(3): 213–217.

Laison E, Lusk E (1985) Evaluating handwashing technique. Journal of Advanced Nursing 10(6): 547–552.

Leiper A (1995) Late effects of total body irradiation. Archives of Disease in Childhood 72(5): 382–385.

Leiper A, Stanhope R, Kitching C, Chessells JM (1987) Precocious and premature puberty associated with treatment of acute lymphoblastic leukaemia. Archives of Disease in Childhood 62(11): 1107–1112.

Leiper A, Stanhope R, Lau T, Grant D, Blacklock H, Chessells JM, Plowman P (1993) The effect of total body irradiation and bone marrow transplantation during childhood and adolescence on growth and endocrine function. British Journal of Haematology 67(4): 419–426.

Liesner R, Leiper A, Hann IM, Chessells JM (1994) Late effects of intensive treatment for acute myeloid leukaemia and myelodysplasia in childhood. Journal of Clinical Oncology 12(5): 916–924.

Lorenz E, Congdon CC, Uphoff D (1952) Modification of acute radiation injury in mice and guinea pigs by bone marrow injections. Radiology 58(6): 863–877.

Lucarelli G, Polchi P, Galimberti M, Izzc T, Delfini C, Manna M, Agostinelli F, Baronciani D, Giogi C, Angelucci E, Giadini C, Politi P, Manenti F (1985) Marrow transplantation for thalassaemia following busulphan and cyclophosphamide. The Lancet 1(8442): 1355–1357.

Lucarelli G, Galimberti M, Polchi P, Angelucci E, Baronciani D, Giardini C, Politi P, Durazzi SM, Muretto P, Alberinin F (1990) Bone marrow transplantation in patients with thalassemia. New England Journal of Medicine 322(7): 417–421.

Lwin R (1996) Impact of Paediatric Bone Marrow Transplant on Sibling Donors and Sibling Relationship. Unpublished PhD thesis. University College London.

McBride G (1990) Keeping bone marrow donation in the family. British Medical Journal 300(560): 1224–1225.

McDonald GB, Sharma P, Mathews DE, Shulman HM, Thomas ED (1984) Veno-occlusive disease of the liver after bone marrow transplantation: diagnosis, incidence, and predisposing factors. Hepatology 4(1): 116–122.

McDonald GB, Sharma P, Mathews DE, Shulman HM, Thomas ED (1985) The clinical course of 53 patients with veno-occlusive disease of the liver after marrow transplantation. Transplantation 39(6): 603–606.

McDonnell-Keenan A (1989) Nutritional support of the bone marrow transplant patient. Nursing Clinics of North America 24(2): 383–392.

McGarth PJ, Johnson G, Goodman JT, Schillinger J, Dunn J, Chapman J (1985) CHEOPS: A behavioral scale for rating postoperative pain in children. In Fields HL, Dubner R, Cervero (eds), Advances in Pain Research and Therapy. New York: Raven Press, pp. 395–401.

Magarth I (1994) Bone marrow transplantation for leukaemia: a lame horse for use of high technology medical care. The Lancet 345(8950): 601–602.

Maki DG (1991) Infection caused by intravascular devices: pathogenesis, strategies for prevention. In Maki DG (ed.), Improving Catheter Site Care (International Congress and Symposium series). London: Royal Society of Medicine Services Ltd.

Marcaigh A, Betcher D (1996) Cyclosporine. Journal of Pediatric Oncology Nursing 13(2): 98–100.

Mike V (1982) Incidence of second malignant neoplasms in children: results of an international study. The Lancet 2(8311): 1326–1331.

Molassiotis A, van der Akker T (1995) Psychological stress in nursing and medical staff on bone marrow transplant units. Bone Marrow Transplantation 15(3): 449–454.

Month S (1996) Preventing children from donating may not be in their best interests. British Medical Journal 312(7025): 240.

Morgan G (1993) Bone marrow transplantation for immunodeficiency syndromes. In Trealeven J, Barrett J (eds), Bone Marrow Transplantation in Practice. London: Churchill Livingstone, pp. 119–136.

Morrow L (1990) When one body can save another. Time, June 17.

Nesbit Jr ME, Buckley JD, Feig SA, Jacobsen L, Simmons E, Marks E, Robson M, Bethard W, Gaston E (1994) Chemotherapy for induction of remission of childhood acute myeloid leukaemia followed by marrow transplantation or multiagent chemotherapy: a report from the Children's Cancer Group. Journal of Clinical Oncology 12(1): 127–135.

Nicols K (1992) Understanding support. Nursing Times 88(13): 34–35.

Nitschke R, Humphrey GB, Sexauner C, Catron B, Wander S, Jay S (1982) Therapeutic choices made by parents with end stage cancer. Journal of Pediatrics 101(6): 471–476.

Ord J (1995) Introduction to HLA typing. Personal communication.

Osgood EE, Riddle MC, Mathews TJ (1939) Aplastic anaemia treated with daily transfusions and intravenous marrow. Annals of Internal Medicine 13(2): 357–367.

Patenaude A, Szymanski S, Rappeport J (1979) Psychological costs of bone marrow transplantation in children. American Journal of Orthopsychiatry 49(3): 409–422.

Patterson K (1992) Pain in the pediatric oncology patient. Journal of Pediatric Oncology Nursing 9(3): 119–130.

Patterson K (1993) Bone marrow harvesting and preparation of harvested marrow. In Trealeven J, Barrett J (eds), Bone Marrow Transplantation in Practice. London: Churchill Livingstone, pp. 307–214.

Pegg DE (1966) Allogenic bone marrow transplantation in man. In Pegg DE (ed.), Bone Marrow Transplantation. London: Lloyd-Luke Medical Books.

Peterson MR (1992) At Personal Risk. New York: Norton.

Pike S (1989) Family participation in the care of central venous lines. Nursing 3(38): 22–25.

Pinkerton CR, Cushing P, Sepion B (1994) Bone marrow transplantation. In Pinkerton CR, Cushing P, Sepion B (eds), Childhood Cancer Management. London: Chapman & Hall, pp. 106–125.

Pinkerton R (1993) High dose therapy with autologous bone marrow rescue in solid tumours of childhood. In Treleaven J, Barrett J (eds), Bone Marrow Transplantation in Practice. London: Churchill Livingstone, pp. 105–110.

Poe S, Larson E, McGuire D, Krumm S (1994) A national survey of infection prevention practices on bone marrow transplant units. Oncology Nurses Forum 21(10): 1687–1694.

Pot Mees C (1989) The Psychosocial Effects of Bone Marrow Transplantation in Children. Delft: Eburon.

Prentice HG, Atra A, Cornish JM, Gibson B, Kinset S, Pinkerton R, Potter MN, Will A, Veys P (1996) Donor leukocyte infusion as immunotherapy of acute leukaemia relapsed after allogeneic bone marrow transplant. Protocol of the UKCCSG Paediatric Bone Marrow Transplant Group — Pilot/Dose Finding Study (second draft).

Purandare L (1994) Therapeutic apheresis. Professional Nurse 9(9): 626–631.

Quine WE (1896) The remedial application of bone marrow. Journal of the American Medical Association 26(19): 1012–1013.

R v Cambridge District Health Authority, ex parte B (1995) . The Times, 15 March.

Reiser Y, Martelli M (1995) Bone marrow transplantation across HLA barriers by increasing the number of transplanted cells. Immunology Today 16(9): 437–440.

Richardson J, Webber I (1995) Ethical Issues in Child Health Care. London: CV Mosby.

Richman CM, Weiner RS, Yankee RA (1976) Increase in circulating stem cells following chemotherapy in man. Blood 47(6): 1031–1039.

Roberts A (1994) Systems of life. Blood: 3. Nursing Times 90(28): 31–34.

Robinson K, Abernathy E, Conrad J (1996) Gene therapy of cancer. Seminars in Oncology Nursing 12(2): 142–151.

Roitt I, Male D (1996) Introduction to the immune system. In Roitt I, Brostoff J, Male D (eds), Immunology (fourth edition). London: Mosby.

Rollins J (1990) Childhood cancer: siblings draw and tell. Paediatric Nursing 16(1): 21–35.

Rosenfeld CS, Bolwell B, LeFever A, Taylor R, List A, Fay J, Collins R, Andrews F, Pallansch P, Schuster MW, Resta D, Levitt D, Nemunaitis J (1996) Comparison of four cytokine regimens for mobilization of peripheral blood stem cells: IL-3 alone and combined with GM-CSF or G-CSF. Bone Marrow Transplantation 17(2): 179–183.

Russel N, Gratwohl A, Schmitz N (1996) Annotation — the place of blood stem cells in allogeneic transplantation. British Journal of Haematology 93(4): 747–753.

Ruston C, McEnhill M, Armstrong L (1996) Establishing therapeutic boundaries as patient advocates. Pediatric Nursing 22(3): 185–189.

Sanders J, Pritchard S, Mahoney P, Amos D, Buckner C, Witherspoon P, Deeg H, Doney K, Sullivan K, Appelbaum F, Storb R, Thomas E (1986) Growth and development following marrow transplantation for leukemia. Blood 68(5): 1129–1135.

Sanders J, Sullivan K, Witherspoon R, Doney K, Ansetti C, Beatty P, Peterson F (1989) Long term effects and quality of life in children and adults after bone marrow transplantation. Bone Marrow Transplantation 4(Suppl. 4): 27–29.

Sanders J, Hawley J, Levy W, Gooley T, Buckner C, Deeg H, Doney K, Storb R, Sullivan K, Witherspoon R, Appelbaum F (1996) Pregnancies following high-dose cyclophosphamide with or without high-dose busulfan or total body irradiation and bone marrow transplantation. Blood 87(7): 3045–3052.

Sanders JE, Thomas ED, Buckner DC, Downey K (1987) Marrow transplantation for children with acute lymphoblastic leukemia in second remission. Blood 70(1): 324–326.

Santos GW (1983) History of bone marrow transplantation. Clinical Haematology 12(3): 611–639.

Schmidt G (1992) Prophylaxis of cytomegalovirus infection after bone marrow transplantation. Seminars in Oncology Nursing 8(1): 20–26.

Schon DA (1991) The Reflective Practitioner. Aldershot: Avebury.

Scottish Office (1995) Scotland's Children: A Brief Guide to The Children (Scotland) Act. Scotland: Scottish Office.

Singer J (1992) Role of colony-stimulating factors in bone marrow transplantation. Seminars in Oncology Nursing 8(1): 27–31.

Skinhøj JP, Jacobsen N, Hoiby N, Faber V and the Copenhagen Bone Marrow Transplant Group (1987) Strict protective isolation in allogeneic bone marrow transplantation: effect on infectious complications, fever and graft versus host disease. Scandinavian Journal of Infectious Diseases 19(1): 91–96.

Socinski MA, Sannistra SA, Elias A, Antman KH, Schnipper L, Griffin JD (1988) Granulocyte–macrophage colony stimulating factor expands the circulating haematopoietic progenitor cell compartment in man. The Lancet (8596): 1194–1198.

Sormati M, Dungan S, Rieker P (1994) Pediatric bone marrow transplantation: psychological issues for parents after a child's hospitalisation. Journal of Psychological Oncology 12(4): 23–41.

Souchon V (1992) Nutrition during bone marrow transplantation. In Trealeven J, Barrett J (eds), Bone Marrow Transplantation in Practice. London: Churchill Livingstone, pp. 329–336.

Sullivan KM, Agura E, Anasetti CM (1991) Chronic graft versus host disease: late complications of bone marrow transplantation. Seminars in Hematology 28(2): 250–259.

Taylor M, O'Connor P (1989) Resident parents and shorter hospital stay. Archives of Disease in Childhood 64(2): 274–276.

Terasaki PI, McLelland JD (1964) Mucrodroplet assay of human serum cytotoxins. Nature 204(4962): 998–1000.

Testa NG (1996) Biological characteristics of cells migrating into the blood stream. Bone Marrow Transplantation 17(2): S12–S13.

Thomas ED, Lochte HL, Wan Ching LW, Ferrebee J (1957) Intravenous infusion of bone marrow in patients receiving radiation and chemotherapy. New England Journal of Medicine 257(11): 491.

Trealeven J, Barrett J (1993) Introduction to bone marrow transplantation. In Trealeven J, Barrett J (eds), Bone Marrow Transplantation in Practice. London: Churchill Livingstone, pp. 3–10.

Tyler PA, Ellison RN (1994) Sources of stress and psychological well being in high dependency nursing. Journal of Advanced Nursing 19(3): 469–476.

United Kingdom Central Council for Nursing, Midwifery and Health Visiting (1994) The Future of Professional Practice — the Council's Standards for Education and Practice Following Registration. London: UKCC.

Vaux Z (1996) Peripheral stem cell transplants in children. Paediatric Nursing 8(2): 20–22.

Vellodi A, Comba L, McCathy D (1992) Bone marrow transplantation for unborn errors of metabolism. In Trealeven J, Barrett J (eds), Bone Marrow Transplantation in Practice. London: Churchill Livingstone, pp. 161–176.

Veys P, Sanders F, Calderwood S (1994) The role of graft versus leukaemia in bone marrow transplantation for juvenile chronic myeloid leukaemia. Blood 84(Suppl.): 337A.

Veys P, Hann IM (1997) Bone marrow transplantation for leukaemia. In Plowman PN, Pinkerton R (eds), Paediatric Oncology: Clinical Practice and Controversies (second edition). London: Chapman & Hall Medical, pp. 617–627.

Volelsgang G, Hess A (1994) Graft versus host disease: new directions for a persistent problem. Blood 84(7): 2061–2067.

Vose JM, Armitage JO, Kessinger A (1993) High-dose chemotherapy and autologous transplant with peripheral blood stem cells. Oncology 7(8): 23–29.

Vowels MR, Tang TL, Mameghan H, Honeyman M, Russell S (1991) Bone marrow transplantation in children using closely matched related and unrelated donors. Bone Marrow Transplantation 8(2): 87–92.

Walker F, Roethke SK, Martin G (1994) An overview of the rationale, process and nursing implications of peripheral blood stem cell transplantation. Cancer Nursing 17(2): 141–148.

Welte K (1994) Matched unrelated donors. Seminars in Oncology Nursing 10(1): 20–27.

Whendon M, Ferrell B (1994) Quality of life in adult bone marrow transplant patients: beyond the first year. Seminars in Oncology Nursing 10(1): 42–57.

White A (1994) Parental concerns following a child's discharge from a bone marrow transplant unit. Journal of Paediatric Oncology Nursing 11(3): 93–101.

Wiley FM, Lindamood MM, Pfefferbaum-Levine B (1984) Donor–patient relationship in pediatric bone marrow transplantation. Journal of the Association of Pediatric Oncology Nurses 1(3): 8–15.

Williams HA, Wilson M (1989) Sexuality in children and adolescents with cancer: pediatric oncology nurses' attitudes and behaviors. Journal of Pediatric Oncology Nursing 6(4): 127–132.

Wingard J (1990) Advances in the management of infectious complications after bone marrow transplantation. Bone Marrow Transplantation 6(3): 371–383.

Witherspoon R, Storb R (1993) Bone marrow transplantation. In Lachmann P, Peters K, Rosen Walport M (eds), Clinical Aspects of Immunology (fifth edition). Boston, MA: Blackwell Scientific.

Witherspoon R, Fisher L, Schoch G, Martin P, Sullivan K, Sanders J, Deeg H, Doney K, Thomas F, Storb R (1989) Secondary cancers after bone marrow transplantation for leukemia or aplastic anemia. New England Journal of Medicine 321(12): 784–789.

Wong P, Baker CM (1988) Pain in children: comparison of assessment scales. Pediatric Nurse 14(1): 9–17.

Wujcik D, Ballard B, Camp-Sorrell D (1994) Selected complications of allogeneic bone marrow transplantation. Seminars in Oncology Nursing 10(1): 28–41.

Zerbe M (1992) Relationships between oral mucositis and treatment variables in bone marrow transplants. Cancer Nursing 16(2): 117–122.

Zerbe M, Parkerson S, Ortleib M, Spitzer T (1983) Relationships between oral mucositis and treatment variables in bone marrow transplants. Cancer Nursing 15(3): 196–205.

References
Section Three

Abudu A, Sferopoulos N, Tillman R, Carter S, Grimer R (1996) The surgical treatment and outcome of pathological fractures in localised osteosarcoma. Journal of Bone and Joint Surgery (Br) 78-B(5): 694–698.

Ainsworth H (1989) The nursing care of children undergoing craniotomy. Nursing 3(33): 5–7.

Albright L (1993) Paediatric brain tumours. Clinical Cancer Journal 43(5): 230–232.

Bass M (1993) Novice clinical nurse specialist and role acquisition. Clinical Nurse Specialist 7(3): 148–152.

Bates A (1994) Reducing fast times in paediatric day surgery. Nursing Times 90(48): 38–40.

Belson P (1987) A plea for play. Nursing Times 1(83): 26.

Bending J (1989) TENS in a pain clinic. Physiotherapy 75(5): 292–294.

Benner P (1984) From Novice to Expert. USA: Addison-Wesley.

Berger MS, Baurmgartner B, Geyer JR et al. (1991) The risks of metastases from shunting in children with primary central nervous system tumours. Journal of Neurosurgery 74(6): 872–877.

Biemann Othersen H (1986) Wilms' tumour. In Welch KJ, Randolph JG, Ravita MM, O'Neil JA, Rowe MI (eds), Paediatric Surgery (fourth edition). Chicago/London: Year Book Medical Publishers, pp 293–300.

Bird K, Dearmun A (1995) The impact of illness on the child and family. In Carter B, Dearmun A (eds), Child Health Care Nursing. Oxford: Blackwell Science, pp. 101–115.

Black D (1995) Foreword. In Black D, Judd D (eds), Give Sorrow Words (second edition). London: Whurr.

Black D, Judd D (1995) Give Sorrow Words (second edition). London: Whurr.

Blunden R (1989) An artificial state. Paediatric Nursing 1(1): 12–13.

Bonner K, Siegal KR (1988) Pathology, treatment and management of posterior fossa brain tumors in children. Journal of Neuroscience Nursing 20(2): 84–93.

Bralier L, Trapp A, Yates N (1987) Simon has Cancer. Newcastle upon Tyne: Victoria Publications.

Brimblecome F (1980) Foreword. In Weller BF, Helping Sick Children Play. London: Ballière Tindall.

Brodeur GM, Seeger RC, Barratt A (1988) International criteria for diagnosis, staging and response to treatment in patients with neuroblastoma. Journal of Clinical Oncology 6(12): 1874–1881.

Brown MJ, Dinndorf PA, Perek D et al. (1987) Infectious complications of intra-ventricular reservoirs in cancer patients. Pediatric Infectious Disease 6(2): 182–189.

Brown V (1995) Parents in recovery: parental and staff attitudes. Paediatric Nursing 7(7): 17–19.

Brykczynska G (ed.) (1989) Ethics in Paediatric Nursing. London: Chapman & Hall, p. 7.

Buckman R (1992) How to Break Bad News. London: Papermac.

Burr S (1993) Adolescents and the ward environment. Paediatric Nursing 5(1): 10–13.

Byrne J (1996) The Epidemiology of Brain Tumors in Childhood. Paper presented at the 7th International Symposium for Pediatric Neuro Oncology. Washington DC: Children's National Medical Center.

Canadell J, Forriol F, Cara J (1994) Removal of metaphyseal bone tumours with preservation of the epiphysis. Journal of Bone and Joint Surgery (Br) 76-B(1): 127–132.

Cannon S, Dyson P (1987) Relationship of the site of open biopsy of malignant bone tumours to local recurrence following resection and prosthetic replace-ment. Journal of Bone and Joint Surgery 69(3): 492.

Chalmers J (1988) Tumours of the musculoskeletal system: clinical presentation. Current Orthopaedics 2(3): 135–140.

Corbally M (1993) Supportive care of the paediatric cancer patient. Seminars in Surgical Oncology 9(6): 461–466.

Craft M (1993) Siblings of hospitalized children — assessment and intervention. Journal of Paediatric Nursing 8(5): 289–296.

Craft M, Craft J (1989) Perceived changes in siblings of hospitalized children: a comparison of sibling and parent reports. Children's Health Care 18(1): 42–47.

Crow S (1996) Prevention of intravascular infections — ways and means. Journal of Intravenous Nursing 19(4): 175–181.

Daniels L (1995) The psychosocial implications of central venous devices in cancer patients. Journal of Cancer Care 4(1): 141–145.

Day S (1995) Complementary therapies. In Carter B, Dearmun A (eds), Child Health Nursing Care. Oxford: Blackwell Scientific, pp. 237–246.

Department of Education (1993) Special Education Needs: A Guide for Parents. London: HMSO.

Department of Education and the Welsh Office (1994) Code of Practice on the Identification and Assessment of Special Educational Needs. London: Central Office of Information.

Department of Health (1991) The Paediatric Charter. London: HMSO.

Dernham P (1986) Phantom limb pain. Geriatric Nursing 7(1): 34–37.

Dickinson C (1995) The bladder: cystectomy, ideal conduit to treat cancer. Nursing Times 91(42): 34–35.

Dominic (1993) Left out in the cold. Paediatric Nursing 5(3): 28–29.

Dougherty L (1996) The benefits of an i.v. team in hospital practice. Professional Nurse 11(11): 761–763.

Drake J (1993) Ventriculostomy for treatment of hydrocephalus. Neurosurgical Clinics of North America 4(4): 657–666.

Duffner PK, Cohen ME (1992) Changes in the approach to central nervous system tumors in childhood. Pediatric Clinics of North America 39(4): 859–877.

Earl H, Souhami R (1990) Adolescent bone tumours. The Practitioner 234(1494): 816–818.

Education (Northern Ireland) Order (1996) Belfast: HMSO.

Evans M (1993a) Paediatric oncology. In Glasper A, Tucker A (eds), Advances in Child Health Nursing. London: Scutari Press, pp. 217–236.

Evans M (1993b) Teenagers and cancer. Paediatric Nursing 5(1): 14–15.

Favaloro R (1988) Adolescent development and implications for pain management. Paediatric Nursing 14(1): 27–29.

Fedora N (1985) Fighting for my leg . . . and my life. Orthopaedic Nursing 4(5): 39–42.

Friedman M (1987) Intervening with families of school-aged children with cancer. In Leahey M, Wright L (eds), Families and Life Threatening Illness. Pennsylvania: Springhouse Corporation, pp. 219–235.

Gardener R (1992) Psychological care of the neuro-oncology patient and family. British Journal of Nursing 1(11): 553–556.

Genge M (1988) Epidural analgesia in the orthopaedic patient. Orthopaedic Nursing 7(4): 11–19.

Geyer R, Levy M, Berger MS et al. (1980) Infants with medulloblastomas: a single institution review of survival. Neurosurgery 29(5): 701–711.

Gillies M (1992) Teenage traumas. Nursing Times 88(27): 26–29.

Goldman A (1994) (ed.) Care of the Dying Child. Oxford: Oxford University Press.

Grimer R, Carter S (1995) Paediatric surgical oncology 3 — bone tumours. European Journal of Surgical Oncology 21(2): 217–222.

Grimer R, Sneath R (1990) Editorial. Journal of Bone and Joint Surgery (Br) 72-B(5): 754–756.

Hahn K (1987) Therapeutic storytelling: helping children learn and cope. Paediatric Nursing 13(3): 175–178.

Harvey S (1980) The value of play in hospital. Paediatrician 9(8): 191–197.

Hickey J (1992) Neurological and Neurosurgical Nursing. Philadelphia: JB Lippincott.

Hill L (1994) (ed.) Caring For Dying Children and Their Families. London: Chapman & Hall, pp. 67–74.

Hockenberry M, Lane B (1988) Limb salvage procedures in children with osteosarcoma. Cancer Nursing 11(1): 2–8.

Hollis R (1992) Central venous access in children. Paediatric Nursing 4(6): 18–21.

Holt F (1993) The role of the clinical nurse specialist in developing systems of health care delivery. Clinical Nurse Specialist 7(3): 140.

House of Commons Select Committee (1997) Health Inquiry into Services for Children and Young People. London: HMSO.

Houston S, Liquire R (1991) Measuring success. Clinical Nurse Specialist 5(4): 204–209.

Jacques A (1994) Epidural analgesia. British Journal of Nursing 3(14): 734–738.

Johnson B (1995) One family's experience with head injury. Journal of Neuroscience Nursing 27(2): 113–118.

Johnson H (1992) Stoma care for infants, children and young people. Paediatric Nursing 4(4): 8–11.

Jurgens H, Winkler K, Gobel U (1992) Bone tumours. In Plowman P, Pinkerton C (eds), Paediatric Oncology. London: Chapman & Hall, pp. 325–350.

Kaufmann Rauen K, Ho M (1989) Children's use of patient-controlled analgesia after spinal surgery. Paediatric Nursing 15(6): 586–637.

Kehlet H (1994) Editorial. Postoperative pain relief — what is the issue? British Journal of Anaesthesia 72(4): 375–378.

Kemp H (1987) Limb conservation surgery for osteosarcoma and other primary bone tumours. In Souhami R (ed.), Clinical Oncology. London: Ballière Tindall, pp. 111–136.

Kirke E, Howard V, Scott C (1995) Description of posterior fossa syndrome in children after posterior fossa brain tumor surgery. Journal of Pediatric Oncology Nursing 12(4): 181–187.

Lansdown R, Sokel B (1993) Commissioned review. Approaches to pain management in children. ACPP Review and Newsletter 15(3): 105–111.

Lashford L, Lewis I, Fielding S, Flower M, Meller S, Kemshead J, Ackery (1992) Phase I/II study of iodine[131] metaiodobenzylguanidine in chemoresistant neuroblastoma: a United Kingdom Childhood Cancer Study Group investigation. Journal of Clinical Oncology 10(12): 1889–1896.

Lasoff E (1985) When a teenager faces amputation. Registered Nurse 48(2): 44–45.

Leese D (1989) My friend Wiggly. Paediatric Nursing 1(3): 12–13.

Leese D, Barrett M, Windebank K (1997) Central venous catheter use in paediatric oncology patients in the UK: a national multicentre, multidisciplinary study in progress. Journal of Cancer Nursing 1(4): 215–217.

Lew C, La Valley B (1995) The role of stereotactic radiotherapy in the management of children with brain tumors. Journal of Pediatric Oncology Nursing 12(4): 212–222.

Lewer H, Robertson L (1983) Care of the Child; The Essentials of Nursing. London: Macmillan.

Llewellyn N (1993a) Paediatric pain management — an imprecise science. In Glasper A, Tucker A (eds), Advances in Child Health Nursing. London: Scutari Press, pp. 123–140.

Llewellyn N (1993b) The use of PCA for paediatric post-operative pain management. Paediatric Nursing 5(5): 12–15.

Llewellyn N (1996) Pain assessment and the use of morphine. Paediatric Nursing 8(3): 32–35.

Look AT, Hayes FA, Shuster J et al. (1991) Clinical relevance of tumour cell ploidy and N-myc gene amplification in childhood neuroblastoma: a paediatric oncology group study. Journal of Clinical Oncology 9(4): 581–591.

Lowes L (1993) Ethical decision making — theory to practice. Paediatric Nursing 5(9): 10–11.

McCready M, MacDavitt K, O'Sullivan K (1991) Children and pain: easing the hurt. Orthopaedic Nursing 10(6): 33–42.

McGrath P (1990) Pain in children — nature, assessment and treatment. New York: The Guilford Press.

McGrath PA (1989) Evaluating a child's pain. Journal of Pain Symptom Management 4(4): 198–214.

McGuire P (1993) Radiation therapy. In Folet G, Fotchman D, Mooney P (eds), Nursing Care of the Child with Cancer. Philadelphia: PA Saunders.

McGuire Cullen P (1995) Pharmacological care of children with central nervous system tumors. Journal of Pediatric Nursing 12(4): 230–232.

McShane F (1992) Epidural narcotics: mechanism of action and nursing implications. Journal of Postanaesthetic Nursing 7(3): 155–162.

Maki D et al. (1991) Prospective randomised trial of poridone iodine, alcohol and chlorhexadine for prevention of infection associated with central venous and arterial catheters. The Lancet 338(8763): 339–343.

Mankin H, Gebhardt M, Springfield D (1988) Tumours of the musculoskeletal system: investigations. (Mini-symposium). Current Orthopaedics 2(3): 141–144.

Mantle F (1992) Complementary care. Nursing Times 88(18): 44–45.

Mertens W, Bramwell V (1994) Osteosarcoma and other tumours of bone. Current Opinion in Oncology 6(4): 384–390.

Miké V, Meadows A, D'Angio G (1982) Incidence of second malignant neoplasms in children: results of an international study. Lancet 2(8311): 1326–1331.

Moore I (1995) Central nervous system toxicity of cancer therapy in children. Journal of Pediatric Oncology Nursing 12(4): 203–210.

National Association for the Welfare of Children in Hospital (1990) Setting Standards of Adolescents in Hospital. London: NAWCH.

Nirenberg A (1985) The adolescent with osteogenic sarcoma. Orthopaedic Nursing 4(5): 11–15.

Noll R, Pawletko T, Sulzbacher S (1993) Psychosocial support. In Albin AR (ed.), Supportive Care of Children with Cancer. Baltimore, MD/London: Johns Hopkins.

Ornadel D, Souhami R, Whelan J, Nooy M, Ruiz de Elvira C, Pringle J, Lewis I, Steward W, George R, Bridgewater J, Wierzbicki R, Craft A (1994) Doxorubicin and cisplatin with granulocyte colony-stimulating factor as adjuvant chemotherapy for osteosarcoma: phase II trial of the European Osteosarcoma Intergroup. Journal of Clinical Oncology 12(9): 1842–1848.

Packer RJ, Sutton LN, Atkins TE, Radcliffe J, Brunin GR, D'Angio G, Seigel KR, Schut L (1989) A prospective study of cognitive function in children receiving whole brain radiotherapy and chemotherapy: two-year results. Journal of Neurosurgery 70(5): 707–713.

Parsons E (1992) Cultural aspects of pain. Surgical Nurse 5(2): 14–16.

Pasecki R (1992) Update in orthopaedic oncology. Orthopaedic Nursing 11(6): 36–43.

Peck H (1992) 'Please don't tell him the truth.' Paediatric Nursing 4(2): 12–14.

Phipps K (1996) A Retrospective Investigation into Long Term Educational Performance of Children Treated with Medulloblastoma. University of Surrey: Unpublished BSc thesis.

Piasecki P (1987) Bone malignancies. In Groenwald S (ed.), Cancer Nursing: Principles and Practice. Boston, MA: Jones & Bartlett, pp. 417–441.

Pike S (1989) Family participation in the care of central venous lines. Nursing 3(38): 22–24.

Pinkerton CR, Cushing P, Sepion B (1994) Childhood Cancer Management. London: Chapman & Hall.

Plaschkes J (1986) Surgical oncology in children. In Volte PA, Barratt A, Bloom HG, Lemerle K, Neidhardt MK (eds), Cancer in Children (second edition). Berlin/Heidelberg: Springer-Verlag, pp. 46–51.

Plowman P, Pinkerton CR (eds) (1992) Paediatric Oncology — Clinical Practice and Controversies. London: Chapman & Hall.

PONF/UKCCSG (1996) Central Venous Line Audit. Unpublished data from private correspondence.

Porter D, Holden S, Steel C, Cohen B, Wallace M, Reid R (1992) A significant proportion of patients with osteosarcoma may belong to Li-Fraumeni cancer families. Journal of Bone and Joint Surgery (Br) 74-B(6): 883–886.

Pringle J (1987) Pathology of bone tumours. In Souhami R (ed.), Clinical Oncology. London: Ballière Tindall, pp. 21–63.

Roberts P, Chan D, Grimer R, Sneath R, Scales J (1991) Prosthetic replacement of the distal femur for primary bone tumours. Journal of Bone and Joint Surgery (Br) 73-B(5): 762–769.

Rodin L (1985) Will This Hurt? London: Royal College of Nursing.

Rounseville C (1992) Phantom limb pain; the ghost that haunts the amputee. Orthopaedic Nursing 11(2): 67–71.

Ryan J, Shiminski-Maher T (1993) Neuro-oncology nurses: undaunted, hopeful and enthusiastic. Journal of Paediatric Oncology 12(4): 179–180.

Ryan J, Shiminski-Maher T (1995) Hydrocephalus and shunts in children with brain tumors. Journal of Pediatric Oncology Nursing 12(4): 223–229.

Salisbury J, Byers P (1994) Osteoblastic and cartilaginous neoplasms. In Salisbury J, Woods C, Byers P (eds), Diseases of Bones and Joints. London: Chapman & Hall, pp. 315–334.

Salkeld J (1992) (compiled) Childhood Brain Tumours — A Guide for Parents. London: Great Ormond Street Hospital for Sick Children's Trust/Institute of Child Health.

Sanger M, Copeland D (1989) Handbook of Pediatric Oncology. USA: Little Brown & Co.

Schwartz C, Constine L, Putnam T, Cohen H (1993) Paediatric solid tumours. In Rubin P (ed.), Clinical Oncology (seventh edition). Philadelphia: WB Saunders, pp. 282–288.

Scottish Office, Education and Industry Department (1996) Children and Young Persons with Special Educational Needs. Assessment and Recording. Edinburgh: HMSO.

Sensky T (1996) Eliciting lay beliefs across cultures — principles and methodology. British Journal of Cancer 74 (Suppl. XXIX): S63–S65.

Sepion B (1990) Investigations, staging and diagnosis — implications for nurses. In Thompson J (ed.), The Child with Cancer — Nursing Care. London: Scutari Press, pp. 47–59.

Seynour J (1996) Self catheterisation. Nursing Times 92(5): 40–48.

Shapiro C (1995) Central venous access catheters. Surgical Oncology Clinics of North America 4(3): 493–451.

Shiminski-Maher T (1993) Physician–patient–parent communication problems. Paediatric Neurosurgery 19(2): 104–108.

Shiminski-Maher T, Shields M (1995) Pediatric brain tumors: diagnosis and management. Journal of Pediatric Oncology Nursing 12(4): 188–198.

Sidey A (1995) Enteral feeding in community settings. Paediatric Nursing 7(6): 21–24.

Souhami R, Tobias J (1986) Bone and soft tissue sarcomas. In Souhami R, Tobias J (eds), Cancer and Its Management. London: Blackwell Scientific, pp. 433–452.

Sparacino P (1992) Advanced practice: the clinical nurse specialist. Nursing Practice 5(4): 2–4.

Spears N (1994) *In vitro* growth of oocyte. Human Reproduction 9(6): 969–976.

Spicer RD (1995) The management of soft tissue sarcomas in children. European Journal of Surgical Oncology 21(4): 317–320.

Spross J, Hope A (1985) Alterations in comfort — pain related to cancer. Orthopaedic Nursing 4(5): 48–52.

Stedeford A (1984) Facing Death; Patients, Families and Professionals. London: William Heineman Medical.

Stiller C (1988) Centralisation of treatment rates and survival rates for cancer. Archives of Disease in Childhood 63(1): 23–26.

Stoker D, Cobb J, Pringle J (1991) Needle biopsy of musculoskeletal lesions. Journal of Bone and Joint Surgery (Br) 73-B(3): 498–500.

Storr G (1988) The clinical nurse specialist: from the outside looking in. Journal of Advanced Nursing 13(1): 228–234.

Tait DM (1992) Minimization and management of morbidity from radiotherapy. In Plowman PN, Pinkerton CR (eds), Paediatric Oncology — Clinical Practice and Controversies. London: Chapman & Hall, p. 592.

Taylor B (1996) Parents as partners in care. Paediatric Nursing 8(4): 24–27.

Taylor J, Muller D (1995) Nursing Adolescents. London: Blackwell Scientific.

Tebbi C, Erpenbeck A (1996) Cancer. In Rickert V (ed.), Adolescent Nutrition. USA: Chapman & Hall, pp. 479–502.

Thomson J, Avizonis V, Fuller D, Walker M, Nilson D, Menlove R (1992) Late effects following cranial nervous system irradiation in a paediatric population. Neuropaediatrics 23(5): 228–234.

Tobias JS, Hayward RD (1989) Brain and spinal cord tumours in children. In Thomas DAF (ed.), Neuro-oncology. London: Edward Arnold.

Triche RS (1992) Tumour pathology. In Plowman PN, Pinkerton CR (eds), Paediatric Oncology — Clinical Practice and Controversies. London: Chapman & Hall, pp. 51–72.

Turner L (1989) Creating the right atmosphere. Nursing Times 85(32): 34–35.

Tweedle DA, Windebank KP, Barrett AM, Leese DC, Cowing R (1997) Central venous catheter use in UKCCSG oncology centres. Archives of Disease in Childhood 77(1): 58–59.

Uchida A, Araki N, Shinto Y, Yoshikawa H, Kurisaki E, Ono K (1990) The use of hydroxyapatite ceramic in bone tumour surgery. Journal of Bone and Joint Surgery (Br) 72-B(2): 298–302.

UKCCSG (1996) Biopsy of Paediatric Solid Tumours. Unpublished paper.

Unwin P, Cannon S, Grimer R, Kemp H, Sneath R, Walker P (1996) Aseptic loosening in cemented custom-made prosthetic replacements for bone tumours of the lower limb. Journal of Bone and Joint Surgery (Br) 78-B(1): 5–13.

Vos A (1995) Primary liver tumours in children. European Journal of Surgical Oncology 21(4): 101–105.

White C (1995) Life crises for children and their families. In Carter B, Dearmun A (eds), Child Health Care Nursing. London: Blackwell Scientific, pp. 116–129.

Wiener E, Lawrence W, Hays DM (1991) Complete response or not complete response? Second look operations are the answer in children with rhabdomyosarcoma. Proceedings of the American Society of Clinical Oncology 10: 316.

Willett K, Simmons C, Bentley G (1988) The effect of suction drains after total hip replacement. Journal of Bone and Joint Surgery (Br) 70-B(4): 607–710.

Wilson K (1993) Education for the hospitalised child. Paediatric Nursing 5(4): 24–25.

Winder A (1994) Achieving independence. Nursing Times 90(22): 50–52.

Wisoff JM, Epstein FJ (1994) Management of hydrocephalus in children with medulloblastoma: prognostic factors for shunting? Pediatric Neurosurgery 20(4): 240–247.

Woolet H (1981) Imparting the diagnosis of life threatening illness in children. British Medical Journal 298(6688): 1623–1626.

Zoeller G, Pekran A, Lakomek M, Ringert RH (1995) Staging problems in the pre-operative chemotherapy of Wilms' tumour. British Journal of Urology 76(4): 501–503.

References
Section Four

Anderson V, Smibert E, Ekert H, Godber T (1994) Intellectual, educational, and behavioural sequelae after cranial radiation and chemotherapy. Archives of Disease in Childhood 70(6): 176–183.

Aquino VM, Smyr CB, Hagg R, McHara KM, Prestridge L, Sandler ES (1995) Enteral nutritional support by gastrostomy tube in children with cancer. Journal of Pediatrics 127(1): 58–62.

Ash P (1980) The influence of radiation on fertility in man. British Journal of Radiology 53(2): 271–278.

Atra A, Ward HC, Aitken K, Boyle M, Dicks-Mireaux C, Duffy PG, Mitchell CD, Plowman PN, Ransley PG, Pritchard J (1994) Conservative surgery in multimodal therapy for pelvic rhabdomyosarcoma in children. British Journal of Cancer 70(5): 1001–1008.

Baldwin PD (1983) Epidural spinal cord compression secondary to metastatic disease: a review of the literature. Cancer Nursing 6(6): 441–449.

Ball JL, Moore AD (1980) Essential Physics for Radiographers. Oxford: Blackwell Scientific.

Barbarin OA (1987) Psychosocial risks and invulnerability: a review of the theoretical and empirical bases of preventative family-focused services for survivors of childhood cancer. Journal of Psychosocial Oncology 5(1): 25–41.

Barkham A (1993) Radiotherapy skin reactions and treatments. Professional Nurse 8(11): 732–736.

Baron MC (1991) Advances in the care of children with brain tumours. Journal of Neuroscience Nursing 23(1): 39–43.

Bentzen SM, Overgaard M (1995) Actual versus ideal treatment time in radiotherapy for head and neck cancer. International Journal of Radiation Oncology, Biology & Physics 31(3): 687–688.

Berger B (1992) Neurologic Aspects of Pediatrics. Boston, MA: Butterworth–Heinemann.

Biti G, Cellai E, Magrini SM, Papi M, Ponticelli P, Boddi V (1994) Second solid tumours and leukaemia after treatment for Hodgkin's disease: an analysis of 1121 patients from a single institution. International Journal of Radiation Oncology, Biology & Physics 29(1): 25–31.

Blatt J, Sherin SR, Niebrugger D (1985) Leydig cell function in boys following treatment for testicular relapse of acute lymphoblastic leukaemia. Journal of Clinical Oncology 3(9): 1227–1231.

Bleyer WA (1981) Neurologic sequelae of methotrexate and ionising radiation: a new classification. Cancer Treatment 65(1): 89–98.

Bleyer WA, Griffin TW (1980) White matter necrosis, mineralising angiopathy and intellectual abilities in survivors of childhood leukaemia. In Gilbert NA, Keegan AR (eds), Radiation Damage to the Nervous System. New York: Raven Press.

Bloom JR, Gorsky RD, Fobair P et al. (1990) Physical performance at work and at leisure: validation of a measure of biological energy in survivors of Hodgkin's disease. Journal of Psychosocial Oncology 8(1): 49–63.

Bokemeyer C, Schmoll HJ (1995) Treatment of testicular cancer and the development of secondary malignancies. Journal of Clinical Oncology 13(1): 283–292.

Bozzola M, Giorgianai G, Locatelli F et al. (1993) Growth in children after bone marrow transplantation. Hormone Research 39(3–4): 122–126.

Brauner R, Czernichow R, Cramer P (1983) Leydig cell function in children after direct testicular irradiation for acute lymphoblastic leukemia. New England Journal of Medicine 309(1): 25–28.

Brunner DW, Iwamoto R, Keane K, Strohl R (eds) (1992) Manual for Radiation Oncology Nursing Practice and Education. Pittsburgh: Oncology Nursing Society.

Bucholtz JD (1992) Issues concerning the sedation of children for radiotherapy. Oncology Nurses Forum 19(4): 649–655.

Byrne J, Mulvihill MH, Myers R et al. (1987) Effects of treatment on fertility in long term survivors of childhood and adolescent cancer. New England Journal of Medicine 317(21): 1315–1321.

Byrne TN (1992) Spinal cord compression from epidural metastases. New England Journal of Medicine 327(9): 614–619.

Calissendorff B, Bolme P, el Azuzi M (1991) The development of cataracts in children as a late side-effect of bone marrow transplanation. Bone Marrow Transplantation 7(6): 427–429.

Campbell I, Illingworth M (1992) Can patients wash during radiotherapy to the breast or chest wall? A randomised controlled trial. Clinical Oncology 4(2): 78–82.

Campbell J, Lane C (1996) Skin care protocol for radiotherapy patients. Professional Nurse 12(2): 105–108.

Campbell S (1987) Mouth care in cancer patients. Nursing Times 22(83): 59–60.

Carl W (1983) Oral complications in cancer patients. American Family Physician 27(2): 161–170.

Carl W (1995) Oral complications of local and systemic cancer treatment. Current Opinion in Oncology 7(4): 320–321.

Cassady JR, Lebowitz RL, Jaffe N, Hoffman A (1981) Effect of low dose irradiation in renal enlargement in children following nephrectomy for Wilms' tumour. Acta Radiologica Oncology 20(1): 5–8.

Chesler MA, Barbarin OA (1987) Childhood Cancer and The Family. New York: Brunner/Mazel.

Christie D, Battin M, Leiper AD, Chessells JM, Vargha-Khadem F, Neville BG (1994) Neuropsychological and neurological outcome after relapse of lymphoblastic leukaemia. Archives of Disease in Childhood 70(4): 275–280.

Christie D, Leiper AD, Chessells JM, Vargha-Khadem F (1995) Intellectual performance after presymptomatic cranial radiotherapy for leukaemia: effects of age and sex. Archives of Disease in Childhood 73(1): 136–140.

Cicognani A, Cacciari E, Rosito P, Mancini AF, Carla G, Mandini M, Paulucci C (1994) Longitudinal growth and final height in long term survivors of childhood leukemia. European Journal of Pediatrics 153(10): 726–730.

Clifton DK, Bremner WJ (1983) The effect of testicular x-irradiation on spermatogenesis in man. Journal of Andrology 4(6): 387–392.

Coleman S (1995) An overview of the oral complications of adult patients with malignant haematological conditions who have undergone radiotherapy and chemotherapy. Journal of Advanced Nursing 22(6): 1085–1091.

Commeau Lew C (1992) Special needs of children. In Hassey-Dow K, Hilderley LJ (eds), Nursing Care in Radiation Oncology. Philadelphia: WB Saunders, pp. 177–203.

Constine L, Cann D, Woolf P, Mick G, McCormick K, Rubin P (1989) Radiation induced hypothalamic and pituitary injury in children following treatment for CNS malignancies. Pediatric Research 25(1): 149a.

Constine LS (1991) Late effects of radiation therapy. Pediatrician 18(1): 37–48.

Constine LS, Rubin P (1988) Total body irradiation; normal tissue effects. In Bleehan NM (ed.), Radiobiology in Radiotherapy. London: Springer, pp. 95–122.

Constine LW, Donaldson SS, McDougall IR (1984) Thyroid dysfunction after radiotherapy in children with Hodgkin's disease. Cancer 53(4): 878–883.

Coons T (1995) Monoclonal antibodies: the promise and the reality. Radiologic Technology 67(1): 39–64.

Cooper CO, Heron TE, Heward WL (1987) Applied Behavioral Analysis. Columbus, OH: Merrill.

Cosset JM, Socie G, Dubray B, Girinsky T, Fourquet A, Gluckman E (1994) Single dose versus fractionated total body irradiation before bone marrow transplantation. International Journal of Radiation Oncology, Biology & Physics 30(2): 177–192.

Crellin AM, Marks A, Maher EJ (1989) Why don't British radiologists give single fractions of radiotherapy for bony metastases? Clinical Oncology 1(2): 63–66.

Cristy M (1981) Active bone marrow distribution as a function of age in humans. Physics in Medicine and Biology 26(3): 389–400.

Crowne EC, Wallace WHB, Moore C et al. (1992) A novel variant of growth hormone insufficiency following low dose cranial radiation. Clinical Endocrinology 36(1): 9–68.

Cust MP, Gangar KF, Hillard TC, Whitehead MI (1990) A risk–benefit assessment of estrogen therapy in postmenopausal women. Drug Safety 5(5): 345–358.

Daeffler R (1981) Oral hygiene measures for patients with cancer. Cancer Nursing 4(1): 29–35.

Dalhllof G, Barr M, Bolme P (1988) Disturbances in dental development after total body irradiation on bone marrow transplant recipients. Oral Surgery, Oral Medicine, Oral Pathology 65(1): 41–44.

D'Angio GJ, Green DM (1995) Induced malignancies. In Abeloff MD, Armitage JO, Lichter AS, Niederhuber JE (eds), Clinical Oncology. New York: Churchill Livingstone, pp. 833–849.

Davies HA, Didcock EA, Didi M (1994) Disproportionate short stature after cranial irradiation and combination therapy for leukaemia. Archives of Disease in Childhood 70(6): 472–475.

Davies MC, Hall ML, Jacobs HS (1989) Ovarian failure after total body irradiation. British Medical Journal 299(6714): 1494–1497.

Department of Health (1985a) The Ionising Radiation Regulations. London: HMSO.

Department of Health (1985b) The Protection of Persons Against Ionising Radiation Arising from Any Work Activity. London: HMSO.

Department of Health (1987) Restriction of the use of crystal violet. Pharmacy Journal 239(4): 665.

Derengowski S, O'Brien E (1996) Critical care of the pediatric oncology patient. AACN Clinical Issues 7(1): 109–119.

Devine EC, Westlake SK (1995) The effects of psychoeducational care provided to adults with cancer. Oncology Nurses Forum 22(9): 1369–1381.

Didcock E, Davies HA, Didi M, Ogilvy-Stuart AL, Wales JKH, Shalet SM (1995) Pubertal growth in young adult survivors of childhood leukaemia. Journal of Clinical Oncology 13(10): 2503–2507.

Dietz K, Flaherty AM (1990) Oncological emergencies. In Groenwald SL (ed), Cancer Nursing: Principles and Practice (second edition). Boston, MA: Jones & Bartlett, pp. 644–668.

Donaldson SS, Kaplan HS (1982) Complications of treatment of Hodgkin's disease in children. Cancer Treatment Reports 66(4): 977–989.

Doyle K (1984) The young child. In McIntire S, Cioppa A (eds), Cancer Nursing — A Developmental Approach. New York: John Wiley, pp. 46–55.

Dreifke L, DeMeyer E (1992) Information guide for patients receiving total body irradiation before bone marrow transplantation. Cancer Nursing 15(3): 206–210.

Dudjak L (1987) Mouth care for mucositis due to radiation therapy. Cancer Nursing 10(3): 131–133.

Dudjak L (1992) Alteration in dose fractionations and treatment volumes. In Hassey-Dow K, Hilderley LJ (eds), Nursing Care in Radiation Oncology. Philadelphia: WB Saunders, pp. 285–290.

Dunbar SF, Loeffler JS (1994) Stereotactic radiation therapy. In Mauch PM, Loeffler JS (eds), Radiation Oncology, Technology and Biology. Philadelphia: WB Saunders, pp. 237–257.

Duncan G, Duncan EW, Maher EJ (1993) Patterns of palliative radiotherapy in Canada. Clinical Oncology 5(2): 92–97.

Dunne-Daly CF (1994) Nursing care and adverse reactions of external radiation therapy: a self learning module. Cancer Nursing 17(3): 236–256.

Edbaugh H (1988) Becoming an Ex: The Process of Role Exit. Chicago: University of Chicago Press.

Edge WG, Morgan M (1977) Ketamine and paediatric radiotherapy. Anaesthetic Intensive Care 5(2): 153–156.

Eilers J, Berger A, Peterson M (1988) Development, testing, and application of the oral assessment guide. Oncology Nurses Forum 15(3): 325–330.

Emami B, Lyman J, Brown A, Coia L et al. (1991) Tolerance of normal tissues to therapeutic irradiation. International Journal of Radiation Oncology, Biology & Physics 21(1): 109–122.

Everhart C (1991) Overcoming childhood cancer misconceptions among long term survivors. Journal of Pediatric Oncology Nursing 8(1): 46–48.

Faithful S (1991) Patients' experiences following cranial radiotherapy: a study of the somnolence syndrome. Journal of Advanced Nursing.16(8): 930–946.

Faithful S (1992) The diary method for nursing research; a study of somnolence syndrome. European Journal of Cancer Care 1(2): 13–18.

Faithful S (1995) 'Just grin and bear it and hope it will go away'; coping with the urinary symptoms from pelvic radiotherapy. European Journal of Cancer Care 4(4): 158–165.

Feber T (1995) Mouth care for patients receiving oral irradiation. Professional Nurse 10(10): 666–670.

Fergusson J, Ruccione K, Hobbie WL (1986) The effects of the treatment of cancer in childhood on growth and development. Journal of the Association of Pediatric Oncology Nurses 3(4): 13–21.

Flentje M, Weirich A, Potter R, Ludwig R (1994) Hepatotoxicity in irradiated nephroblastoma patients during post-operative treatment according to SIOP 9. Radiation Oncology 31(3): 222–228.

Flietkau R, Iro H, Sailer D, Sauer R (1991) Percutaneous endoscopically guided gastrostomy in patients with head and neck cancer. Recent Results in Cancer Research 121: 269–282.

Fontanesi J, Rao BN, Fleming ID, Bowman LC, Pratt CB, Furman WL, Coffey DH, Kun LE (1994) Pediatric brachytherapy, the St Jude Children's Research Hospital experience. Cancer 74(2): 733–739.

Fox PC, van der Verv PF, Baum BJ, Mandel ID (1986) Pilocarpine for the treatment of xerostomia associated with salivary gland dysfunction. Oral Surgery 161(3): 243–248.

Fraser MC, Tucker MA (1988) Late effects of cancer therapy: chemotherapy related malignancies. Oncology Nurses Forum 1(1): 67–77.

Freeman J, Johnston P, Voke K (1973) Somnolence after prophylactic cranial irradiation in children with acute leukaemia. British Medical Journal 4(891): 523–525.

Fritz G, Williams J (1988) Issues of adolescent development for survivors of childhood cancer. Journal of the American Academy of Child and Adolescent Psychiatry 27(6): 712–715.

Fritz G, Williams J, Amylon M (1988) After treatment ends: psychosocial sequelae in pediatric cancer survivors. American Journal of Orthopsychiatry 58(4): 552–561.

Fromm M, Littman P, Raney B (1986) Late effects after treatment of twenty children with soft tissue sarcomas of the head and neck. Cancer 57(10): 2070–2076.

Fu KK, Pajak TF, Marcial VA, Ortiz HG, Rotman M et al. (1995) Late effects of hyperfractionated radiotherapy for advanced head and neck cancer: long term follow up. International Journal of Radiation Oncology, Biology & Physics 32(3): 577–588.

Furlong TG, Gallucci BB (1994) Pattern of occurrence and clinical presentation of neurological complications in bone marrow transplant patients. Cancer Nursing 17(1): 27–36.

Gallagher J (1995) Management of cutaneous symptoms. Seminars in Oncology Nursing 11(4): 239–247.

Gaze MN (1996) The role of radiotherapy in the management of neuroblastoma. In Tobias JS, Thomas PRM (eds), Current Radiation Oncology (Volume 2). London: Edward Arnold, pp. 218–240.

Gelfand MJ (1993) Meta-iodobenzylguanidine in children. Seminars in Nuclear Medicine 23(3): 231–242.

Gibbs S (1991) Action on the environment; validation hazards. Nursing Times 87(27): 46–47.

Gilbert HA, Kaplan P, Naussbaum H et al. (1977) Evaluation of radiation therapy for bone metastases, pain relief and quality of life. American Journal of Roentgenology 129(6): 1095–1096.

Ginsberg M (1961) A study of oral hygiene nursing care. American Journal of Nursing 61(10): 67–69.

Glover DJ, Glick JH (1991) Oncology emergencies. In Holleb AI, Fink DJ, Murphy GP (eds), American Cancer Society Textbook of Clinical Oncology. Atlanta, GA: American Cancer Society, pp. 276–283.

Goff JR, Anderson JR, Cooper PF (1980) Distractability and memory deficits in long term survivors of acute lymphoblastic leukaemia. Development, Behavior and Pediatrics 1(4): 158–163.

Goldman A (1992) Care of the dying child. In Plowman PN, Pinkerton CR (eds), Paediatric Oncology: Clinical Practice and Controversies. London: Chapman & Hall, pp. 618–630.

Goldwein JW (1987) Radiation myelopathy: a review. Medical and Pediatric Oncology 15(1): 89–95.

Gomez EG (1995) A teaching booklet for patients receiving mantle field irradiation. Oncology Nurses Forum 22(10): 121–126.

Goodman M (1989) Managing the side effects of chemotherapy. Seminars in Oncology Nursing 5(1): 43–45.

Goolden AW, Goldman JM, Kam KC, Dunn PA et al. (1983) Fractionation of whole body irradiation before bone marrow transplantation of patients with leukaemia. British Journal of Radiology 56(66): 245–250.

Graham KM, Pecoraro DA, Ventura M, Meyer CC (1993) Reducing the incidence of stomatitis using a quality assessment and improvement approach. Cancer Nursing 16(2): 117–122.

Gray RE, Doan BD, Shermer P, Fitzgerald AV, Berry MP, Jenkin D, Doherty MA (1992) Surviving childhood cancer: a descriptive approach to understanding the impact of life threatening illness. Psycho-oncology 4(11): 35–245.

Graydon JE, Bubela N, Irvine D, Vincent L (1995) Fatigue reducing strategies used by patients receiving treatment for cancer. Cancer Nursing 18(1): 23–28.

Green DM (1989) Long Term Complications of Therapy for Cancer in Childhood and Adolescence. Baltimore, MD: Johns Hopkins University Press.

Green DM (1993) Effects of treatment for childhood cancer on vital organ systems. Cancer 71(10) (Suppl.): 3299–3305.

Greifzu S (1990) Oral care is a part of cancer care. RN 53(6): 43.

Guerra P, Colombo L, Maira G (1990) Therapeutic possibilities of ^{131}ImIBG in metastatic carcinoid tumours. Tumour 76(5): 485–487.

Hagopian GA (1991) The effects of a weekly radiation therapy newsletter on patients. Oncology Nurses Forum 18(7): 1199–1203.

Hagopian GA (1996) The effects of informational audiotapes on knowledge and self-care behaviours of patients undergoing radiation therapy. Oncology Nurses Forum 23(4): 697–700.

Hall EJ (1986) Radiation biology. Cancer 55(6): 2051–2057.

Halperin E, Kun L, Constine L, Tarbell N (1989) Pediatric Radiation Oncology. New York: Raven Press.

Hanigan MJ, Walker GA (1992) Nutritional support of the child with cancer. Journal of Pediatric Oncology Nursing 9(3): 110–118.

Hasse GM, Meagher DP, McNeely LK, Daniel WE, Poole MA, Blake M, Odom LF (1994) Electron beam intraoperative radiation therapy for pediatric neoplasms. Cancer 74(2): 740–747.

Hassey-Dow K (1992) Principles of brachytherapy. In Hassey-Dow K, Hilderley LJ (eds), Nursing Care in Radiation Oncology. Philadelphia: WB Saunders, pp. 16–33.

Hatton-Smith CK (1994) The last bastion of ritualised practice? Professional Nurse 9(5): 304–308.

Hawkins MM (1990) Second primary tumours following radiotherapy for childhood cancer. International Journal of Radiation Oncology, Biology & Physics 19(5): 1297–1301.

Haylock PJ, Hart LK (1979) Fatigue in patients receiving localised radiation. Cancer Nursing 2(2): 161–167.

Henriksson R, Franzen L, Edbom C, Littbrand B (1995) Sulcrafate: prophylaxis of mucosal damage during cancer therapy. Scandinavian Journal of Gastroenterology 210: 45–47.

Hewitt CC, Gaylor DW (1985) Chronic toxicity and carcinogenicity studies of gentian violet in mice. Fundamental and Applied Toxicology 5(7): 902–912.

Heyn R, Ragob A, Raney B et al. (1986) Late effects of therapy in orbital rhabdomyosarcoma. Cancer 57(9): 1738–1743.

Hilderley L (1983) Skin care in radiation therapy. Oncology Nurses Forum 10(1): 51–56.

Hilderley L (1992a) Radiation oncology: historical background and principles of teletherapy. In Hassey-Dow K, Hilderley L (eds), Nursing Care in Radiation Oncology. Philadelphia: WB Saunders, pp. 3–16.

Hilderley L (1992b) Pain and fatigue. In Hassey-Dow K, Hilderley L (eds), Nursing Care in Radiation Oncology. Philadelphia: WB Saunders, pp. 57–69.

Hillard TC, Whitcroft S, Ellerington MC, Whitehead MI (1991) The long term risks and benefits of hormone replacement therapy. Journal of Clinical Pharmacological Therapy 16(4): 231–245.

Hobbie WL, Schwartz C (1989) Endocrine late effects among survivors of cancer. Seminars in Oncology Nursing 5(1): 14–21.

Hobbie W, Ruccione K, Moore I, Truesdell S (1993) Late effects in long term survivors. In Foley FV, Fochtman D, Hardin-Mooney K (eds), Nursing Care of the Child with Cancer. Philadelphia: WB Saunders, pp. 466–497.

Hockenberry M (1986) Impact of cancer. In Hockenberry M, Coody D (eds), Pediatric Oncology and Hematology — Perspectives on Care. St Louis, MO: CV Mosby, pp. 419–428.

Hoefnagel CA, De-Kraker J, Valdes-Olnos RA, Voute PA (1994) I[131] mIBG as a first line treatment in high risk neuroblastoma patients. Nuclear Medicine Communication 15(9): 712–717.

Hoffman B (1992) Legal remedies to job and insurance discrimination against former childhood cancer patients. In Green DM, D'Angio GJ (eds), Late Effects of Treatment for Childhood Cancer. New York: Wiley Liss, pp. 165–171.

Hogan CM (1990) Advances in the management of nausea and vomiting. Nursing Clinics of North America 25(20): 175–197.

Holmes S (1986) Radiotherapy: planning nutritional support. Nursing Times 829(160): 26–29.

Holmes S (1991) Support can boost the body's defences: nutrition in cancer care. Professional Nurse 7(2): 83–84.

Horowitz ME, Pizzo PA (eds) (1991) The Pediatric Clinics of North America: Solid Tumours in Children. Philadelphia: WB Saunders.

Horowitz ME, Neff JR, Kun LE (1991) Ewing's sarcoma: radiotherapy versus surgery for local control. In Horowitz ME, Pizzo PA (eds), The Pediatric Clinics of North America: Solid Tumours in Children. Philadelphia: WB Saunders.

Hughes LL, Baruzzi MJ, Ribeiro RC, Ayers GD, Rao B, Parham DM, Pratt CB, Kun LE (1994) Paratesticular rhabdomyosarcoma: delayed effects of multi-modality therapy and implications for current management. Cancer 73(2): 476–482.

Hungerford JL, Toma NMG, Plowman PN, Kingston JE (1995) External beam radiotherapy for retinoblastoma: I Whole eye technique. British Journal of Ophthalmology 79(2): 109–111.

Hurwitz JI, Kaplan DM, Kaiser E (1962) Designing an instrument to assess parental coping mechanisms. Social Casework 10(3): 527–532.

Husebye E, Hauer-Jensen M, Kjorstad K, Skar V (1994) Severe late radiation enteropathy is characterised by impaired motility of proximal small intestine. Digestive Disease and Science 39(11): 2341–2349.

Hymovich DP, Roehnart JE (1989) Psychosocial consequences of childhood cancer. Seminars in Oncology Nursing 5(1): 56–62.

Ilhan I, Sarialioglu F, Ozbarlas N, Buyukpamukcu M, Akyuz C, Kutluk T (1995) Late cardiac effects after treatment for childhood Hodgkin's disease with chemotherapy and low dose radiotherapy. Postgraduate Medical Journal 71(833): 164–167.

Ingham J, Beveridge A, Cooney NJ (1993) The management of spinal cord compression in patients with advanced malignancy. Journal of Pain and Symptom Management 8(1): 1–6.

Inoue HK, Nakamura M, Ono N, Kawashima Y, Hirato M, Ohye C (1993) Long term clinical effects of radiation therapy for primitive gliomas and medulloblas-tomas: a role for radiosurgery. Stereotactic Functional Neurosurgery 61 (Suppl. 1): 51–58.

Iwamoto R (1992) Altered nutrition. In Hassey-Dow K, Hilderley LJ (eds), Nursing Care in Radiation Oncology. Philadelphia: WB Saunders, pp. 69–96.

Iwamoto R (1994) Radiation therapy. In Otto SE (ed.), Oncology Nursing (second edition). St Louis, MO: CV Mosby, pp. 298–331.

Jenkin D, Greenberg M, Hoffman H, Hendrick B, Humphreys R, Vatter A (1995) Brain tumours in children: long term survival after radiation treatment. International Journal of Radiation Oncology, Biology & Physics 31(3): 445–451.

Jenney MEM, Kissen GDN (1996) Late effects after treatment of childhood leukaemia and lymphoma. Clinical Paediatrics 3(4): 715–735.

Jones G, Larkkarman E (1987) Tolerance revisited. International Journal of Radiation Oncology, Biology & Physics 13(2): 290–291.

Kanner R (1987) Epidural spinal cord compression. In Dutchetr JP, Weirnik PH (eds), Handbook of Hematologic and Oncologic Emergencies. New York: Plenum Medical Book Co., pp. 763–770.

Kaplan MM, Garrick MB, Gelber R, Li FP et al. (1983) Risk factors for thyroid abnormalities after neck irradiation for childhood cancer. American Journal of Medicine 74(2): 272–280.

Kaste SC, Hopkins KP, Jenkins JJ (1994) Abnormal odontogenesis in children treated with radiation and chemotherapy, imaging findings. American Journal of Roentgenology 162(6): 1407–1411.

Kazak AE (1994) Implications of survival: paediatric oncology patients and their families. In Bearison DJ, Mulhern RK (eds), Paediatric Oncology: Psychological Perspectives on Children with Cancer. Oxford: Oxford University Press, pp. 171–193.

Kenny SA (1990) The effect of two oral care protocols on the incidence of stomatitis in haematology patients. Cancer Nursing 13(6): 345–353.

King KB (1985) Patients' descriptions of the experience of receiving radiation therapy. Oncology Nurses Forum 12(4): 55–61.

Kirkbride P (1995) The role of radiation therapy in palliative care. Journal of Palliative Care 11(1): 19–26.

Kissen GDN (1996) Late effects of treatment on paediatric oncology. In Selby P, Bailey C (eds), Cancer and the Adolescent. London: BMJ Publications, pp. 226–242.

Kissen GDN, Wallace WHB (1993) Long Term Follow-up Guidelines. London: UKCCSG.

Knight-Morse L (1992a) Spinal cord compression. In Hassey-Dow K, Hilderley LJ (eds), Nursing Care in Radiation Oncology. Philadelphia: WB Saunders, pp. 237–248.

Knight-Morse L (1992b) Superior vena cava syndrome. In Hassey-Dow K, Hilderley LJ (eds), Nursing Care in Radiation Oncology. Philadelphia: WB Saunders, pp. 227–236.

Koocher GP, O'Malley J (1981) The Damocles Syndrome. New York: McGraw-Hill.

Koocher GP, O'Malley J, Gogan J, Foster G (1980) Psychological adjustment among pediatric cancer survivors. Journal of Child Psychology and Psychiatry 21(2): 163–173.

Kooy HM (1993) Three dimensional treatment planning for stereotactic radiosurgery of intra-cranial lesions. International Journal of Radiation Oncology, Biology & Physics 21(3): 683–693.

Kornblinth PL, Cassidy JR (1985) Central nervous system emergencies; spinal cord compression. In Devita VT, Hellman S, Rosenberg SA (eds), Cancer, Principles and Practice of Oncology (second edition). Philadelphia: JB Lippincott, pp. 217–223.

Kroll SS, Woo SY, Santin A, Zietz H, Ried HL, Jaffe N, Larsom DL (1994) Long term effects of radiotherapy administered in childhood for the treatment of malignant diseases. Annals of Surgical Oncology 1(6): 173–179.

Kun LE, Moulder JE (1993) General principles of radiotherapy. In Pizzo PA, Poplack DG (eds), Principles and Practices of Pediatric Oncology (second edition). Philadelphia: JB Lippincott, pp. 289–323.

Kupst MJ (1994) Coping with paediatric cancer; theoretical and research. In Bearison DJ, Mulhern RK (eds), Paediatric Oncology: Psychological Perspectives on Children with Cancer. Oxford: Oxford University Press, pp. 35–61.

Kupst MJ, Schulman JL (1988) Long term coping with pediatric leukemia; a six year follow up study. Journal of Pediatrics 13(1): 7–22.

Lancaster J (1993) Women's experiences of gynaecological cancer treated with radiation. Curationis — South African Journal of Nursing 16(1): 37–42.

Lansky SB, Ritter-Sterr C, List, MA, Hart MJ (1993) Psychiatric and psychological support of the child and adolescent with cancer. In Pizzo PA, Poplack DG (eds), Principles and Practice of Pediatric Oncology (second edition). Philadelphia: JB Lippincott, pp. 1127–1141.

Larson DL, Kroll S, Jaffe N, Serure A, Goepfert H (1990) Long term effects of radiotherapy in childhood and adolescence. American Journal of Surgery 160(4): 348–351.

Lawton J, Twoomey M (1991) Breast care; skin reactions to radiotherapy. Nursing Standard 6(10): 53–54.

Leandro J, Dyck J, Poppe D, Shore R, Airhart C, Greenberg M, Gilday D, Smallhorn J, Benson L (1994) Cardiac dysfunction late after cardiotoxic therapy for childhood cancer. American Journal of Cardiology 71(11): 1152–1156.

Lee PA (1993) Disorders of puberty. In Lifshitz F (ed.), Pediatric Endocrinology (second edition — revised). New York: Marcel Dekker, pp. 217–249.

Leiper AD (1990) Management of growth failure in the treatment of malignant disease. Paediatric Haematology and Oncology 7(4): 365–371.

Leiper AD, Stanhope R, Kiching P, Chessels JM (1987) Precocious and premature puberty associated with treatment of acute lymphoblastic leukaemia. Archives of Disease in Childhood 69(11): 1107–1112.

Lew CM, LaValley B (1995) The role of stereotactic radiation therapy in the management of children with brain tumors. Journal of Pediatric Oncology Nursing 12(4): 212–222.

Lilley MD, Shalet SM, Beardwell CG (1990) Radiation and hypothalamic-pituitary function. Ballieres Clinical Endocrinology and Metabolism 4(1): 147–175.

Lindsey R (1993) Criteria for successful estrogen therapy in osteoporosis. Osteoporosis International 3 (Suppl. 2): 9–12.

Lipshultz SE, Sallan SE (1993) Cardiovascular abnormalities in long term survivors of childhood malignancy. Journal of Clinical Oncology 11(7): 1199–1203.

Little J (1996) Head and neck cancer: oral care during radiotherapy. Nursing Standard 10(22): 39–42.

Littman P, Meadows A, Polgar G, Borns PR, Rubin E (1984a) Pulmonary function in survivors of Wilms' tumour. Cancer 32(2): 2773–2776.

Littman P, Rosenstock J, Gale G, Kirsch R, Meadows A, Sather H (1984b) The somnolence syndrome in leukaemic children following reduced daily dose fractions of cranial irradiation. International Journal of Radiation Oncology, Biology & Physics 10(2): 1851–1853.

Livesey EA, Hindmarsh PC, Brook CGD, Whitton AC, Bloom HGJ, Tobias JS, Godlee JN, Britton J (1990) Endocrine disorders following treatment of childhood brain tumours. British Journal of Cancer 61(4): 622–625.

Locatelli F, Giorgiani G, Pession A, Bozzola M (1993) Late effects in children after bone marrow transplantation: a review. Haematologica 78(5): 319–328.

McCarthy CP (1992) Altered patterns of elimination. In Hassey-Dow K, Hilderley LJ (eds), Nursing Care in Radiation Oncology. Philadelphia: WB Saunders, pp. 317–332.

McCoy AM, Mierzejewski A (1993) Acute oncological disorders. In Kinney MR, Packa DR, Dunbar SB (eds), AACN Clinical Reference for Critical Care Nursing (third edition). St Louis, MO: CV Mosby, pp. 436–472.

McDonald A (1992) Altered protective mechanisms. In Hassey-Dow K, Hilderley LJ (eds), Nursing Care in Radiation Oncology. Philadelphia: WB Saunders, pp. 96–126.

McDonald E, Marino C (1992) Dry mouth; common but treatable. Geriatric Medicine 22(6): 43.

Maguire P (1993) Radiation therapy. In Foley GV, Fochtman D, Mooney KH (eds), Nursing Care of the Child with Cancer (second edition). Philadelphia: WB Saunders, pp. 117–130.

Maher EJ, Timothy A, Squire CJ et al. (1993) Audit: the use of radiotherapy in NSCLC in the UK. Clinical Oncology 5(2): 72–79.

Maiche A, Isokangs OP, Grohn P (1994) Skin protection by sulcrafate cream during electron beam therapy. Acta Oncologica 33(2): 201–203.

Mairs RJ, Gaze MN, Barratt A (1991) The uptake and retention of I^{131} mIBG by neuroblastoma cell line. British Journal of Cancer 64(2): 293–295.

Mandell L, Walker W, Steinhez P, Fuks Z (1989) Reduced incidence of the somnolence syndrome in leukaemic children with steroid coverage during prophylactic cranial radiation therapy. Cancer 63(10): 1978–1988.

Mandell LR, Hazra-Tapan T, Henry L (1986/87) Cancer patients and radiotherapy: close encounters of the third kind. Loss, Grief and Care 1(1–2): 79–86.

Marcus RB, McGrath B, O'Conner K, Scarborough M (1994) Long term effects on the musculoskeletal and integumentary system and the breast. In Schwartz CL, Constine LS, Hobbie WL, Ruccione KS (eds), Survivors of Childhood Cancer. St Louis, MO: CV Mosby, pp. 263–292.

Marks JE, Wong J (1985) The risk of cerebral radionecrosis in relation to dose, time and fractionation. Progress in Experimental Tumor Research 29: 210.

Martinez-Clement J, Castel-Sanchez V, Esquembre-Menor C, Verdeguer-Miralles A, Ferris-Tortajada J (1994) Scale for assessing quality of life of children survivors of cranial posterior fossa tumours. Journal of Neuro-oncology 22(1): 67–76.

Matejka M, Nell A, Kment G, Schien A, Leukauf M, Porteder H et al. (1990) Local benefit of prostaglandin E_2 in radiochemotherapy-induced oral mucositis. British Journal of Oral and Maxilofacial Surgery 28(1): 89–91.

Meadows AT, Fenton GJ (1994) Follow up care of patients at risk for the development of second malignant neoplasms. In Schwartz CL, Constine LS, Hobbie WL, Ruccione KS (eds), Survivors of Childhood Cancer. St Louis, MO: CV Mosby, pp. 319–328.

Meadows AT, Hobbie WL (1986) The medical consequences of cure. Cancer 58 (Suppl. 2): 524–528.

Meadows AT, Silber J (1985) Delayed consequences of therapy for childhood cancer. CA 35(5): 271–286.

Medical Research Council (1991) Randomised trials of palliative radiotherapy with ten or two fractions. British Journal of Cancer 63(2): 265–270.

Meric F, Hirschi RB, Mahboubi S, Womer RB, Goldwein J, Ross AJ IIIrd, Schnaufer L (1994) Prevention of radiation enteritis in children, using a pelvic mesh sling. Journal of Paediatric Surgery 29(7): 917–921.

Mitchell WG, Fishman LS, Miller JH, Nelson M, Zeltzer PM, Soni D, Siegel SM (1991) Stroke as a late sequela of cranial irradiation for childhood brain tumours. Journal of Child Neurology 6(2): 128–133.

Moore IM (1995) Central nervous system toxicity of cancer therapy in children. Journal of Pediatric Oncology Nursing 12(4): 203–210.

Moore IM, Kramer JH, Wara W et al. (1991) Cognitive function in children with leukaemia: effect of radiation dose and time since irradiation. Cancer 68(9): 1913–1917.

Morgan GW, Freeman AP, McLean RG, Jarvie BH, Giles RW (1985) Late cardiac, thyroid and pulmonary sequelae of mantle radiotherapy for Hodgkin's disease. International Journal of Radiation, Oncology & Biology 11(11): 1925-1931.

Morris JG, Grattan-Smith P, Panegyres PK, O'Neill P, Soo YS, Langlands AO (1994) Delayed cerebral radiation necrosis. Quarterly Journal of Medicine 87(2): 119–129.

Moss W, Cox J (1989) Radiation Oncology; Rationale, Technique and Results (sixth edition). St Louis, MO: CV Mosby.

Mulhern R, Wassermann A, Friedman A, Fairclough D (1989) Social competence and behavioral adjustment of children who are long term survivors of cancer. Pediatrics 83(1): 18–25.

Mulhern R, Hancock J, Fairclough D, Kun L (1992) Neuropsychological status of children treated for brain tumors: a critical review and integrative analysis. Medical and Pediatric Oncology 20: 181–191.

Mullen F (1984) Re-entry: the educational needs of the cancer survivor. Health Education Quarterly 10 (Suppl.): 88–94.

Nayel H, el-Ghonelmy E, el-Haddad S (1992) Impact of nutritional supplementation on treatment delay and morbidity in patients with head and neck tumours treated with irradiation. Nutrition 8(1): 13–18.

Neal A, Hoskin P (1994) Clinical Oncology. London: Edward Arnold.

Ochs J, Mulhern R, Fairclough D et al. (1991) Comparison of neuropsychologic functioning and clinical indicators of neurotoxicity in long term survivors of childhood leukaemia given cranial irradiation or parenteral methotrexate: a prospective study. Journal of Clinical Oncology 9(1): 145–151.

Ogilvy-Stuart AL, Clark DJ, Wallace WHB et al. (1992) Endocrine defects after fractionated TBI. Archives of Disease in Childhood 67(9): 1107–1110.

Ogilvy-Stuart AL, Clayton PE, Shalet SM (1994a) Cranial irradiation and early puberty. Journal of Clinical Endocrinology and Metabolism 78(6): 1282–1286.

Ogilvy-Stuart AL, Wallace WH, Shalet SM (1994b) Radiation and neuro-regulatory control of growth hormone secretion. Clinical Endocrinology 41(2): 163–168.

Oski FA, DeAngelais CD, Feigin RD (1990) Principles and Practice of Pediatrics. Philadelphia; PA: JB Lippincott & Co.

Otto SE (ed.) (1994) Oncology Nursing (second edition). St Louis, MO: CV Mosby, p. 427.

Pachnis A, Gaze M, Levitt G, Michalski A, Pritchard J (eds) (1996) Some stage III FH Wilms' patients may not need radiotherapy. UKCCSK Scientific meeting, Liverpool 7 November.

Packer RJ, Meadows AT, Rorke LB (1987) Long term sequelae of cancer treatment on the central nervous system in childhood. Medical Paediatric Oncology 15(2): 241–253.

Packer RJ, Bleyer WA, Pochedly C (eds) (1992) Paediatric Neuro-oncology: New Trends in Clinical Research. Reading: Harwood Academic Press.

Parker BR, Castellino RA (1977) Pediatric Oncologic Radiology. St Louis, MO: CV Mosby.

Pedrick RJ, Hoppe RT (1986) Recovery of spermatogenesis following pelvic irradiation for Hodgkin's disease. International Journal of Radiation Oncology, Biology and Physics 12: 117–121.

Perch SJ, Machtay M, Markiewicz DA, Kligerman MM (1995) Decreased acute toxicity by using midline mucosa sparing blocks during radiation therapy for carcinoma of the oral cavity, oropharynx, and nasopharynx. Radiology 197(3): 863–866.

Pervan V (1993) Understanding anti-emetics. Nursing Times 89(10): 36–38.

Pinkerton CR, Cushing P, Sepion B (1994) Childhood Cancer Management: A Practical Handbook. London: Chapman & Hall.

Piper B (1988) Fatigue in cancer patients: current perspectives on measurement and management. In American Cancer Society, Nursing Management of Current Problems; State of the Art. Proceedings of the fifth national conference of cancer nursing. New York: American Cancer Society, pp. 217–224.

Pizer BL, Kemshead JT (1994) The potential of targeted radiotherapy in the treatment of central nervous system leukaemia. Leukaemia and Lymphoma 15(3–4): 281–289.

Pizer B, Papanastassiou V, Hancock J, Cassano W, Coakham H, Kemshead J (1991) A pilot study of monoclonal antibody targeted radiotherapy in the treatment of central nervous system leukaemia in children. British Journal of Haematology 77(4): 466–472.

Pizzo PA, Poplack DG (1993) Principles and Practices of Pediatric Oncology. Philadelphia: JB Lippincott.

Plowman PH (1983) The effects of conventionally fractionated, extended portal radiotherapy on the human peripheral blood count. International Journal of Radiation Oncology, Biology & Physics 9(6): 829–839.

Plowman PH (1992) Tumours of the central nervous system. In Plowman PN, Pinkerton CR (eds), Paediatric Oncology: Clinical Practice and Controversies. London: Chapman & Hall, pp. 240–268.

Plowman PN, Pinkerton CR (eds) (1992) Paediatric Oncology: Clinical Practice and Controversies. London: Chapman & Hall.

Porta C, Moroni M, Nastasi G (1994) Allopurinal mouthwashes in the treatment of 5-Fluorouracil induced stomatitis. American Journal of Clinical Oncology 17(3) 246–247.

Potijola-Sintonen S, Tottermann KJ, Salmo M, Siltanen P (1987) Late cardiac effects of mediastinal radiotherapy in patients with Hodgkin's disease. Cancer 60(1): 31–37.

Price P, Hoskin PJ, Austin A, Palmer SJ, Yarnold JR (1986) Prospective and randomised trial of single and multifraction radiotherapy schedules in the treatment of painful bony metastases. Radiotherapy and Oncology 6(4): 247–255.

Priestman TJ (1990) Results of a randomised double blind comparative study of ondansetron and metoclopramide in the prevention of nausea and vomiting following high dose upper abdominal irradiation. Journal of Clinical Oncology 2(1): 71–75.

Probert JC, Parker BR, Kaplan IIK (1973) Growth retardation in children after megavoltage irradiation of the spine. Cancer 32(3): 634–639.

Quick A (1994) Dressing choices. Nursing Times 90(45): 71–72.

Quigley C, Cowell C, Jimenez M (1989) Normal or early development of puberty despite gonadal damage in children treated for acute lymphoblastic leukaemia. New England Journal of Medicine 321(1): 143–151.

Radcliffe J, Bunin GR, Sutton LN, Goldwein JW, Philips PC (1994) Cognitive deficits in long term survivors of childhood medulloblastoma and other noncortical tumours; age dependent effects of whole brain irradiation. International Journal of Developmental Neuroscience 12(4): 327–331.

Rate WR, Butler MS, Robertson WW, D'Angio GJ (1991) Late orthopedic effects in children with Wilms' tumour treated with abdominal irradiation. Medical Pediatric Oncology 19(4): 265–268.

Richter MP, Coia LR (1985) Palliative radiation therapy. Seminars in Oncology 12(4): 375–383.

Robertson WW, Butler MS, D'Angio GJ, Rate WR (1991) Leg length discrepancy following irradiation for childhood tumours. Journal of Pediatric Orthopedics 11(3): 284–287.

Rodriguez CS, Ash CR (1996) Associated late effects (IV). Cancer Nursing 19(6): 455–468.

Rose M (1989) Health promotion and risk prevention: applications for cancer survivors. Oncology Nurses Forum 16(3): 335–340.

Rose MA, Schrader-Bogen CL, Korlath G, Priem J, Larson LR (1996) Identifying patient symptoms after radiotherapy using a nurse managed telephone interview. Oncology Nurses Forum 23(1): 99–102.

Rubin P (1984) Late effects of chemotherapy and radiation therapy: a new hypothesis. International Journal of Radiation Oncology, Biology & Physics 10(1): 5–34.

Rubin P, Van Houtte P, Constine L (1982) Radiation sensitivity and organ tolerances in pediatric oncology: a new hypothesis. Frontiers in Radiation Therapy and Oncology 16(1): 62–82.

Ruccione KS (1994) Issues in survivorship. In Schwartz CL, Constine LS, Hobbie WL, Ruccione KS (eds), Survivors of Childhood Cancer. St Louis, MO: CV Mosby, pp. 329–339.

Saunders JR, Brown MS, Hirata BW, Jaques DA (1991) Percutaneous endoscopic gastrostomy in patients with head and neck malignancies. American Journal of Surgery 162(4): 381–383.

Schafer SL (1994) Oncologic complications. In Otto S (ed.), Oncology Nursing. St Louis, MO: C.V. Mosby, pp. 406–439.

Scheibel-Jost P, Pfeil J, Niethard FU, Fromm B, Willich E, Kuttig H (1991) Spinal growth after irradiation for Wilms' tumour. International Orthopedics 15(4): 387–391.

Sedgewick DM, Howard GC, Fergusson A (1994) Pathogenesis of acute radiation injury to the rectum. A prospective study in patients. International Journal of Colorectal Diseases 9(1): 23–30.

Semba SE, Mealey BL, Hallmon WW (1994) The head and neck radiotherapy patient: part 1 oral manifestation of radiotherapy. Compendium 15(2): 250–260.

Sentft M, Fietkau R, Iro H, Sailer D, Sauer R (1993) The influence of supportive nutritional therapy via percutaneous endoscopically guided gastrostomy on the quality of life of cancer patients. Supportive Care in Cancer 1(5): 272–275.

Servodidio CA, Abramson DH (1993) Acute and long term effects of radiation therapy to the eye in children. Cancer Nursing 16(5): 371–381.

Shalet SM (1996) Cytotoxic induced damage. In Selby P, Bailey C (eds), Cancer and the Adolescent. London: BMJ Publications, pp. 148–160.

Shalet SM, Horner A, Ahmed SR, Morris-Jones PH (1995) Leydig cell damage after testicular irradiation for lymphoblastic leukaemia. Medical Paediatric Oncology 13(1): 65–68.

Shank B, Andreeff M, Li D (1983) Cell survival kinetics in peripheral blood and bone marrow transplantation. International Journal of Radiation Oncology, Biology & Physics 9(11): 1613–1623.

Shaw NJ, Eden OB, Jenney ME, Stevens RF, Morris-Jones PH, Craft AW, Castillo L (1991) Pulmonary function in survivors of Wilms' tumour. Pediatric Hematology & Oncology 8(2): 131–137.

Sheline GE, Wara WM, Smith V (1980) Therapeutic irradiation and brain injury. International Journal of Radiation Oncology, Biology & Physics 6(5): 1215–1217.

Shiminski-Maher T (1990) Brain tumours in childhood. Journal of Pediatric Health Care 4: 122–130.

Shminski-Maher T (1993) Physician–patient–parent communication problems. Paediatric Neurosurgery 19(10): 104–108.

Shiminski-Maher T, Wisoff JH (1995) Pediatric brain tumours. Critical Care Nursing Clinics of North America 7(1): 159–169.

Shuey KM (1994) Heart, lung and endocrine complications of solid tumours. Seminars in Oncology Nursing 10(3): 177–188.

Silverman CL, Goldberg SL (1996) TBI and BMT in advanced lymphomas. In Tobias JS, Thomas PRM (eds), Current Radiation Oncology (Volume 2). London: Edward Arnold, pp. 320–350.

Sittom E (1992) Early and late radiation induced skin alterations: mechanisms of skin changes (part 1). Oncology Nurses Forum 19(5): 801–807.

Sklar C et al. (1982) Thyroid dysfunction among long term survivors of bone marrow transplantation. American Journal of Medicine 73(5): 688–694.

Sklar C, Mertens A, Walter A et al. (1993) Final height after treatment for childhood acute lymphoblastic leukemia: comparison of no cranial irradiation with 1800 and 2400 centigrays of cranial irradiation. Journal of Pediatrics 123(1): 59–64.

Sklar CA, Robinson LL, Nesbit ME, Sather HN, Meadows AT (1990) The effects of radiation on testicular function in long term survivors of childhood acute lymphoblastic leukaemia: a report from the CCSG. Journal of Clinical Oncology 8(12): 1981–1987.

Skowronska-Gardas A (1994) Hyperfractionated radiotherapy for brain stem tumours in children. Radiotherapy Oncology 33(30): 259–261.

Slifer KJ (1996) A video system to help children cooperate with motion control for radiation treatment without sedation. Journal of Paediatric Oncology Nursing 13(2): 91–97.

Slifer KJ, Bucholtz JD, Cataldo MD (1994) Behavioural training of motion control in young children undergoing radiation treatment without sedation. Journal of Paediatric Oncology Nursing 11(2): 55–63.

Slifer KJ, Cataldo MR, Cataldo MD (1993) Behavior analysis of motion control for pediatric neuroimaging. Journal of Applied Behavioral Analysis 26(3): 469–470.

Smith MB, Xue H, Takahashi H, Cangir A, Andrassy RJ (1994) Iodine 131 thyroid ablation in female children and adolescents; long term risk of infertility and birth defects. Annals of Surgical Oncology 1(2): 128–131.

Spencer T (1988) Dry skin and skin moisturizers. Clinics in Dermatology 6(1): 3–5.

Spinetta JJ (1977) Adjustment in children with cancer. Journal of Pediatric Psychology 2(1): 49–51.

Spinetta JJ, Deasy-Spinetta P (1989) Living with Childhood Cancer. St Louis, MO: CV Mosby.

Spirito A, Stark L, Cobelia C, Drigan R, Androkites A, Hewitt K (1990) Social adjustment of children successfully treated for cancer. Journal of Pediatric Psychology 15(3): 359–371.

Steel GG, Wheldon TE (1992) The radiation biology of paediatric tumours. In Plowman PN, Pinkerton CR (eds), Paediatric Oncology; Clinical Practice and Controversies. London: Chapman & Hall, pp. 73–87.

Storb R (1989) Bone marrow transplantation. In DeVita VT, Hellman S, Rosenberg SA (eds), Cancer; Principles and Practice of Oncology. Philadelphia: JB Lippincott, pp. 427–439.

Strohl RA (1990) Radiation therapy; recent advances and nursing implications. Nursing Clinics of North America 25(2): 309–329.

Strohl RA (1992) Ineffective breathing patterns. In Hassey-Dow K, Hilderley L (eds), Nursing Care in Radiation Oncology. Philadelphia: WB Saunders, pp. 160–177.

Sullivan MJ, Abbott GD, Robinson BA (1992) Ondansetron antiemetic therapy for chemotherapy and radiotherapy induced vomiting in children. New Zealand Medical Journal 105(942): 369–371.

Sweet V, Servy EJ, Karow AM (1996) Reproductive issues for men with cancer: technology and nursing management. Oncology Nurses Forum 23(1): 51–58.

Symonds RP, McIlroy P, Khorrami J, Paul J, Pyper E, Alcock SR, McCallum I, Speekenbrink AB, McMurray A, Lindemann E, Thomas M (1996) The reduction of radiation mucositis by selective decontamination antibiotic pastilles: a placebo controlled double blind trial. British Journal of Cancer 74(2): 312–317.

Syndikus I, Tait D, Ashley S, Jannoun L (1994) Long term follow up of young children with brain tumours after irradiation. International Journal of Radiation Oncology, Biology and Physics 30(4): 781–787.

Tarbell N, Newburger P, Pazola K, Sallan S, Schwenn M, Shamberger R (1990) Cancers in children. In Osteen R, Cady B, Rosenthal P (eds), Cancer Manual (eighth edition). Boston, MA: American Cancer Society.

Taylor RE (1996) Cancer in children: radiotherapeutic approaches. British Medical Bulletin 52(4): 873–886.

Tebbi C, Mallon J (1987) Long term psychological outcome among cancer amputees in adolescence and early adulthood. Journal of Psychosocial Oncology 5(1): 69–82.

Teta M, Po M, Kasl S, Miegs J, Myers M, Mulvihill J (1986) Psychological consequences of childhood and adolescent cancer survival. Journal of Chronic Diseases 39(6): 751–759.

Thames HD, Withers HR, Peters LT, Fletcher GH (1982) Changes in early and late radiation responses with altered dose fractionation: implications for dose survival relationships. International Journal of Radiation Oncology, Biology & Physics 9(11): 1613–1623.

Thomas PRM (1996) Medulloblastoma — progress and pitfalls. In Tobias JS, Thomas PRM (eds), Current Radiation Oncology (Volume 2). London: Edward Arnold, pp. 202–218.

Thomas S (1990) Wound Management and Dressings. London: Pharmaceutical Press.

Thompson ES, Afshar F, Plowman PN (1989) Paediatric brachytherapy II: brain implantation. British Journal of Radiotherapy 735(62): 223–229.

Tiesinga LJ, Dassen TWN, Halfens RJG (1996) Fatigue: a summary of the definitions, dimensions and indicators. Nursing Diagnosis 7(2): 51–62.

Tiffany R (1979) Radiotherapy. London: Macmillan.

Tobias JS, Thomas PRM (eds) (1996) Current Radiation Oncology (Volume 2). London: Edward Arnold.

Toma NMG, Hungerford JL, Plowman PN, Kingston JE, Doughty D (1995) External beam radiotherapy for retinoblastoma: II Lens sparing technique. British Journal of Ophthalmology 79(2): 112–117.

Trowbridge J, Carl W (1975) Oral care of the patient having head and neck irradiation. American Journal of Nursing 75(12): 2146–2149.

United Kingdom Children Cancer Study Group (1995) Neuroblastoma working party: phase I pilot study of combined chemotherapy and ImIBG therapy — Nb 95-01. London: UKCCSG.

Uruena M, Stanhope R, Chessels JM et al. (1991) Impaired pubertal growth in acute lymphoblastic leukaemia. Archives of Disease in Childhood 66(12): 1403–1407.

Van Dyk J, Keane TJ, Kan S, Rider WD, Fryer CJH (1981) Radiation penumonitis following single dose irradiation: a re-evaluation based on absolute dose to lung. International Journal of Radiation Oncology, Biology and Physics 11(3): 461–467.

Vermeulen A (1993) Environment, human reproduction, menopause and andropause. Environmental Health Perspectives 101 (Suppl. 2): 91–100.

Waber DP, Tarbell NJ, Kaln CM, Gelber RD, Sallan SE (1992) The relationship of sex and treatment modality to neuropsychologic outcome in childhood acute lymphoblastic leukaemia. Journal of Clinical Oncology 10(5): 810–817.

Wadleigh RG, Redman RS, Graham ML, Krasnow SH, Anderson A, Cohen MJ (1992) Vitamin E in the treatment of chemotherapy induced mucositis. American Journal of Medicine 95(2): 481–484.

Wallace WHB, Shalet SM (1992) Growth and endocrine function following treatment of childhood malignant disease. In Plowman PN, Pinkerton CR (eds), Paediatric Oncology. London: Chapman & Hall, pp. 531–558.

Wallace WHB, Shalet SM, Crowne EC, Morris-Jones PH (1989) Ovarian function following abdominal irradiation in childhood; natural history and progression. Clinical Oncology 1(2): 75–79.

Warzak WJ, Engel LE, Bischoff LG et al. (1991) Developing anxiety reducing procedures for the ventilated dependent pediatric patient. Archives of Physiotherapy and Medical Rehabilitation 72(3): 503–507.

Wasserman AL, Thompson EEL, Wilimas JA et al. (1987) The psychological status of survivors of childhood/adolescent Hodgkin's disease. American Journal of Diseases in Childhood 141(6): 626–631.

Watson R (1989) Care of the mouth. Nursing (UK) 3(44): 20.

Weintraub FN, Hagopian GA (1990) The effect of nursing consultation on anxiety, side effects and self care of patients receiving radiation therapy. Oncology Nurses Forum 17(3): 31–36.

Weiss AH, Kalina RE, Lindsley LK, Pendergrass TW (1994) Visual outcomes of macular retinoblastoma after external beam radiation therapy. Ophthalmology 101(7): 1244–1249.

William R, Karcon I (1978) Sleep Disorders, Diagnosis and Treatment. New York: J Wiley.

Wilson JK, Masaryk TJ (1989) Neurologic emergencies in cancer patients. Seminars in Oncology 16(6): 490–499.

Winningham ML (1992) How exercise mitigates fatigue: implications for people receiving cancer therapy. In Carroll-Johnson RM (ed.), The Biotherapy of Cancer. Pittsburgh: Oncology Nursing Press, pp. 761–768.

Winningham ML, Nail LH, Burke MB, Brophy L et al. (1994) Fatigue and the cancer experience: the state of knowledge. Oncology Nurses Forum 21(1): 23–36.

Wisoff JH, Epstein FJ (1994) Management of hydrocephalus in children with medulloblastoma—prognostic factors for shunting. Pediatric Neurosurgery 20(4): 240–247.

Woods N, Dehner L, Nesbit H et al. (1980) Fatal veno-occlusive disease following high dose chemotherapy and irradiation in bone marrow transplantation. American Journal of Medicine 60: 285–290.

Workman LM (1989) Immunologic late effects in children and adults. Seminars in Oncology Nursing 5(10): 36–42.

Yeung CK, Ward HC, Ransley PG, Duffy PG, Pritchard J (1994) Bladder and kidney function after cure of pelvic rhabdomyosarcoma in childhood. British Journal of Cancer 70(5): 1000–1003.

Young M (1988) Malnutrition and wound healing. Heart and Lung 17(1): 60.

Yule SM, Pearson ADJ, Boddy AV (1996) Fluconazole inhibits cyclophosphamide activation in children. UKCCSG Scientific meeting, Liverpool, 7 November.

Zerbe MB, Parkerson SG, Ortlieg ML, Spitzer T (1992) Relationships between oral mucositis and treatment variables in bone marrow recipients. Cancer Nursing 15(3): 196–205.

Zoubek A, Kronberger M, Puschmann A, Gadner H (1993) Ondansetron in the control of chemotherapy induced and radiotherapy induced emesis in children with malignancies. Anti-cancer Drugs (Suppl. 2): 17–21.

Index

heart *see* cardiac function
hemiparesis 320, 322, 340
hemipelvectomy 371, 387
heparin 115, 240, 262
hepatic function *see* liver and hepatic function
hepatitis 98, 183, 194, 239, 242, 496
hepatoblastoma 282, 292, 301, 428, 436
hepatocellular carcinoma 292
hepatocytes 147, 238
hepatomegaly 239
hepatosplenomegaly 99
Herpes simplex virus (HSV) 107, 194, 214, 232, 236
Hickman line 191–2, 201, 222, 309, 310, 313
high-dose therapies 155–6, 158
high-efficiency particulate air (HEPA) 213–14, 215
hips 370, 376, 377, 381
hirsutism 237
histiocytosis 17, 45
histocompatibility 181, 182, 194, 238
histology
    aid to diagnosis 283, 284
    brain tumours 319–21, 331, 332
        case history 343, 346, 347
    radiotherapy 406, 407, 428–9
    superior vena cava obstruction 464
HIV 98, 164, 183, 496
Hodgkin's disease 293–4, 427–8
    BMT 176
    chemotherapy 16, 17, 20, 35, 44
        late effects 145, 146, 152
    general surgery 293–4
    radiotherapy 397, 427–8, 435, 475, 483, 488
    superior vena cava obstruction 464
home setting for chemotherapy 54–8
hormones 3, 15, 18, 20, 476–7, 478–9
    cranial irradiation 355–6
    growth (GH) 472–3, 475, 476–7, 482, 488
    radiotherapy 428
        late effects 472–3, 475–9, 482–3, 485, 488, 497
    replacement therapy 485
human leukocyte antigens (HLA) system 179–81
    BMT 174–6, 178–81, 182, 194, 250, 252

GVHD 235
humerus 363, 370
Hunter's syndrome 177
Hurler's syndrome 177
hyaluronidase 40
hydration 351–2
    brain tumours 351–2
    chemotherapy 30, 50–1, 56
    side effects 83, 117, 120, 121, 123, 124
    general surgery 286, 305
    PBSCT 260
    radiotherapy 447, 454, 461
    see also dehydration; fluid balance; hyperhydration
hydrocephalus 323–5
    brain tumours 320, 321, 322, 323–5, 326, 338
    case history 341, 346
hydrocortisone 40, 97, 211, 233, 300
    anaphylaxis 116
    radiotherapy side effects 441, 444
hydronephrosis 491
hydroxyurea 5
hyoscine-N-butyl bromide (buscopan) 91, 211
hyperhydration 196, 211, 212, 232, 324
hyperkalaemia 117, 118, 119, 121–2
hyperphosphataemia 117, 118, 122
hyperpyrexia 197, 330, 377
    see also fever
hypersensitivity 61, 62, 105
hypertension 148, 211, 286, 299, 302, 490
    cyclosporin 237–8
hyperuricaemia 117, 118, 120–1
hypnosis 81, 381
hypoalbuminaemia 8, 239
hypocalcaemia 117, 122, 263
hypophosphataemia 147
hypoplasia 481, 483
hypotension 50, 158, 166, 211, 298
    antiemetics 78
    acute tumour lysis syndrome (ATLS) 117
    septic shock 110
hypothalamus 330, 340, 355
    neurosurgery 319, 320, 321
    radiotherapy 475, 476, 477, 483